Respiratory
Pharmacology and
Pharmacotherapy

Series Editors:

Dr. David Raeburn
Discovery Biology
Rhône-Poulenc Rorer Ltd
Dagenham Research Centre
Dagenham
Essex RM10 7XS
England

Dr. Mark A. Giembycz
Department of Thoracic Medicine
National Heart and Lung Institute
Imperial College of Science, Technology and Medicine
London SW3 6LY
England

Molecular Biology of the Lung
Volume II: Asthma and Cancer

Edited by
R. A. Stockley

Springer Basel AG

Editor:

Prof. Robert A. Stockley
University Hospital Birmingham
Department of Respiratory Medicine
Edgbaston, Birmingham B15 2TH
UK

Library of Congress Cataloging-in-Publication Data

Molecular biology of the lung / edited by
  R.A. Stockley
      p.   cm. – (Respiratory pharmacology and pharmacotherapy)
  Contents: V. 1. Emphysema and infection – V. 2. Asthma and
  cancer.
    ISBN 978-3-0348-9773-0   ISBN 978-3-0348-8784-7 (eBook)
    DOI 10.1007/978-3-0348-8784-7

    1. Lungs–Diseases–Molecular aspects.   I. Stockley, Robert A.   II. Series.
    [DNLM: 1. Lung Diseases, Obstructive–immunology.   2. Pulmonary
  Emphysema.   3. Asthma.   WF 600M719 1999]
  RC756.M67   1999
  616.2' 4 – dc21
  DNLM/DLC
  for Library of Congress   99–36983
                                                                          CIP

Die Deutsche Bibliothek – CIP-Einheitsaufnahme

Molecular biology of the lung / ed by R. A. Stockley. – Basel ;
Boston ; Berlin : Birkhäuser
    (Respiratory pharmacology and pharmacotherapy)
    ISBN 978-3-0348-9773-0

    Vol. 2 Asthma and cancer. – 1999
    ISBN 978-3-0348-9773-0

Contents

List of Contributors VII

1. Gene Therapy
   Joanne T. Douglas and David T. Curiel 1

Asthma

2. Genetics of Asthma
   Andrew J. Walley and William O. C. M. Cookson 23

3. Transcription Factors and Inflammatory Lung Disease
   Peter J. Barnes and Ian M. Adcock 41

4. Regulation of the Cytokine Gene Cluster on Chromosome 5q
   David J. Cousins, Dontcho Z. Staynov and Tak H. Lee 71

5. Cytokine Expression in Asthma
   C. J. Corrigan 85

6. β-Adrenoceptors
   Peter J. Barnes and Judith C. W. Mak 101

7. Regulation of Eosinophil Migration
   Peter J. Jose, Anne Burke-Gaffney and Timothy J. Williams . . . 125

8. Proteinase Allergens of House Dust Mites: Molecular Biology,
   Biochemistry and Possible Functional Significance of Their
   Enzyme Activity
   Clive Robinson, Hong Wan, Helen L. Winton, David R. Garrod,
   Geoffrey A. Stewart and Philip J. Thompson 145

Cancer

9. Gene Expression in Lung Cancer
   Tariq Sethi. 165

10. Gene Therapy for Cancer: Prospects for the Treatment of
    Lung Tumours
    Nicola K. Green, Moira G. Gilligan, David J. Kerr,
    Peter F. Searle and Lawrence S. Young 183

Index 203

List of Contributors

Ian M. Adcock, Department of Thoracic Medicine, National Heart and Lung Institute, Imperial College School of Medicine, London SW3 6LY, UK; e-mail: ian.adcock@ic.ac.uk

Peter J. Barnes, Department of Thoracic Medicine, National Heart and Lung Institute, Imperial College School of Medicine, Dovehouse St, London SW3 6LY, UK; p.j.barnes@ic.ac.uk

Anne Burke-Gaffney, Leukocyte Biology, Biomedical Sciences Division, Imperial College School of Medicine, Dovehouse Street, London SW3 6LY, UK

William O.C.M. Cookson, Nuffield Department of Clinical Medicine, John Radcliffe Hospital, Oxford OX3 9DU, UK

C.J. Corrigan, Department of Respiratory Medicine, National Heart & Lung Institute, Imperial College School of Medicine, Charing Cross Hospital, Fulham Palace Road, London W6 8RF, UK

David J. Cousins, Department of Respiratory Medicine and Allergy, GKT Medical School, King's College, Guy's Hospital, London SE1 9RT, UK

David T. Curiel, Division of Pulmonary and Critical Care Medicine, Department of Medicine and Gene Therapy Program, University of Alabama at Birmingham, 1824 Sixth Avenue South, Birmingham, Alabama 35294, USA

Joanne T. Douglas, Division of Pulmonary and Critical Care Medicine, Department of Medicine and Gene Therapy Program, University of Alabama at Birmingham, Birmingham, Alabama 35294, USA

David R. Garrod, School of Biological Sciences, University of Manchester, Manchester M13 9PT, UK

Moira G. Gilligan, CRC Institute for Cancer Studies, University of Birmingham, Edgbaston, Birmingham B15 2T, UK

Nicola K. Green, CRC Institute for Cancer Studies, University of Birmingham, Edgbaston, Birmingham B15 2T, UK

Peter J. Jose, Leukocyte Biology, Biomedical Sciences Division, Imperial College School of Medicine, Dovehouse Street, London SW3 6LY, UK

David J. Kerr, CRC Institute for Cancer Studies, University of Birmingham, Edgbaston, Birmingham B15 2T, UK

Tak H. Lee, Department of Respiratory Medicine and Allergy, GKT Medical School, King's College, Guy's Hospital, London SE1 9RT, UK; e-mail: t.lee@umds.ac.uk

Judith C.W. Mak, Department of Thoracic Medicine, National Heart and Lung Institute, Imperial College School of Medicine, Dovehouse Street, London SW3 6LY, UK

Clive Robinson, Department of Pharmacology & Clinical Pharmacology, St George's Hospital Medical School, Cranmer Terrace, London SW17 0RE, UK; e-mail: c.robinson@sghms.ac.uk

Peter F. Searle, CRC Institute for Cancer Studies, University of Birmingham, Edgbaston, Birmingham B15 2T, UK

Tariq Sethi, Respiratory Medicine Unit, Department of Medicine (RIE), University of Edinburgh, The Rayne Laboratory, Teviot Place, Edinburgh EH3 9YW, Scotland, UK

Dontcho Z. Staynov, Department of Allergy and Respiratory Medicine, United Medical and Dental Schools, Guy's Hospital, London SE1 9RT, UK

Geoffrey A. Stewart, Department of Microbiology, University of Western Australia, Nedlands 6907, Western Australia

Philip J. Thompson, Department of Medicine, University of Western Australia, Nedlands 6907, Western Australia

Andrew J. Walley, Nuffield Department of Clinical Medicine, John Radcliffe Hospital, Oxford OX3 9DU, UK;
e-mail: awalley@radius.jr2.ox.ac.uk

Hong Wan, Department of Pharmacology & Clinical Pharmacology, St George's Hospital Medical School, Cranmer Terrace, London SW17 0RE, UK

Timothy J. Williams, Leukocyte Biology, Biomedical Sciences Division, Imperial College School of Medicine, Dovehouse Street, London SW3 6LY, UK

Helen L. Winton, Department of Pharmacology & Clinical Pharmacology, St George's Hospital Medical School, Cranmer Terrace, London SW17 0RE, UK

Lawrence S. Young, CRC Institute for Cancer Studies, University of Birmingham, Edgbaston, Birmingham B15 2T, UK

Molecular Biology of the Lung
Vol. 2: Asthma and Cancer
ed. by R. A. Stockley
© 1999 Birkhäuser Verlag Basel/Switzerland

CHAPTER 1
Gene Therapy

Joanne T. Douglas and David T. Curiel

Division of Pulmonary and Critical Care Medicine, Department of Medicine and Gene Therapy Program, University of Alabama at Birmingham, Birmingham, AL, USA

1   Introduction
2   The Lung As a Target For Gene Therapy
3   Vector Systems For Gene Delivery to the Lung
3.1   Viral Vectors
3.2   Nonviral Vectors
4   Gene Therapy For Diseases of the Lung
4.1   Inherited Pulmonary Diseases
4.1.1   Cystic fibrosis
4.1.2 α_1-Antitrypsin deficiency
4.1.3   Surfactant protein B deficiency
4.2   Thoracic Malignancies
4.2.1   Genetic immunopotentiation
4.2.2   Molecular chemotherapy
4.2.3   Mutation compensation
4.3   Acquired Pulmonary Diseases
4.3.1   Inflammatory diseases
4.3.2   Infectious diseases
4.3.3   Pulmonary vascular diseases
5   Future Challenges
        Acknowledgements
        References

1. Introduction

Gene therapy was originally conceived as an approach to the treatment of classic monogenic inherited disorders for which it was proposed that transfer of a normal copy of a single defective gene would revert the disease phenotype. However, as the field has evolved, it has been recognized that gene transfer is a rational option for the treatment of both acquired diseases, such as cancer, and infectious diseases, such as AIDS, which have defined genetic components. In addition, the elucidation of the molecular basis of the host defense mechanisms against viral or bacterial pathogens suggests that these pathways could be exploited for therapeutic purposes using gene transfer technology. Therefore, gene therapy is now broadly defined as the transfer of genetic material to the cells of an individual for therapeutic purposes.

For a disease to be considered a candidate for gene therapy, it must meet certain criteria which were initially proposed by Anderson [1]. First, it is necessary to understand the molecular basis of an inherited or acquired genetic disease, or of the host response to an infectious disease. Second, in recognition of the fact that gene therapy is still a radical therapeutic intervention, the disease should represent a significant cause of morbidity and/or mortality for which, moreover, there is no conventional treatment. Last, both scientific and clinical data must be obtainable in a gene therapy study.

2. The Lung As a Target For Gene Therapy

Although many disease states are potentially suitable for gene therapy approaches, diseases of the lung have to date represented a disproportionately large fraction of the approved human gene therapy clinical protocols [2]. This reflects the fact that the lung possesses several advantages which make it a particularly attractive target organ for gene therapy. The genes for two inherited pulmonary disorders, cystic fibrosis (CF) and α_1-antitrypsin deficiency, have been identified. These diseases are the two most common fatal inherited disorders of white Europeans and cannot be cured by current therapeutic regimens. Cystic fibrosis and α_1-antitrypsin deficiency are thus attractive targets for gene therapy. Similar considerations apply to lung cancer, which is a common disease for which the molecular basis is currently being elucidated and for which conventional therapy is also ineffective. Carcinoma of the lung is the major lethal cancer, its incidence is increasing, and overall mortality from this disease has only minimally improved over the past two decades. Similarly, there is no effective therapy for malignant mesothelioma, which represents a model of localized malignancy without a major metastatic component. Hence, there are a number of pulmonary diseases that meet the criteria justifying a gene therapy approach.

In addition, there are practical considerations which make the lung an attractive target for gene therapy. As a general principle, delivery of the therapeutic gene to the target cell represents a significant limitation to gene therapy applications. In certain disorders, this problem has been overcome by genetically modifying cells *ex vivo* and then reimplanting the corrected cells into the target disease organ. However, this approach is limited to those relatively few cases in which the target cells can be maintained in culture for prolonged periods of time and then reinfused after gene transfer. Therefore, direct *in vivo* gene delivery is mandated for most diseases. The lung differs from other solid organs in possessing a number of advantages which render it accessible for *in vivo* gene delivery. To date, most gene therapy approaches to lung disorders have involved gene delivery via the airway, which provides a direct approach to lung epithelia and should restrict the therapeutic gene almost entirely to the target organ. Airway access to the lung also forms the basis of the novel approach of *in utero* gene transfer [3]. This strategy is based on the hypothesis that expanding stem cells of epithelial origin in the developing lung are accessible via the amniotic fluid, providing the opportunity for permanent gene replacement. Thus, genes administered to a fetus by injection into the amniotic fluid can be delivered to somatic stem cells of the lung epithelia by means of fetal breathing movements. Alternatively, the dual vascular supply of the lung affords a unique opportunity to achieve gene delivery via the pulmonary circulation, thereby permitting gene therapy for pulmonary vascular diseases. In addition, the circulation could be exploited to access primary or metastatic lung tumors. These practical aspects favor the development of gene therapy strategies for diseases of the lung.

3. Vector Systems For Gene Delivery to the Lung

One of the barriers to the implementation of gene therapy strategies for any disease is the requirement for a vector that can deliver the therapeutic gene specifically to the target organ, where it will be expressed at the appropriate level for the length of time necessary to confer a therapeutic benefit. A number of vector systems, both viral and nonviral, have been employed for gene delivery to the lung, each of which is associated with particular advantages and disadvantages; at present, there is no single vector that meets the criteria of specificity, efficiency, and safety of gene expression.

3.1. Viral Vectors

Recombinant viral vectors are designed to exploit the efficient strategies that viruses have evolved to infect cells and deliver their genetic material. For safety reasons, all viral vectors that have been approved for clinical gene therapy trials have been disabled by deletion of part of their genome, so that they are no longer competent to replicate in the target cell.

The first viral vectors to be employed for gene therapy were derived from murine retroviruses [4]. The retrovirus live cycle includes a stage in which the RNA genome is converted into double-stranded DNA which randomly integrates into the host chromosomal DNA. Thus, retroviral vectors have been exploited in gene therapy strategies to achieve stable transduction of the target cell with transmission of the therapeutic gene to all progeny. However, a major disadvantage of these vectors is that they are extremely labile in the presence of serum complement, which has restricted their use to *ex vivo* protocols. In addition, the requirement for the target cells to be actively proliferating at the time of retroviral infection results in poor transduction of the lungs, where the rate of cellular proliferation is low. A further problem, which has hampered the use of retroviral vectors, is the fact that they can be produced only in relatively low titers.

Recombinant adenoviral vectors have been the most widely employed vehicles for gene delivery to the lung because of their natural tropism for the respiratory tract [5]. Adenoviral vectors can accomplish highly efficient gene transfer to a range of cell types *in vivo*, including both dividing and nondividing cells. Another major advantage of adenoviral vectors is that, unlike retroviruses, they can be concentrated to high titers. However, the present generation of adenoviral vectors suffers from a number of limitations which have prevented the realization of their full potential. One problem associated with the use of adenoviral vectors for gene therapy is that host cellular and humoral immune responses result in transient expression of the delivered therapeutic gene and preclude readministration of the same vector. To circumvent this immunological problem, investigators are developing new (so-called "second generation") vectors which have been engineered to minimize the expression of viral antigens. A further disadvantage in certain disease contexts is that the adenoviral genome is not integrated into the host genome, so that expression of the therapeutic gene is only transient. In addition, it has recently been reported that adenoviral vectors do not efficiently infect the columnar and more differentiated cells of the airway [6].

The third major class of viral vectors under consideration for gene delivery to the lung is based on the adeno-associated virus (AAV), a nonpathogenic parvovirus with a single-stranded DNA genome [7]. Like the adenovirus, AAV is naturally tropic for the airway epithelium. Attractive features of AAV vectors are the ability to integrate into the host genome and to transduce a variety of cell types, including both dividing and nondividing cells. Practical disadvantages include the facts that AAV vectors can be produced only at very low titers and that the size of the therapeutic gene that can be accommodated is limited to 4.5 kilobase-pairs (kb). In addition, whereas the parental AAV can achieve site-specific integration, this capacity is not retained by AAV-based vectors, which raises the possibility of insertional mutagenesis.

3.2. Nonviral Vectors

A number of nonviral vector systems have been developed for gene transfer. In these approaches the therapeutic gene is either administered to the target cell in the form of so-called "naked DNA" or is complexed with other macromolecules in order to achieve cellular entry. Nonviral vectors possess the potential advantage of increased safety and reduced immunogenicity compared with viral vectors, but their employment has been restricted by a relatively low efficiency of gene transfer *in vivo*.

Artificial lipid bilayers, or liposomes, have been widely used to translocate DNA into the cytosol via membrane fusion or endocytosis [8]. Cationic lipids complex with anionic plasmid DNA via charge/charge interactions and have been shown to increase the transfection efficiency of naked DNA by 100- to 1000-fold. In contrast, anionic liposomes encapsulate plasmid DNA within a lipid vesicle. Liposomes possess the important attribute of systemic stability and can therefore be employed *in vivo*. Strategies to improve liposomes have focused extensively on new lipids and formulations, whereas antibodies or ligands have been incorporated into the design to permit targeting to specific cell types.

Molecular conjugate vectors have been developed specifically to accomplish the delivery of heterologous genes to target cells via the receptor-mediated endocytosis pathway [9]. The basic design of molecular conjugates consists of plasmid DNA complexed to polylysine and a macromolecular ligand which can be internalized by the target cell. However, this class of vector is incapable of efficient gene transfer *in vivo*, because the polylysine component renders the conjugate unstable in the presence of serum.

4. Gene Therapy For Diseases of the Lung

4.1. Inherited Pulmonary Diseases

4.1.1. Cystic fibrosis: Cystic fibrosis (CF) is an autosomal recessive disease affecting about 1 in 3000 white European births. In 1989, the genetic defect responsible for CF was identified as mutations in the gene encoding the cystic fibrosis transmembrane conductance regulator (CFTR), a cAMP-mediated chloride channel which also regulates a number of other cationic and anionic channels. The major cause of morbidity and mortality in CF is pulmonary disease characterized by viscous mucus secretion, chronic bacterial infection, airway inflammation, and premature death at around 29 years of age. The lung has therefore been the primary target organ in CF gene therapy, whereby investigators seek to restore the normal phenotype by introduction of the wild-type (normal) CFTR gene into airway epithelial cells.

The feasibility of gene replacement therapy for CF was first shown in *in vitro* experiments which demonstrated that the introduction of the wild-type CFTR gene into cultured CF airway epithelial cells leads to restoration of normal Cl⁻ transport [10, 11]. A number of studies have investigated the relationship between the efficiency of gene transfer (the fraction of cells transduced) and the degree of functional correction. In separate *in vitro* studies, Johnson et al. have indicated that, whereas expression of CFTR in as few as 6–10% of CF airway epithelial cells can restore normal Cl⁻ transport properties to an entire epithelial sheet, gene transfer to all the cells may be necessary to correct the sodium hyperabsorption characteristic of CF [12, 13]. These results have been confirmed in an animal model in which the CFTR gene was delivered by an adenoviral vector to human

CF bronchial xenografts grown in *nu/nu* mice: 5% gene transfer completely restored Cl⁻ transport but had a variable effect on sodium hyperabsorption [14]. Thus, if sodium hyperabsorption across surface epithelia plays a
major role in the pathogenesis of CF lung disease, highly efficient gene
transfer may be necessary to restore normal airway function.

These studies have provided the rationale for the delivery of the CFTR
gene to intact airways, first in animal models and, subsequently, in human
clinical trials based on nasal and/or lung-directed gene transfer. The goal of
this work is the efficient delivery of the CFTR gene to the appropriate
target cells without causing toxicity or inflammation. In addition, as the airway surface epithelium regenerates slowly over time, long-term expression
of the CFTR gene will either require integration into a population of stem
cells or readministration of the vector. The preclinical studies and human
CF gene therapy trials have been described extensively elsewhere [15] and
are therefore not reviewed in detail in this chapter.

Current approaches to CF gene therapy have primarily employed adenoviruses, adeno-associated viruses, and liposomes to achieve gene transfer
via the lumen. Each of these vectors can transfer the CFTR gene to airway
epithelia *in vivo*, resulting in at least partial correction of the Cl⁻ transport
defect. However, a number of problems have been identified with these
systems, which will need to be overcome if gene therapy is to become of
clinical utility in the treatment of CF. Initial human trials have revealed that
the efficiency of gene transfer to uninjured airway epithelia by the current
generation of vectors is low. In the case of adenoviral vectors, the ineffi-
ciency of gene transfer to fully differentiated epithelial cells has been correlated with a paucity of the cellular receptors required for adenovirus internalization [16]. A second major concern relates to the safety of the vectors.
Several studies have shown that the number of adenoviral particles required for efficient gene transfer is associated with direct viral toxicity, mani-
festing as both local and systemic inflammation. A further problem with
the use of adenoviral vectors for CF gene therapy is that host cellular and
humoral immune responses result in transient expression of the delivered
gene and preclude readministration of the vector. Several groups are developing strategies to overcome these immune responses to adenoviral vectors, based on an understanding of the underlying biological mechanisms.
One approach has been to modify the adenoviral vector itself to minimize
the expression of viral proteins. Various immunomodulatory regimens are
also being investigated as strategies to prolong expression of the therapeutic
gene and/or permit readministration of the adenoviral vector. Thus, further
advances with CF gene therapy will be dependent on improvements to the
efficiency and safety profiles of the vectors used to deliver the CFTR gene.

4.1.2. α₁-Antitrypsin deficiency: After CF, α_1-antitrypsin (α_1AT) deficiency
is the second most common lethal hereditary disorder in white Europeans,
with an incidence of about 1 in 3000 births. The α_1-antitrypsin protein is a

52 kDa serum glycoprotein which is synthesized and secreted primarily from the liver. Its major site of action is the lower respiratory tract of the lung, where passive diffusion of α_1-antitrypsin into the alveoli confers protection against neutrophil elastase-mediated proteolysis. A deficiency in the serum levels, and consequently in the epithelial lining fluid (ELF) levels, of α_1-antitrypsin permits unimpeded elastolytic destruction of the lung, creating the chronic condition defined as emphysema – permanent enlargement of the airspaces distal to the terminal bronchioles, accompanied by destruction of the alveolar wall. Patients with α_1-antitrypsin deficiency usually develop emphysema in their fifth decade.

The 12.2 kb α_1-antitrypsin gene has a high level of polymorphism, with over 70 alleles described. The normal variant, designated the M allele, is present in most individuals, although other alleles are associated with a variety of deficiency phenotypes, including impaired function of the α_1-antitrypsin protein, reduced amounts or unstable α_1-antitrypsin protein, or intracellular destruction of the newly synthesized protein. The α_1-antitrypsin gene is codominantly expressed which means that the presence of a normal M allele maintains serum levels of α_1-antitrypsin above 10 µmol/l, the threshold associated with the risk of pulmonary emphysema.

The traditional treatment of α_1-antitrypsin deficiency has focused on intravenous weekly to monthly infusions of α_1-antitrypsin to maintain adequate serum levels. This approach suffers from a number of limitations, including the high costs and inconvenience of long-term treatment, together with the risks associated with the use of products derived from human plasma. Thus, α_1-antitrypsin deficiency is also an attractive candidate for gene therapy. In addition to meeting the criteria necessary for a gene therapy approach, the disease offers several practical advantages. First, α_1-antitrypsin can be expressed by a variety of cell types and does not require any specialized processing. Second, it can be secreted into the serum from numerous sites and then localize to the respiratory tract. Furthermore, no disease is associated with serum α_1-antitrypsin levels above a clear threshold so that strict gene regulation does not seem to be necesary.

The feasibility of gene therapy for α_1-antitrypsin deficiency was established by Garver et al. who transformed mouse fibroblasts *ex vivo* with a retroviral vector carrying the α_1-antitrypsin cDNA and then transplanted the modified cells into the peritoneal cavities of nude mice [17]. Human α_1-antitrypsin was detected in both the sera and the epithelial surface of the lungs for one month. Other investigators have subsequently targeted *in vivo* expression of α_1-antitrypsin to either the liver, its normal site of synthesis, or the lung, its site of protection.

Various gene delivery systems have been employed to transfer the human α_1-antitrypsin gene to the liver *in vivo*. Kay et al. employed a retroviral vector expressing α_1-antitrypsin to transduce hepatocytes harvested from dogs and then reinfused the modified cells back into the animal via the portal vein. Serum α_1-antitrypsin was detected for one month [18]. In an alternative approach, they induced liver regeneration in a mouse model by performing partial hepatectomies and then transduced hepatocytes *in situ* by infusion of retroviral vectors via the portal vein [19]. This resulted in the transduction of $1-2\%$ of hepatocytes, whereas expression of α_1-antitrypsin persisted for up to 6 months. In another approach, Jaffe et al. infused an adenoviral vector containing α_1-antitrypsin into the portal circulation of rats, producing detectable serum levels for 4 weeks [20]. However, in all these cases the serum α_1-antitrypsin levels were far below what would be required for physiologic correction of deficiency.

The low levels of α_1-antitrypsin expression achieved by the liver have led other investigators to develop strategies to target the lower respiratory tract directly. As the levels of α_1-antitrypsin required to maintain effective anti-elastase activity in the ELF are much lower than serum levels, it was hypothesized that local production of α_1-antitrypsin by genetic modification of airway epithelial cells might confer a therapeutic benefit. After direct *in vivo* intratracheal administration into cotton rats of an adenoviral vector expressing α_1-antitrypsin, it was synthesized and secreted by lung tissue, and was detected in the ELF for at least a week [21]. However, the issue of adenoviral vector-induced inflammation means that repetitive delivery will not be a feasible solution to the problem of transient expression. To address this limitation, Canonico et al. used an alternative vector system, liposomes, to deliver the α_1-antitrypsin cDNA directly into the lungs of New Zealand white rabbits by either the aerosol or intravenous routes at weekly intervals for 4 weeks [22]. Protein expression persisted for this period, with no evidence of toxicity. This work has been developed into an approved phase I human gene therapy trial.

Therefore, although α_1-antitrypsin deficiency is an ideal candidate disease for gene therapy, the present generation of vectors is inadequate to achieve sustained serum levels of α_1-antitrypsin of a sufficient magnitude to achieve physiologic correction. Although the approach of local production of α_1-antitrypsin at the site of disease pathogenesis may overcome this limitation, this strategy is again dependent on the availability of suitable vector systems.

4.1.3. Surfactant protein B deficiency: Human surfactant protein B (SP-B) is a phospholipid-associated polypeptide of 79 amino acids expressed by respiratory epithelial cells. SP-B is essential for lung function, enhancing the spreading and stability of surfactant phospholipids that reduce surface tension at the alveolar air-liquid interface. SP-B deficiency is an inherited disease of full-term newborn infants which leads to lethal respiratory failure within the first year of life. This disorder therefore represents a logical candidate for gene therapy, in which the human SP-B cDNA would be transferred to the epithelium of the lower respiratory tract. To this end, two groups have demonstrated pulmonary expression of SP-B after adenoviral-mediated gene transfer to the respiratory epithelium of rodents [23, 24]. A

number of investigators have hypothesized that, as SP-B deficiency mani-
fests in the perinatal period, prenatal or fetal gene therapy might be required to minimize morbidity. In this approach, it will be necessary to optimize the timing of gene transfer to maximize gene expression in the
airways, while minimizing the inflammatory response that can be mounted
by the immune system of the developing fetus.

4.2. Thoracic Malignancies

Lung cancer is the most common cause of cancer death in the USA and its
incidence is increasing in other countries. Standard treatment regimens for
lung cancer, including chemotherapy and radiotherapy, have achieved only
marginal improvements in patient survival, suggesting that the benefits
afforded by any novel therapeutic approach are likely to be significant.
Similarly, there is no effective conventional therapy for another thoracic
neoplasm, malignant mesothelioma, which, although less common than
lung cancer, has been studied because it represents a compartmentalized
model of disease, localized to the pleural space. The elucidation of the
molecular mechanisms underlying neoplastic transformation and progression means that cancer can be regarded as a genetic disease, resulting from
the accumulation of a series of acquired genetic lesions, involving aberrant
expression of dominant oncogenes or loss of expression of recessive tumor-
suppressor genes. Therefore, gene therapy represents a rational approach to
the treatment of lung cancer and mesothelioma.

Gene therapy strategies for cancer can be divided into three broad categories: genetic immunopotentiation, molecular chemotherapy, and mutation compensation. Genetic immunopotentiation is defined as the introduction of genetic modifications into host cells in order to augment the
immunologically mediated destruction of tumor cells. In the approach of
molecular chemotherapy, the aim is to eradicate cancer cells by the selective delivery or expression of a toxin gene. Strategies to achieve mutation
compensation are designed to rectify the molecular lesions in the cancer
cell responsible for malignant transformation.

4.2.1. Genetic immunopotentiation: The strategy of genetic immunopotentiation is based on two principles. First, during carcinogenesis, cells
develop protein structural changes which should allow the normally functioning immune system to recognize tumor cells as foreign and destroy
them. In this regard, a number of tumor-associated antigens have been identified. Second, tumor cells acquire immunologic adaptations which allow
them effectively to avoid immune destruction. Various mechanisms by
which tumor cells evade immune surveillance have been identified or proposed, including: inability of tumor-specific antigens to induce an effective
host T cell response; defects of antigen processing or low expression of

major histocompatibility complex (MHC) class I molecules; lack of co-stimulatory signals; tumor secretion of immunosuppressive factors; and defects in signal transduction by host T cells.

Based on these principles, a number of approaches have been developed, including; (1) the transfer of various cytokine genes into cancer cells to modify the tumor's interactions with the host immune system by stimulating T cell and natural killer (NK) cell proliferation and activity; (2) augmenting antigen presentation or attracting effector cells; (3) increasing the immunogenicity of tumor cells by introduction of genes to augment MHC class I antigen presentation or direct introduction of foreign MHC class I molecules; (4) introduction of genes to provide co-stimulatory signals to augment T cell proliferation; and (5) the use of agents that inhibit the production of suppressive factors. The resulting immune response has the potential to detect and kill nongene-modified tumor cells bearing the same tumor-specific antigen, even though these may be distant from the site of gene transfer, as in the case of metastases. In addition, the technique of "genetic vaccination", which involves the use of DNA expression vectors encoding tumor-specific epitopes, has the potential to induce substantial immunity with little or no toxicity.

A number of cytokines have been tested in genetic immunopotentiation approaches to lung cancer in animal models (reviewed in Lee and Carbone [25]). In most work to date, tumor cells have been transfected with the gene of interest *ex vivo* and then reintroduced into the host animal. More recent studies have attempted to directly transduce tumor cells *in situ*. Induction of antitumor cytotoxic T lymphocytes has been demonstrated after transduction of lung tumor cells with genes expressing several cytokines, including interleukin 2 (IL-2), IL-4, IL-6, IL-7, IL-12, interferon-γ (IFN-γ), tumor necrosis factor α (TNF-α), and granulocyte-macrophage colony-stimulating factor (GM-CSF). Reduction of metastatic potential and/or suppression of tumorigenicity has also been reported in these animal studies. These data therefore support the hypothesis that locally released cytokines from tumor cells can help the host immune system detect previously unrecognized tumor-specific antigens and induce the ability to kill the tumor cells. Based on these results, a number of human clinical trials have been initiated using cytokine gene-modified cells. In another approach to the treatment of lung cancer by genetic immunopotentiation, Plaskin et al. have shown that expression of a transfected MHC gene converted a highly metastatic Lewis lung carcinoma cell to a non- or low-metastatic phenotype and protected against metastatic spread [26].

4.2.2. Molecular chemotherapy: The approach of molecular chemotherapy involves the tumor cell-specific expression of an enzyme which converts a normally nontoxic drug into a toxic substance. Thus, tumor cells that express the activating enzyme will be killed upon administration of the prodrug, whereas cells lacking the enzyme will not be harmed. Several enzyme/prodrug combinations have been proposed, including cytosine deaminase/5-fluorocytosine, cytochrome P450 2B1/cyclophosphamide and xanthine-guanine phosphoribosyltransferase/6-thioxynthine. To date, the most widely investigated system has involved the introduction of the gene encoding herpes simplex virus thymidine kinase (HSV-TK) into mammalian cells. This enzyme, which is not normally present in mammalian cells, converts the nontoxic nucleoside analog, gancyclovir (GCV) into a monophosphorylated form which is then converted by the normal mammalian thymidine kinase enzymes into a triphosphorylated form which blocks DNA synthesis and leads to cell death. The approach possesses the advantage that toxic metabolites can be transferred via gap junctions to neighboring, non-transduced cells, resulting in cell death. This "bystander effect" means that it is not necessary to transduce all the cells in a solid tumor in order to get relatively complete killing.

The rationale for the use of the HSV-TK/GCV system in the treatment of thoracic neoplasms has been provided by Smythe et al. who used an adenoviral vector to transfer the HSV-TK gene to cell lines derived from human malignant mesotheliomas and nonsmall cell lung cancers [27]. Expression of HSV-TK rendered cells sensitive to doses of GCV that were 2–3 logs lower than uninfected cells or those infected with a control virus. These investigators performed initial animal experiments to test this strategy using localized models of malignancy formed by growing human lung cancer and mesothelioma cancer tumors within the peritoneal cavities of severe combined immune-deficient (SCID) mice. After GCV therapy, macroscopic tumor was eradicated in 90% of animals and microscopic tumor was undetectable in 80% of animals [28]. Similar reductions in tumor burden have also been seen in systems that more closely mimic the human disease, for which syngeneic models of malignant mesothelioma were developed in the pleural space of rats and nonhuman primates and treated with intrapleurally administered adenovirus expressing HSV-TK [29, 30]. These results have led to the initiation of a clinical trial employing intrapleural delivery of the adenoviral vector to transfer HSV-TK to patients with malignant mesothelioma. However, preliminary results have served to underline the inadequacy of current vector systems for gene therapy. Thus, although it was believed that the compartmentalized nature of malignant mesothelioma would restrict expression of HSV-TK to the target cancer cells, extrathoracic viral dissemination has been observed. In addition, intrapleural administration of the adenoviral vectors has been associated with a low level of efficiency of gene transfer to the disease cells. This indicates that future advances will be dependent on improvements in vector technology, including modifications to permit cell-specific targeting and to increase the efficieny of gene transfer.

4.2.3. Mutation compensation: The identification of the molecular basis of thoracic malignancies means that it may be possible specifically to correct the underlying genetic lesions. These mutations are of two general types: loss of function of tumor-suppressor genes or gain of function of dominant oncogenes. Mutation compensation strategies therefore involve either replacement of a defective tumor-suppressor gene or ablation of a dominant oncogene at the level of its DNA, mRNA, or protein. The formation of triplex DNA by oligonucleotides targeted to the promoter regions of dominant oncogenes has been shown to result in specific and selective inhibition of transcription *in vitro*. Antisense oligonucleotides function by binding to the target mRNA and blocking further processing of the genetic information by triggering the degradation of the target mRNA by RNase H. A second class of anti-mRNA agents is made up of the ribozymes, which are small oligoribonucleotides capable of catalyzing RNA-cleavage reactions at specific sites. Alternatively, oncogenes can be functionally inactivated at the protein level by the use of intracellular single-chain antibodies or by the heterologous expression of a mutant protein, which can inhibit the normal function of the native gene product in a cell – the so-called dominant negative mutation strategy.

Mutations in the p53 tumor-suppressor gene are the most common genetic lesions in human tumors and occur with high frequency in non-small cell lung cancer, thereby representing an important target for gene therapy. Restoration of wild-type p53 gene expression after delivery of the p53 gene by retroviral or adenoviral vectors has been shown to result in growth arrest of a number of human lung cancer cell lines *in vitro* (reviewed in [31]). In an orthotopic murine model of human lung cancer, direct intratracheal administration of retroviral or adenoviral vectors carrying wild-type p53 led to suppression of tumor growth. Replacement of p53 in p53-deleted lung cancer cell lines has also been shown to increase chemosensitivity to cisplatin, a DNA-active agent. Based on these preclinical studies, human phase I clinical trials have been initiated by Dr Jack Roth at the University of Texas M.D. Anderson Cancer Center. In the first trial, a retroviral vector containing the wild-type p53 gene was used to mediate transfer of wild-type p53 into human non-small cell lung cancers by direct injection. No clinically significant vector-related toxic effects were noted up to 5 months after treatment. A second trial involves bronchoscopic adenovirus-mediated delivery of p53 with or without cisplatin. Hence, the current state of vector development has limited this mutation-compensation strategy to the treatment of localized tumors without any attempt to treat metastatic disease.

Activation of the dominant K-*ras* oncogene as a result of a point mutation is commonly found in lung cancer and is therefore a rational target for mutation-compensation strategies (reviewed in [31]). Roth's group has employed both a plasmid and a retroviral vector to deliver an antisense K-*ras* fragment and reduce the growth rate of lung cancer cells *in vitro* and the tumorigenicity in a murine model. This successful use of antisense K-*ras* RNA to achieve targeted therapeutic tumor regression *in vivo* has been translated into a clinical protocol for the regional treatment of human lung cancer.

As the growth of tumors depends on dysregulation of the cell cycle, specific cell cycle regulatory proteins present rational targets for cancer gene therapy. In this regard, the regulatory protein cyclin D1 is overexpressed in lung cancer. An antisense cyclin D1 construct inhibited the expression of cyclin D in mouse lung cancer cells, significantly reducing both their *in vitro* proliferation and tumorigenicity in nude mice relative to control cells [32].

Mutation compensation strategies have also been employed to target various growth factor receptors which are aberrantly expressed in lung cancer. For example, the insulin-like growth factor I receptor (IGF-Ir) is often overexpressed in lung cancer and therefore provides a good target for gene therapy strategies. Delivery of an adenovirus expressing an antisense IGF-Ir has been shown to decrease the IGF-Ir number by about 50% in human lung cancer cell lines *in vitro*, whereas, in a murine model of established intraperitoneal human lung cancer, intraperitoneal treatment by this vector resulted in prolonged survival [33]. The transmembrane protein kinase receptor erbB-2 (also called Her-2 or neu) is also overexpressed in several human malignancies including lung cancer. As an alternative to using antisense constructs, Grim et al. have shown that intracellular expression of an anti-erbB-2 single-chain antibody delivered by an adenoviral vector can cause specific cytotoxicity in lung cancer cells *in vitro* [34]. In this approach, production of the single-chain antibody within the cell appears to prevent cell surface expression of the erbB-2 receptor.

A number of mutation compensation strategies therefore exist to accomplish the ablation of aberrantly expressed dominant oncogenes. The challenges facing the practical implementation of these approaches in the clinic include the need to improve the efficiency of vector systems, in order to increase the percentage of cells that are transduced by the therapeutic gene. The issue of vector delivery is also pertinent because if metastatic disease is to be treated, intravenous administration of the vector will be required. In this context, there is a stringent demand for specificity of gene delivery to the tumor cells, in order both to avoid vector wastage after transduction of nontarget cells and, more importantly, to prevent toxicity associated with expression of the therapeutic genes in normal cells.

4.3. Acquired Pulmonary Diseases

4.3.1. Inflammatory diseases: Gene therapy is also being considered as a rational therapeutic option for the treatment of both chronic and acute inflammatory diseases of the lung. Candidate disorders include idiopathic pulmonary fibrosis (IPF), asthma, emphysema, and acute diseases such as acute respiratory distress syndrome (ARDS) and radiation-induced pulmonary inflammation. In these cases, disease is not the result of a single genetic defect, but may be a direct or indirect consequence of multiple genetic detects or of interactions between genetic and environmental factors or the response to a toxic stimulus. Therapeutic intervention must therefore be based on an understanding of the molecular pathogenesis of the inflammatory response.

In general, the progression of inflammatory lung diseases involves a cascade of events presenting multiple opportunities for intervention at the molecular level by gene therapy-based approaches. Rational targets include: the manipulation of the levels of either pro- or anti-inflammatory cytokines; down-regulation of cell surface adhesion molecules; enhancement of host antioxidant defenses; increasing the levels of endogenous antiproteases; and upregulation of the production of anti-inflammatory prostanoids [35]. Genetic intervention at any of these levels clearly offers many possibilities for the treatment of inflammatory pulmonary diseases and will also provide information of more general relevance to the field of gene therapy. Selected examples of these approaches will be discussed here.

Expression of TNF-α is increased in IPF and other inflammatory lung diseases. Systemic delivery of soluble TNF-α receptor has been shown to be effective in reducing inflammation in a mouse model of pulmonary fibrosis [36]. Kolls et al. have demonstrated a similar response in mice treated intravenously with an adenoviral vector encoding a soluble TNF-α receptor [37], whereas intravenous injection of antibodies against TNF-α has blocked the onset of other inflammatory diseases in animal models. In an alternative approach, local delivery of the soluble TNF-α receptor gene has attenuated the local inflammatory response in the mouse [38]. Local and/or systemic delivery of inhibitors of other proinflammatory cytokines could similarly be employed in a gene therapy approach. Many cytokines are potential targets for knockout in the treatment of pulmonary inflammatory diseases, including IL-1, IL-4 and IL-5, platelet-derived growth factor [39], transforming growth factor β, and GM-CSF [40]. In a specific approach to ARDS, the cytokine macrophage inhibitory factor (MIF), has recently been identified as a key mediator sustaining the pulmonary inflammatory response, suggesting that an anti-MIF strategy would represent a logical therapeutic intervention [41]. In contrast, IL-10 is an anti-inflammatory cytokine able to suppress expression of a variety of cytokines by macrophages. Thus, IL-10 might be of general therapeutic utility in blocking the immune response at the site of pulmonary inflammation.

Cell surface adhesion molecules such as intercellular adhesion molecule-1 (ICAM-1) and endothelial leukocyte adhesion molecule (E-selectin) serve as ligands for inflammatory cell adhesion and activation. Expression of these molecules on the surface of pulmonary vascular endothelial cells is upregulated in chronic and acute inflammatory conditions. Hence, a number of investigators are employing gene therapy strategies designed to knock-out cell adhesion molecules. In support of this approach, the lack of ICAM-1 in transgenic mice has been shown completely to abrogate the development of pulmonary inflammation during murine lupus [42]. Inflammatory cell infiltration into the lung in response to exposure to ionizing radiation has been demonstrated to be attenuated in mice treated with an anti-ICAM-1 blocking antibody [43].

In an approach to the treatment of acute lung injury, Erzurum et al. have shown that adenovirus-mediated delivery of the catalase gene to pulmonary endothelium can provide augmented vascular antioxidant defenses which would be of therapeutic utility for diseases such as ARDS [44]. Another class of enzymes, antiproteases, also has potential for use in the treatment of chronic and acute lung inflammation. Activated neutrophils sequestered in the lungs release neutrophil elastase (NE) which can degrade almost every connective tissue component of the lung. Canonico et al. have shown that the release of neutrophil chemoattractants from human airway epithelial cells exposed to NE was prevented if the cells were transfected with the human α_1-antitrypsin cDNA before elastase exposure [45]. This suggests that the general anti-inflammatory properties of antiproteases could be exploited for gene therapy.

Prostacyclin (PGI$_2$) and prostaglandin E$_2$ (PGE$_2$) exhibit anti-inflammatory effects which could be used to treat chronic or acute inflammatory lung diseases. Patients with IPF have a diminished capacity to synthesize these prostanoids as a result of a deficiency of PG synthase. Conary et al. demonstrated expression of PGI$_2$ and PGE$_2$ in the lungs of rabbits 24 hours after delivery, via the pulmonary artery, of the PG synthase gene complexed to cationic liposomes [46]. In isolated, perfused rabbit lungs transfected with the PG synthase gene, the pressor response to endotoxin was markedly attenuated. In addition, pulmonary edema was markedly decreased in lungs from animals receiving the synthase gene compared with controls. The data obtained in this model of acute lung injury therefore suggest that up-regulation of PGI$_2$ and PGE$_2$ protects the lungs from endotoxin.

Hence, the identification of the molecular mechanisms underlying the disease process can suggest gene therapy strategies for the treatment of inflammatory lung disorders.

4.3.2. Infectious diseases: In a similar manner, understanding of the host defense mechanisms against the viral or bacterial pathogens responsible for pulmonary infectious diseases can lead to the exploitation of these pathways for therapeutic purposes. To date, the gene therapy strategies proposed for the treatment of inflammatory lung diseases are based on the transfer of proinflammatory cytokines to enhance the host immune responses to the pathogens.

One of the first lines of host defense against bacterial invasion of the lower respiratory tract is provided by alveolar macrophages. The cytokine elaboration by these cells is critical to recruitment of inflammatory cells, which are necessary to clear the bacteria from the lung. Thus cytokines have been proposed as therapeutic agents for a variety of pulmonary infections. To avoid the complications of toxicity, which are associated with the intravenous administration of cytokines such as TNF, IL-2 and IL-12, researchers are investigating the local, compartmentalized delivery of specific cytokines as a rational approach to the treatment of focal diseases such as pneumonia. Greenberger et al. have demonstrated that intratracheal delivery of an adenoviral vector expressing the proinflammatory cytokine IL-12 enhanced both bacterial clearance and survival in mice challenged with *Klebsiella pneumoniae* [47]. In this work, treatment with anti-IFN-γ antibodies or soluble TNF receptor partially and completely attenuated the survival benefits observed in animals receiving the adenovirally delivered IL-12, respectively.

Lei et al. [48] have investigated the treatment of pneumonia by adenovirus-mediated delivery of murine IFN-γ, a critical cytokine in pulmonary host defenses against both intracellular and extracellular pathogens. After intratracheal inoculation in rats, this vector resulted in prolonged expression of functional IFN-γ *in vivo*, as demonstrated by enhanced host defenses against *Pseudomonas aeruginosa* and *Klebsiella pneumoniae* [48]. Transfer of the IFN-γ gene has also been employed by this group in an attempt to enhance cell-mediated immunity against tuberculosis (TB). In this case, adenovirus-mediated delivery of the murine IFN gene resulted in a significant attenuation of growth of TB in mice given a low-dose aerosol challenge with the organism.

Thus, the compartmentalized overexpression of proinflammatory cytokines has been demonstrated to be of utility in animal models of bacterial pulmonary infections.

4.3.3. Pulmonary vascular diseases: To date, most therapeutic gene transfer to the lung has involved delivery via the airways in order to reach epithelial cell targets. However, the delivery of genes via the pulmonary circulation would be a useful approach to the treatment of diseases affecting vascular function, including pulmonary hypertension, pulmonary thrombosis disorders, and vasculitis. In addition, the pulmonary circulation could be used to access primary or metastatic lung tumors. The pulmonary circulation could also be exploited to provide an indirect route for delivery of genes to the airways. Hence, there are many disease states for which it might prove beneficial to deliver genes via the pulmonary circulation.

The feasibility of gene transfer to the lung vasculature *in vivo* has been demonstrated with a number of vector systems. Lemarchand et al. achieved gene delivery to the lung of sheep by surgically isolating the pulmonary artery and veins, inserting a catheter into the cranial segment and infusing an adenviral vector [49]. In contrast, Rodman et al. have employed percutaneous catheter-mediated delivery of both liposomes and adenoviral vectors to transfer reporter genes to the pulmonary circulation in rats [50]. In this study, the efficiency of gene transfer by the adenovirus was more than 50-fold that achieved by the liposomes. The detection of extrapulmonary expression of the transgenes suggests that future developments should include targeting strategies to achieve cell-specific expression of therapeutic genes.

5. Future Challenges

Although tremendous progress has been made in the ability to transfer genes to cells successfully, the field of gene therapy is still in its infancy. Although many therapeutic genes have been identified for the treatment of both inherited and acquired diseases of the lung, there remain several unresolved problems limiting the practical translation of these gene therapy strategies at the present time. Thus, a number of researchers are attempting to increase the transduction efficiency of viral and nonviral vectors in order to permit gene transfer to a greater percentage of cells. To this end, strategies are also being explored which would enable viral vectors to replicate specifically within the targets cells, to permit gene transfer within a solid tumor, for example. Other investigators are seeking to develop vector-targeting strategies, which will be important to permit gene transfer to disseminated cancer cells as well as to permit cell-specific gene delivery in compartmentalized models of disease. Methods to regulate the expression of therapeutic genes are being explored and it is expected that a lot of attention will be focused on the identification of promoters that can selectively activate genes only within the target disease cells. Other key areas of future research include modifying viral vectors to reduce toxicity and immunogenicity. Some improvements will be specific to individual vector systems, for example, modifications to adenoviral vectors to permit long-term gene expression, which will be important for certain diseases. The lung will continue to serve as a model system in the field of gene therapy in which the requirements for advances in vector development are identified and novel vectors are evaluated. As vector technology evolves, it should become possible to realize the full potential of gene therapy as a valid therapeutic option for pulmonary diseases.

Acknowledgements

The authors gratefully acknowledge support from the National Institutes of Health (R01 HL 50255), the American Lung Association (both to DTC), and the American Heart Association (DTC and JTD).

References

1 Anderson WF (1984) Prospects for human gene therapy. *Science* 226: 401–409
2 National Institutes of Health Recombinant DNA Advisory Committee (1997) Human gene therapy protocols. *Hum Gene Therapy* 8: 1981–2003

3 Sekhon HS, Larson JE (1995) *In utero* gene transfer into the pulmonary epithelium. *Nature Med* 1: 1201–1203

4 Vile RG, Russell SJ (1995) Retroviruses as vectors. *B Med Bull* 51: 12–30

5 Trapnell B, Gorziglia M (1994) Gene therapy using adenoviral vectors. *Curr Opin Biotech* 5: 617–625

6 Grubb BR, Pickles RJ, Ye H, Yankaskas JR, Vick RN, Engelhardt JF, Wilson JM, Johnson LG, Boucher RC (1994) Inefficient gene transfer by adenovirus vector to cystic fibrosis airway epithelia of mice and humans. *Nature* 371: 802–806

7 Muzyczka N (1992) Use of adeno-assocaited virus as a general transduction vector for mammalian cells. *Curr Top Microbiol Immunol* 158: 97–128

8 Lee RJ, Huang L (1997) Lipidic vector systems for gene transfer. *Crit Rev Ther Drug Carrier Systems* 14: 173–206

9 Cristiano RJ, Curiel DT (1996) Strategies to accomplish gene delivery via the receptor-mediated endocytosis pathway. *Cancer Gene Therapy* 3: 49–57

10 Drumm ML, Pope HA, Cliff WH, Rommens JM, Marvin SA, Tsui Lc, Collins FS, Frizzell RA, Wilson JM (1990) Correction of the cystic fibrosis defect *in vitro* by retrovirus-mediated gene transfer. *Cell* 62: 1227–1233

11 Rich DP, Anderson MP, Gregory RJ, Cheng SH, Paul S, Jefferson DM, McCann JD, Klinger KW, Smith AE, Welsh MJ (1990) Expression of cystic fibrosis transmembrane conductance regulator corrects defective chloride channel regulation in cystic fibrosis airway epithelial cells. *Nature* 347: 358–363

12 Johnson LG, Olsen JC, Sarkadi B, Moore KL, Swanstrom R, Boucher RC (1992) Efficiency of gene transfer for restoration of normal airway epithelial function in cystic fibrosis. *Nature Genet* 2: 21–25

13 Johnson LG, Boyles SE, Wilson J, Boucher RC (1995) Normalization of raised sodium absorption and raised calcium-mediated chloride secretion by adenovirus-mediated expression of cystic fibrosis transmembrane conductance regulator in primary human cystic fibrosis airway epithelial cells. *J Clin Invest* 95: 1377–1382

14 Goldman MJ, Yang Y, Wilson JM (1995) Gene therapy in a xenograft model of cystic fibrosis lung corrects chloride transport more effectively than the sodium defect. *Nature Genet* 9: 126–131

15 Wilson JM (1995) Gene therapy for cystic fibrosis: challenges and future directions. *J Clin Invest* 96: 2547–2554

16 Goldman M, Su Q, Wilson JM (1996) Gradient of RGD-dependent entry of adenoviral vector in nasal and intrapulmonary epithelia: implications for gene therapy of cystic fibrosis. *Gene Therapy* 3: 811–818

17 Garver RI Jr, Chytil A, Courtney M, Crystal RG (1987) Clonal gene therapy: transplanted mouse fibroblast clones express human α_1-antitrypsin gene *in vivo*. *Science* 237: 762–764

18 Kay MA, Baley P, Rothenberg S, Leland F, Fleming L, Ponder KP, Liu T, Finegold M, Darlington G, Pokorny W et al. (1992) Expression of human α_1-antitrypsin in dogs after autologous transplantation of retroviral transduced hepatocytes. *Proc Natl Acad Sci USA* 89: 89–93

19 Kay MA, Li Q, Liu TJ, Leland F, Toman C, Finegold M, Woo SL (1992) Hepatic gene therapy: persistent expression of human α_1-antitrypsin in mice after direct gene delivery *in vivo*. *Hum Gene Therapy* 3: 641–647

20 Jaffe HA, Danel C, Longenecker G, Metzger M, Setoguchi Y, Rosenfeld MA, Gant TW, Thorgeirsson SS, Stratford-Perricaudet LD, Perricaudet M et al. (1992) Adenovirus-mediated *in vivo* gene transfer and expression in normal rat liver. *Nature Genet* 1: 372–378

21 Rosenfeld MA, Siegfried W, Yoshimura K, Yoneyama K, Fukayama M, Stier LE, Paakko PK, Gilardi P, Stratford-Perricaudet LD, Perricaudet M et al. (1991) Adenovirus-mediated transfer of a recombinant α_1-antitrypsin gene to the lung epithelium *in vivo*. *Science* 252: 431–434

22 Canonico AE, Plitman JD, Conary JT, Meyrick BO, Brigham KL (1994) No lung toxicity after repeated aerosol or intravenous delivery of plasmid-cationic liposome complexes. *J Appl Phys* 77: 415–419

23 Yei S, Bachurski CJ, Weaver TE, Wert SE, Trapnell BC, Whitsett JA (1994) Adenoviral-mediated gene transfer of human surfactant protein B to respiratory epithelial cells. *Am J Respir Cell Mol Biol* 11: 329–336

24 Korst RJ, Bewig B, Crystal RG (1995) *In vitro* and *in vivo* transfer and expression of human surfactant SP-A- and SP-B-associated protein cDNAs mediated by replication-deficient, recombinant adenoviral vectors. *Hum Gene Therapy* 6: 277–287

25 Lee C-T, Carbone DP (1997) Gene therapy for lung cancer. In: KL Brigham (ed): *Gene therapy for lung cancer.* Marcel Dekker, New York, 323–345

26 Plaskin D, Gelber C, Feldman M, Eisenbach L (1988) Reversal of the metastatic phenotype in Lewis lung carcinomas after transfection with syngeneic H-2Kb gene. *Proc Natl Acad Sci USA* 85: 4463–4467

27 Smythe WR, Hwang HC, Amin KM, Eck SL, Davidson BL, Wilson JM, Kaiser LR, Albelda SM (1994) Use of recombinant adenovirus to transfer the herpes simplex virus thymidine kinase (HSVtk) gene to thoracic neoplasms: an effective *in vitro* drug sensitization system. *Cancer Res* 54: 2055–2059

28 Hwang HC, Smythe WR, Elshami AA, Kucharczuk JC, Amin KM, Williams JP, Litzky LA, Kaiser LR, Albelda SM (1995) Gene therapy using adenovirus carrying the herpes simplex-thymidine kinase gene to treat *in vivo* models of human malignant mesothelioma and lung cancer. *Am J Respir Cell Mol Biol* 13: 7–16

29 Elshami AA, Kucharczuk JC, Zhang HB, Smythe WR, Hwang HC, Litzky LA, Kaiser LR, Albelda SM (1996) Treatment of pleural mesothelioma in an immunocompetent rat model utilizing adenoviral transfer of the herpes simplex virus thymidine kinase gene. *Hum Gene Therapy* 7: 141–148

30 Kucharczuk JC, Raper S, Elshami AA, Amin KM, Sterman DH, Wheeldon EB, Wilson JM, Litzky LA, Kaiser LR, Albelda SM (1996) Safety of intrapleurally administered recombinant adenovirus carrying herpes simplex thymidine kinase DNA followed by ganciclovir therapy in nonhuman primates. *Hum Gene Therapy* 7: 2225–2233

31 Roth JA, Cristiano RJ (1997) Gene therapy for cancer: what have we done and where are we going? *J Natl Cancer Inst* 89: 21–39

32 Schrump DS, Chen A, Consoli U (1996) Inhibition of lung cancer proliferation by antisence cyclin D. *Cancer Gene Therapy* 3: 131–135

33 Lee CT, Wu S, Gabrilovich D, Chen H, Nadaf-Rahrov S, Ciernik IF, Carbone DB (1996) Antitumor effects of an adenovirus expressing antisense insulin-like growth factor I receptor on human lung cancer cell lines. *Cancer Res* 56: 3038–3041

34 Grim J, Deshane J, Feng M, Lieber A, Kay M, Curiel DT (1996) erbB-2 knockout employing an intracellular single-chain antibody (sFv) accomplishes specific toxicity in erbB-2-expressing lung cancer cells. *Am J Respir Cell Mol Biol* 15: 348–354

35 Brigham KL (1997) Gene therapy for acute diseases of the lung. In: KL Brigham (ed): *Gene therapy for acute diseases of the lung.* Marcel Dekker, New York, 309–322

36 Piguet PF, Vesin C (1994) Treatment by recombinant soluble TNF receptor of pulmonary fibrosis induced by bleomycin or silica in mice. *Eur Respir J* 7: 515–518

37 Kolls J, Peppel K, Silva M, Beutler B (1994) Prolonged and effective blockade of tumor necrosis factor activity through adenovirus-mediated gene transfer. *Proc Natl Acad Sci USA* 91: 215–219

38 Rogy MA, Auffenberg T, Espat NJ, Philip R, Remick D, Wollenberg GK, Copeland EMR, Moldawer LL (1995) Human tumor necrosis factor receptor (p55) and interleukin 10 gene transfer in the mouse reduces mortality to lethal endotoxemia and also attenuates local inflammatory responses. *J Exp Med* 181: 2289–2293

39 Ohta K, Nakano J, Nishizawa M, Kaneta M, Nakagome K, Makino K, Suzuki N, Nakajima M, Kawashima R, Mano K et al. (1997) Suppressive effect of antisense DNA of platelet-derived growth factor on murine pulmonary fibrosis with silica particles. *Chest* 111: 105S

40 Xing Z, Tremblay GM, Sime PJ, Gauldie J (1997) Overexpression of granulocyte-macrophage colony-stimulating factor induces pulmonary granulation tissue formation and fibrosis by induction of transforming growth factor-beta 1 and myofibroblast accumulation. *Am J Pathol* 150: 59–66

41 Donnelly SC, Haslett C, Reid PT, Grant IS, Wallace WAH, Metz CN, Bruce LJ, Bucala R (1997) Regulatory role for macrophage migration inhibitory factor in acute respiratory distress syndrome. *Nature Med* 3: 320–323

42 Lloyd CM, Gonzalo J-A, Salant DJ, Just J, Gutierrez-Ramos J-C (1997) Intercellular adhesion molecule-1 deficiency prolongs survival and protects against the development of pulmonary inflammation during murine lupus. *J Clin Invest* 100: 963–971

43 Hallahan DE, Virudachalam S (1997) Intercellular adhesion molecule 1 knockout abrogates radiation induced pulmonary inflammation. *Proc Natl Acad Sci USA* 94: 6432–6437

44 Erzurum SC, Lemarchand P, Rosenfeld MA, Yoo J-H, Crystal RG (1993) Protection of human endothelial cells from oxidant injury by adenovirus-mediated transfer of the human catalase cDNA. *Nuleic Acids Res* 21: 1607–1612

45 Canonico AE, Brigham KL, Carmichael LC, Plitman JD, King GA, Blackwell TR, Christman JW (1996) Plasmid-liposome transfer of the α_1-antitrypsin gene to cystic fibrosis bronchial epithelial cells prevents elastase-induced cell detachment and cytokine release. *Am J Respir Cell Mol Biol* 14: 348–355

46 Conary JT, Parker RE, Christman BW, Faulks RD, King GA, Meyrick BO, Brigham KL (1994) Protection of rabbit lungs from endotoxin injury by *in vivo* hyperexpression of the prostaglandin G/H synthase gene. *J Clin Invest* 93: 1834–1840

47 Greenberger MJ, Kunkel SL, Strieter RM, Lukacs NW, Bramson J, Gauldie J, Graham FL, Hitt M, Danforth JM, Standiford TJ (1996) IL-12 gene therapy protects mice in lethal Klebsiella pneumonia. *J Immunol* 157: 3006–3012

48 Lei DH, Lancaster JR, Joshi MS, Nelson S, Stoltz D, Bagby GJ, Odom G, Shellito JE, Kolls JK (1997) Activation of alveolar macrophages and lung host defenses using transfer of the interferon-gamma gene. *Am J Physiol Lung Cell Mol Physiol* 16: L852–L859

49 Lemarchand P, Jones J, Danel C, Yamada I, Mastrangeli A, Crystal RG (1994) *In vivo* adenovirus-mediated gene transfer to the lungs via the pulmonary artery. *J Applied Physiol* 76: 2840–2845

50 Rodman DM, San H, Simari R, Stephan D, Tanner F, Yang Z, Nabel GJ, Nabel EG (1997) *In vivo* gene delivery to the pulmonary circulation in rats: transgene distribution and vascular inflammatory response. *Am J Respir Cell Mol Biol* 16: 640–649

Asthma

Molecular Biology of the Lung
Vol. 2: Asthma and Cancer
ed. by R. A. Stockley
© 1999 Birkhäuser Verlag Basel/Switzerland

Chapter 2
Genetics of Asthma

Andrew J. Walley and William O. C. M. Cookson

Nuffield Department of Clinical Medicine, John Radcliffe Hospital, Oxford, UK

1   Introduction
2   Finding Genes
3   Genes Influencing Asthma
3.1   Class 1 Asthma Genes: Genes Influencing IgE-Mediated Inflammation
3.1.1   Chromosome 5q23–31
3.1.2   Chromosome 11q12–13
3.1.3   Chromosome 12q15–q24.1
3.2   Class 2 Asthma Genes: Genes Influencing the Specific IgE Response
3.2.1   Human Leukocyte Antigens
3.2.2   The T cell receptor
3.3   Class 3 Asthma Genes: Genes Influencing Bronchial Responsiveness
3.4   Class 4 Asthma Genes: Genes Influencing Non-IgE-Mediated Inflammation
4   Whole Genome Screens for Atopy and Asthma in Humans
5   Whole Genome Screens for Quantitative Trait Loci Underlying Atopy
        and Asthma in Mice
6   Conclusions
        References

1. Introduction

Asthma is strongly familial and so results partly from genetic factors. Defining these factors improves the understanding of the aetiology and pathophysiology of the disease. The involvement of particular genes may allow the prediction of distinct clinical courses and responses to therapy, and the early identification of children at genetic risk of asthma will then be possible. Although the estimate of risk may be relatively imprecise, the prevention of illness by environmental or other intervention in susceptible children is both feasible and desirable. Genetic discoveries will, in the long run, lead to new pharmacological treatments for asthma.

In contrast to single gene disorders such as cystic fibrosis or Duchenne muscular dystrophy, genes predisposing to asthma will not usually contain mutations. Rather they will be variants of normal genes (polymorphisms), whose evolutionary advantage has been lost in the current Western environment. It is also important to remember that the environmental component to asthma and atopy is at least as strong as the genetic component. In children 95% of asthma is allergic, or atopic and atopic asthma is clinically the most easily recognized and defined, and has the most obvious familial clustering. Although other types of asthma, such as aspirin-sensi-

tive asthma (ASA), are neither familial nor atopic, they are still likely to
result from the interaction between genetic and environmental factors.

2. Finding Genes

Genes causing disease may be found either by the process known as positional cloning [1, 2] or by the direct examination of candidate genes.

Positional cloning relies on the phenomenon of genetic linkage. Genes are arranged in a linear array of DNA throughout the genome which is divided into the 23 pairs of chromosomes. During the first stage of meiosis, replicated chromosomes pair up in the cell, break at certain points, form a small number of links to the other member of the pair, and recombine to form two entirely novel chromosome pairs, containing elements of each of the original chromosome pair – a process known as crossing over. After crossover and recombination, there is a second round of cell division without DNA replication, resulting in a single copy of the 23 chromosomes in each gamete (the ovum or sperm). The full set of 46 chromosomes is only restored when a sperm fertilizes an ovum to produce the zygote, from which the fetus develops.

The number of crossovers occuring along a given chromosome is small, often numbering only one or two. As a result of this, large segments of DNA remain intact during meiosis, and genes or segments of DNA that are close together will tend to be passed on to the next generation together. If they are very close they will remain together through many generations. This process, the co-inheritance of stretches of adjacent genes, is known as genetic linkage.

Positional cloning relies on the demonstration of genetic linkage of disease and genetic markers of known chromosomal localization. Once linkage is established, the linked region can be dissected by further genetic mapping with a dense array of closely linked markers. Genetic mapping is followed by physical mapping, the assembly of overlapping DNA clones covering the linked regions, and the eventual identification and sequencing of genes from the DNA.

The positional cloning approach has the advantage of not requiring preexisting knowledge of the pathophysiology of the disease. However, the power to detect linkage in complex genetic diseases is very limited, so that several thousand two-generation families may be necessary to detect linkage to a gene affecting 10% of individuals with disease. Genetic linkage has traditionally been assessed statistically by the lod score. The lod score is the logarithm of the **od**ds that two markers are linked rather than unlinked, for a given estimate of the genetic distance between them. This elegant statistic was the main tool for the localization of single gene disorders such as cystic fibrosis. It has not functioned well in complex disorders because it requires precise knowledge of the model of inheritance, which includes the gene frequency of the disorder, the mendelian inheritance pattern and its penetrance at different ages. For this reason, non-parametric statistics, based on the phenotypes of siblings but ignoring parental phenotypes, are now preferred. Genetic linkage in complex disorders, however assessed, often replicates poorly, at least in the early stages [3]. This is because linkage to a heterogeneous trait is normally only found fortuitously, in samples that contain an exceptional proportion of individuals or families influenced by that particular gene. Simulation experiments have shown that, in these circumstances, many studies may be necessary before replication occurs.

Candidate genes are genes whose known functions suggest that they may have a role in the pathophysiology of a disease. For a candidate, or any gene, to be responsible for the difference between asthmatic and non-asthmatic subjects, there must be at least two varieties: functional and variant. The variant gene may be non-functional or it may function differently.

The role of candidate genes may be assessed by defining polymorphisms within them, and testing for associations with disease. Associations may be found even if the polymorphisms do not alter the function of a gene. This is because when a new mutation or variant first arises in a gene, it will be physically associated or linked with polymorphisms (alleles) of other sequences on the same chromosome. This association of alleles on a chromosome is somewhat clumsily named linkage disequilibrium [4]. Within a gene, linkage disequilibrium of alleles persists for hundreds of generations, so that non-functional alleles will serve as surrogates for the functional alleles nearby. However, establishing whether a polymorphism affects function can be difficult, particularly if it occurs in a non-coding region of a gene.

The enormous increase in understanding of the complex cytokine networks that influence atopy and inflammation means that a plausible case could be made for a large number of different candidates. Successful identification of genes predisposing to asthma is therefore likely to depend on a combination of positional cloning and candidate gene strategies.

3. Genes Influencing Asthma

Many different kinds of genes may be involved in atopy and asthma. These can arbitrarily be divided into four classes: (1) genes predisposing in general to immunoglobulin E (IgE)-mediated inflammation; (2) genes influencing the specific IgE response; (3) genes influencing bronchial hyperresponsiveness independently of atopy; and (4) genes influencing non-IgE-mediated inflammation.

3.1. Class 1 Asthma Genes: Genes Influencing IgE-Mediated Inflammation

Genetic loci influencing total serum IgE levels and the atopic state have been identified on chromosomes 5, 11 and 12, by a combination of genetic linkage and candidate gene approaches.

3.1.1. Chromosome 5q23–31: Linkage of the total serum IgE concentration to markers on chromosome 5q31–33 has been demonstrated by Marsh et al. [5]. Eleven Amish pedigrees made up of 20 nuclear families were selected on the basis of having at least one child with detectable specific IgE to a mixture of 20 common inhalant allergens. Linkage was strongest in the region containing the cytokine cluster. The result was replicated by Myers et al. [6] in Dutch asthmatic families. Using different models of inheritance they concluded, from their data, that there were two unlinked loci on chromosome 5 regulating total serum IgE levels [7]. Further evidence for linkage of the chromosome 5 region with asthma phenotypes was provided by Postma et al. [8] who studied 303 children and grandchildren of asthmatic probands and found linkage of chromosome 5 markers with total serum IgE and bronchial hyperresponsiveness. Doull et al. [9] took the analysis one step further by examining microsatellite markers located in the cytokine cluster region on chromosome 5 for allelic associations between them and atopy and bronchial hyperresponsiveness. They demonstrated a significant allelic association ($p = 0.003$) between the 118 allele of the interleukin-9 microsatellite and total serum IgE. At least one study has contradicted these results with four large Minnesota families being investigated for linkage with none to total serum IgE being detected across the region [10].

We have recently presented results on linkage and allelic associations between chromosome 5q markers and atopic asthma phenotypes in 80 nuclear families from a larger general population sample [11]. We demonstrated weak linkage to total serum IgE or to bronchial hyperresponsiveness ($p < 0.01$) though there was a highly significant strong linkage to eosinophilia (marker D5S658, $p = 0.00091$). Using allelic associations we were able to demonstrate significant associations to microsatellite alleles with allele frequencies greater than 2%. The most significant results were as follows: D5S1995 and total serum IgE ($p = 0.0035$), IL4RP1 and eosinophil count ($p = 0.0011$), and interleukin-9 (IL-9) and bronchial hyperresponsiveness ($p = 0.00042$). The IL-9 association appears to be to a different allele from that reported by Doull et al. [9].

Interest has concentrated upon the chromosome 5q23–31 region because of the plethora of candidate genes in this region. These include IL-3, IL-4, IL-5, IL-9, IL-12b and IL-13, interferon regulatory factor 1 (IFR1), the glucocorticoid (GRL), β_2-adrenergic (ADRB2), colony-stimulating factor 1 (CFS1R) and platelet-derived growth factor (PDGFR) receptors, and granulocyte–macrophage colony-stimulating factor (GM-CSF). As yet there is only evidence for one polymorphism being functional, in the IL-4 promoter [12]. We have investigated this polymorphism for associations with atopy and asthma phenotypes in two populations [13]. In a general Caucasian population sample of 1004 people, a weak association was detected of specific IgE to house dust mite (*Dermatophagoides pteronyssinus*) ($p = 0.013$). However, in the second population, which was a case-control study in which asthmatic atopic probands were compared with unrelated age- and sex-matched, non-atopic, non-asthmatic individuals, there were no significant associations between the polymorphism and either total or specific IgE.

3.1.2. Chromosome 11q12–13: The first suggested linkage of atopy was to the marker D11S97 on chromosome 11q13 [14]. After some controversy [15], linkage has been confirmed consistently [16–20]. It is now obvious that the early difficulty in replicating the linkage to chromosome 11 was the result of the inappropriate use of the lod statistic, and the testing of very small sample sizes. This linkage was also confounded by the high prevalence of atopy, and because the linkage was predominately seen in maternal meioses [21, 22]. In the largest study described, linkage was exclusively maternal [21]. The reasons for the maternal linkage are not known, and it is not clear that this maternal phenomenon corresponds to the phenotypic maternal inheritance of atopy that has previously been noted.

Recognition of the maternal linkage allowed fine mapping of the atopy locus, to within 1 lod unit support interval of 7 cM [22, 23]. This interval was centromeric to and excluded the original D11S97 marker to which linkage was first observed. A lymphocyte surface marker, *CD20*, was noted to be within the interval. *CD20* shows sequence homology to the β chain of the high affinity receptor for IgE (*FcεRIβ*), and has been localized close to that gene on mouse chromosome 19 [24]. The human *FcεRIβ* gene was subsequently found to be on chromosome 11q13, in close genetic linkage to atopy [22].

Two coding polymorphisms were initially identified within the gene: *FcεRIβ Leu181*, and *FcεRIβ Leu181/Leu183* [25]. These variants, situated at the start of exon 6, both showed strong associations with atopy when maternally inherited, and seemed to be quite common. However, a study of 1000 subjects found the population prevalence of *FcεRIβ Leu181/Leu183* to be only 4%, and that of *FcεRIβ Leu 181* was not found at all [26].

Subsequently, both variants have been very difficult to assay reliably, and their status is currently uncertain. The detection of a third homologous gene, *Htm4*, in close proximity to *FcεRIβ* and *CD20* [27], suggests the possibility that homologous sequences in unknown genes or pseudogenes confound the detection of these variants.

A further variant in the receptor, *FcεRIβ E237G*, has recently been described. It is also associated with atopy and bronchial hyperresponsiveness [28]. It is present in about 5% of the UK and other European populations and has also been found in 20% of asthmatic Japanese people [29]. The glutamine to glycine change coded by this variant mkes a substantial polarity change in the intracellular part of the protein, which is likely to have functional implications. Functional studies are still, however, ongoing.

3.1.3. Chromosome 12q15–q24.1: This region on chromosome 12 has attracted some attention because of the presence of several candidate genes within the area, namely: interferon-γ (*IFNG*), mast cell growth factor (*MGF*), leukotriene-4 hydrolase (*LTA4H*) and insulin-like growth factor-I (*IGFI*). Barnes et al. [30] examined two groups for linkage of chromosome 12 markers with asthma and total serum IgE: the first consisted of 29 Afro-Caribbean multiplex families derived by recruiting the extended families of 29 asthmatic probands, and the second consisted of the 11 Amish kindreds described by Marsh et al. [5] plus 39 additional members, including one new family. Significant linkage was found in the Afro-Caribbean group to asthma (D12S379, $p = 0.001$) and total serum IgE (D12S360, $p = 0.001$) and in the Amish the result for total serum IgE was similar (D12S360, $p = 0.01$) although at a lower level of significance. Multipoint analysis of asthma in the Afro-Caribbean group also showed a peak of linkage centred on D12S379 ($p = 0.003$). This is 13 cM downstream from the *IFNG* gene and 14 cM upstream from the *IGFI* gene, effectively ruling them out as candidates for the locus affecting these two phenotypes. However, the *MCF* and *LTA4H* genes have only been localized to a 14 cM interval with D12S379 at one end, so they remain possible candidates for these loci.

3.2. Class 2 Asthma Genes: Genes Influencing the Specific IgE Response

Atopic individuals differ in the particular allergens to which they react. This difference is of clinical significance, because asthma and bronchial hyperresponsiveness are associated with allergy to house dust mite (HDM) but not to grass pollens [31, 32]. It is therefore interesting to examine whether particular genes influence the IgE response to specific allergens. In addition, study of these genes could give an insight into the inheritance of normal variation within the immune system, and the functional consequences of such variation.

There are two classes of genes that are probable candidates for constraining specific IgE reactions. These are the genes encoding the human leukocyte antigen (HLA) proteins and the genes for the T cell receptor (TCR). These molecules are central to the handling and recognition of foreign antigens.

Inhaled allergen sources such as HDM are complex mixtures of many proteins. A number of major allergens, i.e. those to which IgE responses are consistently found in most individuals, have been identified from each allergen source. It is likely that genetic associations will be better detected with reactions to purified major allergens, rather than with complex allergen sources. Major allergens include *Der p* I (25.4 kDa) and *Der p* II (14.1 kDa) from the house dust mite *Dermatophagoides pteronyssinus*, *Alt a* I (28 kDa) from the mould *Alternaria alternata*, *Can f* I (25 kDa) from the dog *Canis familiaris, Fel d* I (18 kDa) from the cat *Felis domesticus*, and *Phl p* V (30 kDa) from Timothy grass, *Phleum pratense*.

3.2.1. Human Leukocyte Antigens: The human major histocompatibility complex (MHC) includes genes coding for HLA class II molecules (HLA-DR, -DQ and -DP), which are involved in the recognition and presentation of exogenous peptides.

An HLA influence on the IgE response was first noted by Levine et al. [33], who found an association between HLA class I haplotypes and IgE responses to antigen E derived from ragweed allergen (*Ambrosia artemisifolia*). This association has been subsequently found to result from restriction of the response to a minor component of ragweed antigen (*Amb a* V) by HLA-DR2 [23]. To date the association of *Amb a* V (molecular weight 5 kDa) and HLA-DR2, is the only HLA association to have been consistently confirmed [33–35]. Other suggested associations are of the rye grass antigens *Lol p* I, *Lol p* II and *Lol p* III with HLA-DR3 (in the same 53 allergic subjects) [36, 37], American feverfew (*Parthenium hysterophorus*) and HLA-DR3 in 22 subjects from the Indian subcontinent [38], the IgE response to *Bet v* I, the major allergen of birch pollen, and HLA-DR3 in 37 European subjects [39], and an HLA-DR5 association with another ragweed antigen *Amb a* VI in 38 subjects [40].

Other authors have reported negative associations with particular allergens. These include HLA-DR4 and IgE responses to mountain cedar pollen (37 subjects) [41] and HLA-DR4 and the bee venom melittin (22 subjects) [42]. Non-responsiveness to Japanese cedar pollen may be associated with HLA-DQw8 [43].

To date there is no confirmation of many of these results, and the number of subjects has generally not approached that required to establish an unequivocal HLA association. In addition, there has been no recognition of the problems of reactivity to multiple allergens: significant relationships between HLA-DR alleles and five antigens (*Amb a* V, *Lol p* I, *Lol p* II, *Lol p* III and *Amb a* VI) have been claimed from the same pool of about 200 subjects [34, 36, 37, 40].

To test more definitively whether HLA class II gene products have a general influence on the ability to react to common allergens, we have genotyped for HLA-DR and HLA-DP in a large sample of atopic subjects from the British population [44]. The subjects were tested for IgE responses to the most common major British allergens.

The result showed only weak associations between HLA-DR allele frequencies and IgE responses to common allergens. A possible excess of HLA-DR1 was found in subjects who were responsive to *Fel d* I compared with those who were not (odds ratio or OR = 2; $p = 0.002$), and a possible excess of HLA-DR4 was found in subjects responsive to *Alt a* I (OR = 1.9; $p = 0.006$). Increased sharing of HLA-DR/DP haplotypes was seen in sibling pairs responding to both allergens. *Der p* I, *Der p* II, *Phl p* V and

Can f I were not associated with any definite excess of HLA-DR alleles. No significant correlations were seen with the HLA-DP genotype and reactive to any of the allergens.

Of the possible associations, those of *Alt a* I with HLA-DR4 and of *Fel d* I with HLA-DR1 were supported by a finding of excess sharing of a HLA haplotype in affected sibling pairs. Regression analysis shows that the apparent association of *Phl p* V with HLA-DR4 is caused by the presence of many individuals who have reacted with an IgE response both to *Alt a* I and *Phl p* V. The association of HLA-DR1 and *Fel d* I is the strongest statistically, and is significant, even taking into account the multiple comparisons.

The study was the first to investigate HLA-DP alleles and reactivity to common allergens. As no definite correlations was found between any antigen response and HLA-DP genotypes in a large dataset, HLA-DP genes are unlikely to have a major role in restricting IgE responses to these allergens.

Aspirin-sensitive asthma affects one in ten individuals with adult-onset asthma, but it does not seem to be more common in individuals with atopy. It is not known whether aspirin sensitivity results from immune mechanisms or from interference with biochemical pathways. Possible involvement of MHC genes in aspirin-sensitive asthma has been tested by HLA-DPB1 and HLA-DRB1 genotyping in 59 patients with positive challenge tests for this asthma and in 48 normal and 57 asthmatic controls [45]. The frequency of DPB1*0301 was increased in patients with aspirin-sensitive asthma when compared with normal controls (19.5% vs 5.2%; $OR = 4.4$; 95% confidence interval 95% $CI = 1.6 - 12.1$; $p = 0.002$), and compared with asthmatic controls (4.4%; $OR = 5.3$; 95% $CI = 1.9 - 14.4$; $p = 0.0001$). The frequency of DPB1*0401 in subjects with aspirin-sensitive asthma was decreased when compared with normal controls (28.8% vs 49.0%; $OR = 0.42$; 95% $CI = 0.24 - 0.74$; $p = 0.003$) and asthmatic controls (45.6%; $OR = 0.48$; 95% $CI = 0.28 - 0.83$; $p = 0.008$). The results remained significant when corrected for multiple comparisons. There were no significant HLA-DRB1 associations with ASA. The presence of an HLA association suggests that immune recognition of an unknown antigen may be part of the aetiology of ASA. The relative role of HLA-DP in antigen presentation, compared with HLA-DR and HLA-DQ, is unknown.

The results from the various studies therefore show that HLA-DR alleles do modify the ability to mount an IgE response to particular antigens. However, the odds ratio for the association is usually 2.0 or less. Thus class II HLA restriction seems insufficient to account for individual differences in reactivity to common allergens. It is therefore likely that environmental factors or other loci such as T cell receptor (TCR) genes may be of greater relevance in determining an individual's susceptibility to specific allergens.

3.2.2. The T cell receptor: The TCR is usually made up of one α and one β chain, although 5% of receptors consist of one γ and one δ chain. The α

chain locus is located on chromosome 14q11.2 and contains the δ locus with it. The two other loci are located on chromosome 7, the β chain locus on 7q35 and the γ chain locus on 7p15.

An enormous potential for TCR variety follows from the presence of many variable (V) and junctional (J) segments within the TCR loci. However, the usage of the TCR Vα and Vβ segments by lymphocytes is not random, and may be under genetic control [46–49].

To examine whether the TCR genes influence susceptibility to particular allergens, we have therefore tested for genetic linkage between IgE responses and microsatellites from the TCR-α/δ and TCR-β regions [50]. Two independent sets of families, one British and one Australian, were investigated. As the mode of inheritance was unknown, and because of interactions from the environment and other loci, affected sibling pair methods were used to test for linkage.

No linkage of IgE serotypes to TCR-β was detected, but significant linkage of IgE responses to the house dust mite allergens *Der p* I and *Der p* II, the cat allergen *Fel d* I, and the total serum IgE to TCR-α was seen in both family groups. The results show that a locus in the TCR-α/δ region modulates IgE responses. The close correlation between total and specific IgE makes it difficult to determine whether the locus controls specific IgE reactions to particular allergens or confers generalized IgE responsiveness. Nevertheless, linkage was strongest with highly purified allergens, suggesting that the locus primarily influences specific responses.

Replication of positive results of linkage in a second set of subjects is important in interpreting this study. Differences between the populations for the serotypes showing TCR-α allele sharing may be the result of different allergen exposures because grass pollen responses were much more common in Australian subjects. In addition, British subjects were recruited through clinics, whereas Australian subjects were not selected by symptoms.

No association was seen between particular IgE responses and specific TCR-α microsatellite alleles, implying that the microsatellite is not in immediate proximity to the IgE-modulating elements. The degree of linkage disequilibrium across the TCR-α/δ locus seems low [51], and the microsatellite has been localized only within a 900 kilobase pair (kbp) yeast artificial chromosome [52]. The observed linkage may therefore be with any elements of TCR-α or TCR-δ, or with other genes in the locality.

Several Vα genes have been recognized to be polymorphic [53] and limitation of the response to an allergen may correspond to these polymorphisms. Particular TCR-Vα usage may induce IL-4-dominant helper T cells (Th2), which enhance IgE production [54]. A reported non-random usage of Vα13 usage in *Lol p* I-specific T cell clones gives independent support to the possibility of Vα genes controlling IgE responses [55].

The TCR-δ locus is also a candidate for this linkage. The function of TCR-γ/δ cells is not known, but their location on mucosal surfaces, where allergens initiate IgE responses, could suggest a role in IgE regulation [56].

The genetic restriction of specific IgE responses by TCR-α/δ may be of clinical significance, and may be of general interest in understanding the control of humoral immunity. Further localization of this genetic effect requires the identification of TCR-α/δ elements that show allelic associations with specific IgE responses. Studies are also needed to investigate the interactions between this chromosome 14 linkage and the HLA class II genes.

3.3. Class 3 Asthma Genes: Genes Influencing Bronchial Responsiveness

No genes have as yet been identified that predispose to bronchial hyper-responsiveness independently of atopy, although some work in mice suggests that such genes exist [57]. Variants in the β_2-adrenergic receptor have been identified and it has been suggested that these may be associated with nocturnal asthma [58]. Three polymorphisms were identified in the gene and then two groups consisting of 23 individuals with and 22 without nocturnal asthma were typed for the three polymorphisms. Only an arginine to glycine polymorphism was found to be more frequent in the nocturnal asthmatic group ($p = 0.007$). This R16G polymorphism had previously been shown to increase the rate of agonist-promoted down-regulation of the β_2-adrenergic receptor *in vitro* and so may account for at least part of the nocturnal asthma phenotype.

3.4. Class 4 Asthma Genes: Genes Influencing Non-IgE-Mediated Inflammation

With the rapid advancement of immunology and regular reports of new immunologically active molecules, the number of candidate genes involved in the inflammatory process is large and getting larger all the time. The need to screen for novel polymorphisms to investigate associations with the disease means that progress has been relatively slow. There are, however, a number of genes that now have polymorphisms associated with asthma or atopy phenotypes. Most research has been directed towards cytokines involved in activating T-helper CD4$^+$ cells from Th0 to Th1 or Th2 subtypes. The atopic inflammatory response involves Th2 cells and the main cytokine produced by Th2 cells is IL-4, which stimulates B cells to switch from IgG to IgE production. Th2 cells also produce IL-3, IL-5 and IL-10 and GM-CSF. The genes for all of these cytokines are in the chromosome 5 cytokine cluster with the exception of IL-10, which inhibits switching from Th1 to Th2. IL-10 is located on chromosome 1, but there are no published genetic data as yet linking it with asthma or atopy. If atopy depends upon promoting a Th2 response, the cytokines that are involved in maintaining the Th1 state may also be important. Interferon-γ is the primary cytokine that prolongs the Th1 response and it is interesting that the region containing the *IFNG* gene on chromosome 12 has been linked to high total serum IgE.

Airway inflammation is a characteristic of asthma that may be independent of mechanisms controlling atopy. Tumour necrosis factor α (TNFα) is a potent pro-inflammatory cytokine, which shows constitutional variations in the level of secretion that are linked to polymorphisms in the TNF gene complex [59–61]. We have therefore investigated TNF polymorphisms for association with asthma in 800 normal and abnormal subjects from general population and asthma clinic samples. We found that asthma was significantly increased in subjects with alleles associated with increased secretion of TNFα, most notably the TNFα promoter polymorphism TNF α–308. Considering unrelated subjects only (the parents) from both populations the odds ratio for asthma in individuals who are homozygous for the high secretor allele was 3.9 compared with homozygotes for the low secretor alleles (95% CI = 1.4–11.0; $p = 0.007$) [62]. By analysis of a subset of this population, it was possible to show that asthma was associated with allele 1 of the lymphotoxin-α *Nco*I polymorphism ($p = 0.005$) and allele 2 of the TNFα – 308 polymorphism ($p = 0.004$) and that this association was confined to the LTαNcoI*1/TNF-308*2 haplotype. HLA-DR polymorphisms were excluded as a cause of this association [63].

Other candidate genes include the CC chemokines responsible for the recruitment of cells to the site of inflammation such as eotaxin, RANTES and macrophage inflammatory protein-1β (MIP-1β) [64]. One characteristic feature of the airway inflammation in asthma is the eosinophil infiltrate in the lung and high levels of circulating eosinophils. With the localization and sequencing of genes such as eotaxin and RANTES, whose products have cellular chemoattractant activities, investigation of polymorphisms in the genes has started to produce results. RANTES and eotaxin are located on chromosome 17 but there are no reported polymorphisms to date in the RANTES gene. As asthma is a complex genetic disease, linkage is not as sensitive as association analysis and one single nucleotide polymorphism has been reported very recently in the eotaxin gene. Lilly et al. [65] described a novel polymorphism in the eotaxin gene, resulting in an alanine to threonine change at amino acid 23 in the protein. They then screened 128 asthmatic individuals and 81 healthy controls and found that the polymorphism was significantly associated with asthma ($p < 0.05$). They speculated that the amino acid change was likely to be functional and would be expected to alter the rate of eotaxin secretion from cells.

4. Whole Genome Screens for Atopy and Asthma in Humans

The genes and genetic linkages described above do not account for all asthma or atopy. The chromosome 5 locus would appear not to have major effects on the population as a whole and HLA and TCR-α loci modify the specific response rather than endowing any general predisposition to atopy. Segregation analysis is unable to predict with any accuracy the number and nature of genes contributing to atopy and asthma. To discover whether asthma is a genuine polygenic disorder, we have carried out a complete genome screen in 80 nuclear families, with 300 markers spaced at approximately 10% recombination [66]. We searched for linkage to one qualitative and four quantitative traits associated with asthma: namely atopy, a skin-prick test index, the total serum IgE, the peripheral eosinophil count and bronchial responsiveness. Six potential linkages ($p < 0.001$) were identified on chromosomes 4, 6, 7, 11, 13 and 16, five of which were to quantitative traits. Monte Carlo simulations showed that 1.6 false-positive linkages at this level of significance would be expected from the data. Two linkages, one to chromosome 11q13 and the other to chromosome 6 near the MHC, had been established previously. Three of the new loci (on chromosome 4, 13 and 16) showed evidence of linkage to a second panel of families.

The Collaborative Study on the Genetics of Asthma (CSGA) recently published interim results from a genome screen for asthma susceptibility loci in three ethnically diverse populations [67]. The three populations consisted of 140 nuclear families ascertained through the presence of two asthmatic siblings and made up of 43 African–American, 79 Caucasian and 18 Hispanic families. They reported evidence for linkage to six novel regions ($p < 0.005$) to chromosomes 5p15 and 17p11.1–p11.2 (African–Americans), 11p15 and 19q13 (Caucasian) and 2q33 and 21q21 (Hispanics). None of these linkages was replicated in either of the other two ethnic groups. They also reported linkage ($p < 0.02$) to the previously noted regions on 5q23–31 [5], 6p21.3–23 [62, 63], 12q14–24.2 [30], 13q21.3–qter [66] and 14q11.2–13 [39] in Caucasians, and to 12q14–24.2 in Hispanics. Replication of linkages was not observed among the three groups except for chromosome 12. The analysis carried out did not appear to take into account the multiple testing of many markers in the three populations, and failure to replicate may be because of the low level of statistical significance chosen to declare possible linkage. Alternatively, non-replication may be a consequence of the different genetic backgrounds of the three groups and in addition the environmental backgrounds of the three groups differ. However, the results are derived from only 40% of the total number of sib pairs that will be available when their full study group has been genotyped.

5. Whole Genome Screens for Quantitative Trait Loci Underlying Atopy and Asthma in Mice

Major problems are associated with obtaining sufficient clinical data and samples to carry out a meaningful genome screen. Often compromises have to be made, such as combining study groups that have been ascertained through different routes or who are ethnically dissimilar. However, with a mouse model many of these problems disappear, because there is complete control of environmental factors, full knowledge of pedigrees and no problems with obtaining clinical samples or data. By crossbreeding pure-bred mouse strains with characteristics that are thought to be involved in atopy and asthma, the loci involved in regulating these traits can be detected in relatively small study populations. De Sanctis et al. [57] crossed two strains of mice, A/J and C57BL/6J, which differed in that A/J mice had a threefold increased airway hyperresponsiveness compared with the C57BL/6J mice ($p < 0.0001$). The airway hyperresponsiveness appeared to be inherited as a dominant trait in the F_1 mice and the F_1 generation was then backcrossed to the C57Bl/6J strain to produce a population with a normally distributed variation in airway responsiveness. Analysis of the variance in the F_1 and F_2 generations demonstrated that approximately 50% was the result of genetic background and the rest of environmental factors. They then genotyped 92 phenotypically extreme mice with 157 microsatellite markers and found evidence for linkage of bronchial hyperresponsiveness to three regions of the mouse genome, which they named $Bhr1-3$. To confirm this, all 321 of the backcross progeny were then genotyped with the relevant markers. The nearest candidate genes in the human genome to the mouse regions of linkage were interleukin-1β ($Bhr1$), IL-2b, IL-3b1 and IL-3b2, PDGF β-chain ($Bhr2$), TNFα and mast cell protease genes 6 and 7 ($Bhr3$). Only evidence for the TNFα linkage has been previously reported in humans, underlining the main drawback with mouse studies, namely the difficulty of determining whether a phenotype in the mouse has the same genetic basis as the same phenotype in humans.

With second-stage genome screens in progress in a number of centres, it seems highly likely that a consensus will emerge as to which regions of the human genome can be linked to asthma and its associated phenotypic traits. With the Human Genome Project progressing rapidly, it is easy to foresee combined linkage and sequence data allowing the rapid identification of genes at a peak of linkage. Gene identification is only the start of the long path to drug therapy, because there is still a formidable amount of work to do to move from each gene sequence to the clarification of its role in the development of asthma.

6. Conclusions

The genetic basis for asthma is gradually becoming more certain; the methodological tools for finding genetic linkage and association are now established, and it is likely that all the important genes and their variants will be found in the next 10 years. It should not be forgotten, however, that the environment strongly influences asthma, and that the rising prevalence of asthma in recent decades is probably the result of environmental factors. The increase in prevalence has an important corollary: asthma is preventable. Recognition of children or infants genetically predisposed to asthma is likely to be the first step in strategies for prevention by environmental or other manipulations in the first year of life.

References

1 Collins FS (1992) Positional cloning: let's not call it reverse anymore. *Nature Genet* 1: 3–6
2 Monaco AP (1994) Isolation of genes from cloned DNA. *Curr Opin Genes Dev* 4: 360–365
3 Suarez BK, Hampe CL, Van Eerdewegh P (1994) Problems of replicating linkage claims in psychiatry. In: ES Gershon, CR Cloninger (eds): *Genetic Approaches to Mental Disorders*. American Psychiatric Press Inc, Washington, 23–46
4 Jorde LB (1995) Linkage disequilibrium as a gene-mapping tool. *Am J Hum Genet* 56: 11–14
5 Marsh DG, Neely JD, Breazeale DR, Ghosh B, Freidhoff LR, Erlich-Kautzky E, Schou C, Krishnaswamy G, Beaty TH (1994) Linkage analysis of IL-4 and other chromosome 5q31.1 markers and total serum IgE concentrations. *Science* 264: 1152–1155
6 Myers DA, Postma DS, Panhuysen CIM, Xu J, Amelung PJ, Levitt RC, Bleeker ER (1994) Evidence for a locus regulating total serum IgE levels mapping to chromosome 5. *Genomics* 23: 464–470
7 Xu J, Levitt RC, Panhuysen CIM, Postma DS, Taylor EW, Amelung PJ, Holroyd KJ, Bleecker ER, Meyers DA (1995) Evidence for two unlinked loci regulating total serum IgE levels. *Am J Hum Genet* 57: 425–430
8 Postma DS, Bleecker ER, Amelung PJ, Holroyd KJ, Xu J, Panhuysen CIM, Meyers DA, Levitt RC (1995) Genetic susceptibility to asthma – bronchial hyperresponsiveness coinherited with a major gene for atopy. *N Engl J Med* 333: 894–900
9 Doull IJ, Lawrence S, Watson M, Begishvili T, Beasley RW, Lampe F, Holgate S, Morton NE (1996) Allelic association of gene markers on chromosomes 5q and 11q with atopy and bronchial hyperresponsiveness. *Am J Respir Crit Care Med* 153: 1280–1284
10 Blumenthal MN, Wang Z, Weber JL, Rich SS (1996) Absence of linkage between 5q markers and serum IgE levels in four large atopic families. *Clin Exp Allergy* 26: 892–896
11 Walley AJ, Cookson WOCM (1997) Linkage and allelic association of chromosome 5 microsatellite markers with atopic asthma phenotypes in a general population sample. *Am J Respir Crit Care Med* 155 (4 part 2): A257
12 Rosenwasser LJ, Klemm DJ, Dresback JK, Inamura H, Mascali JJ, Klinnert M, Borish L (1995) Promoter polymorphisms in the chromosome 5 gene cluster in asthma and atopy. *Clin Exp Allergy* 25 (suppl 2): 74–78
13 Walley AJ, Cookson WOCM (1996) Investigation of an interleukin-4 promoter polymorphism for associations with asthma and atopy. *J Med Genet* 33: 689–692
14 Cookson WOCM, Sharp PA, Faux JA, Hopkin JM (1989) Linkage between immunoglobulin E responses underlying asthma and rhinitis and chromosome 11q. *Lancet* i: 1292–1295
15 Marsh DG, Myers DA (1992) A major gene for allergy – fact or fancy? *Nature Genet* 2: 252–254
16 Young RP, Lynch J, Sharp PA, Faux JA, Cookson WOCM, Hopkin JM (1992) Confirmation of genetic linkage between atopic IgE response and chromosome 11q13. *J Med Genet* 29: 236–238
17 Shirakawa T, Morimoto K, Hashimoto T, Furuyama J, Yamamoto M, Takai S (1994) Linkage between severe atopy and chromosome 11q in Japanese families. *Clin Genet* 46: 125–129
18 Collée JM, ten Kate LP, de Vries HG, Kliphuis JW, Bouman K, Scheffer H, Gerritsen J (1993) Allele sharing on chromosome 11q13 in sibs with asthma and atopy. *Lancet* 342: 936
19 Herwerden L, Harrap SB, Wong ZYH, Abramson MJ, Kutin JJ, Forbes AB, Raven J, Lanigan A, Walters EH (1995) Linkage of high affinity receptor gene with bronchial hyperreactivity, even in absence of atopy. *Lancet* 346: 1262–1265

20 Hizawa N, Yamaguchi E, Funuya K, Ohnuma N, Kodama N, Kojima J, Ohe M, Kawakami
    Y (1995) Association between high serum total IgE levels and D11S97 on chromosome
    11q13 in Japanese subjects. *J Med Genet* 32: 363–369
21 Cookson WOCM, Young RP, Sandford AJ, Moffatt MF, Shirakawa T, Sharp PA, Faux JA,
    Julier C, Le Souef PN, Nakumura Y et al. (1992) Maternal inheritance of atopic IgE re-
    sponsiveness on chromosome 11q. *Lancet* 340: 381–384
22 Sandford AJ, Shirakawa T, Moffatt MF, Daniels SE, Ra C, Faux JA, Young RP, Nakamura Y,
    Lathrop GM, Cookson WOCM et al. (1993) Localisation of atopy and the β subunit of the
    high affinity IgE receptor (FcεRI) on chromosome 11q. *Lancet* 341: 332–334
23 Sandford AJ, Moffatt MF, Daniels SE, Nakamura Y, Lathrop GM, Hopkin JM, Cookson
    WOCM (1995) A genetic map of chromosome 11q, including the atopy locus. *Eur J Hum
    Genet* 3: 188–194
24 Hupp K, Siwarski D, Mock BA, Kinet JP (1989) Gene mapping of the three subunits of the
    high affinity FcR for IgE to mouse chromosomes 1 and 19. *J Immunol* 143: 3787–3791
25 Shirakawa TS, Li A, Dubowitz M, Dekker JW, Shaw AE, Faux JA, Ra C, Cookson WOCM,
    Hopkin JM (1994) Association between atopy and variants of the β subunit of the high-
    affinity immunoglobulin E receptor. *Nature Genet* 7: 125–129
26 Hill MR, James AL, Faux JA, Ryan G, Hopkin JM, le Souef P, Musk AW, Cookson WOCM
    (1995) FcεRI-β polymorphism and risk of atopy in a general population sample. *BMJ* 311:
    776–779
27 Adra CN, Lelias J-M, Kobayashi H, Kaghad M, Morrison P, Rowley JD, Lim B (1994)
    Cloning of the cDNA for a haemopoietic cell-specific protein related to CD20 and the beta
    subunit of the high-affinity IgE receptor: Evidence for a family of proteins with four mem-
    brane spanning regions. *Proc Natl Acad Sci USA* 91: 10178–10182
28 Hill MR, Cookson WOCM (1996) A new variant of the β subunit of the high-affinity recep-
    tor for immunoglobulin E (*FcεRI-β E237*G): associations with measures of atopy and bron-
    chial hyper-responsiveness. *Hum Mol Genet* 5: 959–962
29 Shirakawa TS, Mao XQ, Sasaki S, Nomoto TE, Kawai M, Morimoto K, Hopkin JM (1996)
    Association between atopic asthma and a coding variant of FcεRI-β in a Japanese popula-
    tion. *Hum Mol Genet* 5: 1129–1130
30 Barnes KC, Neely JD, Duffy DL, Freidhoff LR, Breazeale DR, Schou C, Naidu RP, Levett
    PN, Renault B, Kucherlapati R et al. (1996) Linkage of asthma and total serum IgE con-
    centration to markers on chromosome 12q: evidence from Afro-Caribbean and Caucasian
    populations. *Genomics* 37: 41–50
31 Cookson WOCM, De Klerk NH, Ryan GR, James AL, Musk AW (1991) Relative risks of
    bronchial hyper-responsiveness associated with skin-prick test responses to common anti-
    gens in young adults. *Clin Exp Allergy* 21: 473–479
32 Sears MR, Herbison GP, Holdaway MD, Hewitt CJ, Flannery EM, Silva PA (1989) The rela-
    tive risks of sensitivity to grass pollen, house dust mite and cat dander in the development
    of childhood asthma. *Clin Exp Allergy* 19: 419–424
33 Levine BB, Stember RH, Fontino M (1972) Ragweed hayfever: genetic control and linkage
    to HL-A haplotypes. *Science* 178: 1201–1203
34 Marsh DG, Meyers DA, Bias WB (1981) The epidemiology and genetics of atopic allergy.
    N Engl J Med 305: 1551–1559
35 Blumenthal MN, Awdeh Z, Alper C, Yunis E (1985) Ra5 immune response, HLA antigens
    and complotypes. *J Allergy Clin Immunol* 75: 155
36 Freidhoff LR, Ehrlich-Kautzky E, Meyers DA, Ansari AA, Bias WB, Marsh DG (1988)
    Association of HLA-DR3 with human immune response to Lol p I and Lol p II allergens in
    allergic subjects. *Tissue Antigens* 31: 211–219
37 Ansari AA, Freidhoff LR, Meyers DA, Bias WB, Marsh DG (1989) Human immune
    responsiveness to *Lolium perenne* pollen allergen Lol p III (rye III) is associated with HLA-
    DR3 and DR5. *Hum Immunol* 25: 59–71 [published erratum appears in *Hum Immunol*
    26: 149]
38 Sriramarao P, Selvakumar B, Damodaran C, Rao BS, Prakash O, Rao PV (1990) Immediate
    hypersensitivity to *Parthenium hysterophorus*. I. Association of HLA antigens and *Par-
    thenium rhinitis*. *Clin Exp Allergy* 20: 555–560
39 Fischer GF, Pickl WF, Fae I, Ebner C, Ferreira F, Breiteneder H, Vikoukal E, Scheiner O,
    Kraft D (1992) Association between IgE response against Bet v I, the major allergen of birch
    pollen, and HLA-DRB alleles. *Hum Immunol* 33: 259–265

40 Marsh DG, Freidhoff LR, Ehrlich-Kautzky E, Bias WB, Roebber M (1987) Immune responsiveness to Ambrosia artemisiifolia (short ragweed) pollen allergen Amb a VI (Ra6) is associated with HLA-DR5 in allergic humans. *Immunogenetics* 26: 230–236

41 Reid MJ, Nish WA, Whisman BA, Goetz DW, Hylander RD, Parker WA Jr, Freeman TM (1992) HLA-DR4-associated nonresponsiveness to mountain cedar allergen. *J Allergy Clin Immunol* 89: 593–598

42 Lympany P, Kemeny DM, Welsh KI, Lee TH (1990) An HLA-associated nonresponsiveness to mellitin: a component of bee venom. *J Allergy Clin Immunol* 86: 160–170

43 Sasazuki T, Nishimura Y, Muto M, Ohta N (1983) HLA-linked genes controlling immune response and disease susceptibility. *Immunol Rev* 70: 51–75

44 Young RP, Dekker JW, Wordsworth BP, Schou P, Pile KD, Matthiesen F, Rosenberg WMC, Bell JI, Hopkin JM, Cookson WOCM (1994) HLA-DR and HLA-DP genotypes and immunoglobulin E responses to common major allergens. *Clin Exp Allergy* 24: 431–439

45 Dekker JW, Nizankowska E, Schmitz-Schumann M, Pile K, Bochenek G, Dyczek A, Cookson WOCM, Szczeklik A (1997) Aspirin-induced asthma and HLA-DRB1 and HLA-DPB1 genotypes. *Clin Exp Allergy* 27: 574–577

46 Loveridge JA, Rosenberg WMC, Kirkwood TBL, Bell JI (1991) The genetic contribution to human T cell receptor repertoire. *Immunology* 74: 246–250

47 Moss PAH, Rosenberg WMC, Zintzaras E, Bell JI (1993) Characterisation of the human T cell receptor α-chain repertoire and demonstration of a genetic influence on Vα usage. *Eur J Immunol* 23: 1153–1159

48 Gulwani-Akolar B, Posnett DN, Janson CH, Grunewald J, Wigzell H, Akolkar P, Gregersen PK, Silver J (1991) T cell receptor V-segment frequencies in peripheral blood T cells correlate with human leukocyte antigen type. *J Exp Med* 174: 1139–1146

49 Robinson MA (1992) Usage of human T cell receptor V β, J β C β and Vα gene segments is not proportional to gene number. *Hum Immunol* 35: 60–67

50 Moffatt MF, Hill MR, Cornélis F, Schou C, Faux JA, Young RP, James AL, Ryan G, le Souef P, Musk AW et al. (1994) Genetic linkage of the TCR-α/δ region to specific Immunoglobulin E responses. *Lancet* 343: 1597–1600

51 Robinson MA, Kindt TJ (1987) Genetic recombination within the human T cell receptor alpha-chain complex. *Proc Natl Acad Sci USA* 84: 9089–9093

52 Cornélis F, Hashimoto L, Loveridge J, MacCarthy A, Buckle V, Julier C, Bell J (1992) Identification of a CA repeat at the TCRA locus using yeast artificial chromosomes: a general method for generating highly polymorphic markers at chosen loci. *Genomics* 13: 820–825

53 Cornélis F, Pile K, Loveridge J, Moos P, Harding C, Julier C, Bell JI (1993) Systematic study of human $\alpha\beta$ T cell receptor V segments shows allelic variations resulting in a large number of distinct TCR haplotypes. *Eur J Immunol* 23: 1277–1283

54 Heinzel FP, Sadick MD, Mutha SS, Locksley RM (1991) Production of interferon gamma, interleukin 2, interleukin 4, and interleukin 10 by CD4+ lymphocytes *in vivo* during healing and progressive murine leishmaniasis. *Proc Natl Acad Sci USA* 88: 7011–7015

55 Mohapatra SS, Mohapatra S, Yang M, Ansari AA, Parronchi P, Maggi E, Romagnani S (1994) Molecular basis of cross-reactivity among allergen-specific human T cells. T cell receptor Vα gene usage and epitope structure. *Immunology* 81: 15–20

56 Holt PG, McMenamin C (1991) IgE and mucosal immunity: studies on the role of intraepithelial Ia+ dendritic cells and δ/γ T lymphocytes in regulation of T cell activation in the lung. *Clin Exp Allergy* 21 (suppl): 148–152

57 De Sanctis GT, Merchant M, Beier DR, Dredge RD, Grobholz JK, Martin TR, Lander ES, Drazen JM (1995) Quantitative locus analysis of airway hyperresponsiveness in A/J and C57BL/6J mice. *Nature Genet* 11: 150–154

58 Turki J, Pak J, Green SA, Martin RJ, Liggett SB (1995) Genetic polymorphisms of the beta-2 adrenergic receptor in nocturnal and non-nocturnal asthma. *J Clin Invest* 95: 1635–1641

59 Jacob CO, Fronek Z, Lewis GD, Koo M, Hansen JA, McDevitt HO (1990) Heritable major histocompatibility complex class II-associated differences in production of tumour necrosis factor α: relevance to genetic predisposition to systemic lupus erythematosis. *Proc Natl Acad Sci USA* 87: 1233–1237

60 Messer G, Spengler U, Jung Mc, Honold G, Blömer K, Pape GR, Riethmüller G, Weiss EH (1991) Polymorphic structure of the Tumour Necrosis Factor (TNF) locus: an NcoI polymorphism in the first intron of the human TNF-β gene correlates with a variant amino acid in position 26 and a reduced level of TNF-β production. *J Exp Med* 173: 209–219

61 Wilson AG, Symons JA, McDowell TL, McDevitt HO, Duff GW (1997) Effects of a polymorphism in the human tumour necrosis factor alpha promoter on transcriptional activation.
Proc Natl Acad Sci USA 94: 3195–3199

62 Moffatt MF, Cookson WOCM (1996) Asthma and tumour necrosis factor polymorphism.
Hum Immunol 47: 160

63 Moffatt MF, Cookson WOCM (1997) Tumour necrosis factor haplotypes and asthma. *Hum
Mol Genet* 6: 551–554

64 Alam R (1997) Updates on cells and cytokines: chemokines in allergic inflammation.
J Allergy Clin Immunol 99: 273–277

65 Lilly CM, Nakamura H, Nakamura T, Weiss S, Luster AD, Drazen JM (1997) A mutation in
the eotaxin gene is associated with the asthma phenotype. *Am J Respir Crit Care Med* 155
(4 part 2): A490

66 Daniels SE, Bhattacharyya S, James A, Leaves NI, Young A, Hill MR, Faux JA, Ryan GF,
le Söuef PN, Lathrop GM et al. (1996) A genome-wide search for quantitative trait loci
underlying asthma. *Nature* 383: 247–250

67 The Collaborative Study on the Genetics of Asthma (1997) A genome-wide search for
asthma susceptibility loci in ethnically diverse populations. *Nature Genet* 15: 389–392

Molecular Biology of the Lung
Vol. 2: Asthma and Cancer
ed. by R. A. Stockley
© 1999 Birkhäuser Verlag Basel/Switzerland

CHAPTER 3
Transcription Factors and Inflammatory Lung Disease

Peter J. Barnes and Ian M. Adcock

Department of Thoracic Medicine, National Heart and Lung Institute, Imperial College, London, UK

1   Introduction
2   Transcription Factors
2.1   Transcription Factor Families
2.2   Methods for Studying Transcription Factors
2.3   Transcription Factor Interactions
2.4   Basal Transcription Machinery
2.5   Specific and Ubiquitous Transcription Factors
3   Nuclear Factor-κB (NF-κB)
3.1   Activation of NF-κB
3.2   Inflammatory and Immune Genes
3.3   Role in Inflammatory Lung Diseases
4   Activator Protein-1 (AP-1)
5   CAAT/Enhancer-Binding Proteins
6   JAK/STAT Family
7   Cyclic AMP Response Element-Binding Protein
8   CREB-Binding Protein
9   Glucocorticoid Receptors (GRs)
9.1   Interaction With Other Transcription factors
9.2   Steroid-Resistant Inflammation
10   Nuclear Factor of Activated T Cells
11   Therapeutic Implications
11.1   New Steroids
11.2   NF-κB Inhibitors
11.3   Drug Interactions
         References

1. Introduction

Inflammation is a central feature of many lung diseases, including asthma, chronic obstructive pulmonary disease (COPD), cystic fibrosis, fibrosing alveolitis and adult or acute respiratory distress syndrome (ARDS). The specific characteristics of the inflammatory response and the site of inflammation differ between these diseases, but all involve the recruitment and activation of inflammatory cells and chances in the structural cells of the lung. These diseases are characterized by an increased expression of many proteins involved in the complex inflammatory cascade. These inflammatory proteins include cytokines, enzymes that produce inflammatory mediators, receptors and adhesion molecules. The increased expression of most of these proteins is the result of increased gene transcription; many of the genes are not expressed in normal cells but are induced in certain cell types in these inflammatory diseases. Changes in gene transcription are regulated by transcription factors, which are proteins that bind to DNA. This suggests that transcription factors may play a key role in the pathophysiology of inflammatory diseases, because they regulate the increased gene expression that may underlie the acute and chronic inflammatory mechanisms that characterize these diseases. Corticosteroids are the most effective therapy in the long-term control of asthma and appear to reduce inflammation in asthmatic airways largely by inhibiting the transcription factors that regulate abnormal gene expression. Corticosteroids may also have a beneficial effect in other inflammatory lung diseases, although this is less marked than in asthma, indicating that different genes and transcription factors are involved.

2. Transcription Factors

Transcription factors are proteins that bind to regulatory sequences, usually in the 5'-upstream promoter region of target genes, to increase (or sometimes decrease) the rate of gene transcription. This may result in increased or decreased protein synthesis and altered cellular function. Transcription factors may be activated by many extracellular influences acting via surface receptors which lead to phosphorylation by several types of kinase [1, 2], or may be directly activated by ligands (such as corticosteroids, thyroid hormone and vitamins). Transcription factors may therefore convert transient environmental signals at the cell surface into long-term changes in gene transcription, thus acting as "nuclear messengers" [3]. Transcription factors may be activated within the nucleus, often with the transcription factor bound to DNA, or within the cytoplasm, resulting in exposure of nuclear localization signals and targeting to the nucleus. Thus transcription factors convert environmental signals into altered gene expression. In the context of inflammatory diseases, transcription factors activated by inflammatory stimuli (such as cytokines or viruses) switch on inflammatory genes, leading to increased synthesis of inflammatory proteins (Figure 1). In this way transcription factors may amplify and perpetuate the inflammatory process and this makes them an important potential target in the development of new anti-inflammatory drugs. It is possible that abnormal functioning of transcription factors may determine disease severity and responsiveness to treatment [4]. Of particular importance is the demonstration that transcription factors may physically interact with each other, resulting in inhibition or enhancement of transcriptional activity.

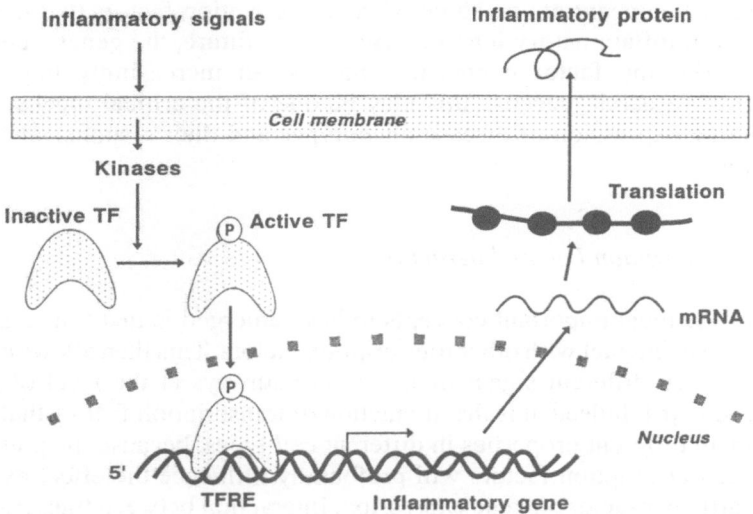

Figure 1. Transcription factors may play a key role in the amplification and perpetuation of inflammatory diseases. Inflammatory signals activate transcription factors (TF) by phosphorylation; these then bind to recognition elements (TFRE) in the promoter regions of inflammatory genes to increase the synthesis of inflammatory proteins.

2.1. Transcription Factor Families

Several families of transcription factors exist and members of each family may share structural characteristics. These families include helix–turn–helix (e.g. POU), zinc finger (e.g. glucocorticoid receptors), basic protein-leucine zipper (cyclic AMP response element-binding factor or CREB, nuclear factor-κB (NF-κB], activator protein-1 [AP-1]) and β-sheet motifs (e.g. HU) [5]. Many transcription factors are common to several cell types (ubiquitous), whereas others are cell specific and determine the phenotypic characteristics of a cell.

2.2. Methods for Studying Transcription Factors

There is relatively little information about the regulation of transcription factors in the airways, particularly in diseases such as asthma. However, molecular methods have been developed for investigation of transcription factor expression and activity. These methods include immunoblotting and immunocytochemistry to detect the transcription factor protein, electrophoretic mobility shift assays to measure transcription factor binding to DNA and DNA footprinting to determine binding to recognition sequences in particular genes. Many transcription factors have now been discovered, but we will concentrate on some of the transcription factors that may be relevant in inflammatory lung diseases. In the future, the genetic control of transcription factor expression may be an increasingly important aspect of research, because this may be one of the critical mechanisms regulating expression of disease phenotypes and their responsiveness to therapy.

2.3. Transcription Factor Interactions

One of the most important concepts to have emerged is that transcription factors may interact with other transcription factors. This then allows cross-talk between different signal transduction pathways at the level of gene expression [6]. Indeed, it is the interaction of transcription factors that may give them different properties in different cell types, because the presence of other transcription factors will profoundly influence the effect exerted by a particular factor on gene expression. Interaction between transcription factors is particularly relevant to the action of drugs, such as corticosteroids and cyclosporin A, which activate or block transcription factors that subsequently modulate other transcription factors.

2.4. Basal Transcription Machinery

Binding of transcription factors to their specific recognition sequences, or activation of the already bound transcription factors in the control regions (promoters) of target genes, is communicated to the basal transcription machinery bound to the TATA box near the start site of transcription. This then leads to activation of the critical enzyme RNA polymerase II, via a chain of basal factors, resulting in increased transcription of the gene and formation of messenger RNA (mRNA), which in turn is then translated into a protein. Binding of transcription factors to their specific binding motifs in the promoter region may alter transcription by interacting directly with components of the basal transcription apparatus or via co-factors that link the transcription factor to the basal transcription apparatus [7] (Figure 2). As DNA loops around histone residues, binding of a transcription factor even far from the TATA boy may interact.

Large proteins that bind to the basal transcription machinery may interact with many transcription factors and thus act as integrators of gene transcription. These co-activator molecules include CREB-binding protein (CBP), which was first recognized as a protein that the transcription factor CREB had to bind to in order to exert its effects [8]. Other co-activator molecules include p300, and these co-activators may bind multiple transcription factors, thus allowing complex interactions between different signalling pathways.

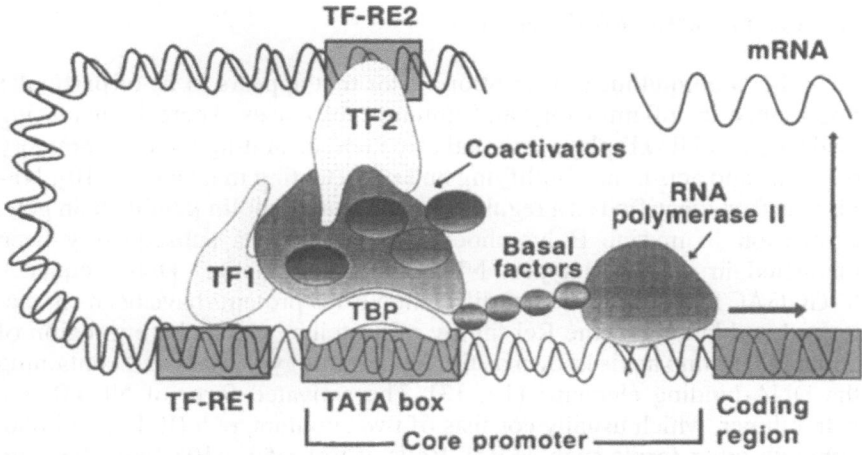

Figure 2. The basal transcription apparatus consists of various proteins that bind to the TATA box at the start site of transcription. These factors include co-activators that bind to transcription factors, some of which may be situated far from the start site as DNA loops around. Transcription factors (TF) bind to specific recognition sequences in the 5'-promoter region (TFRE), resulting in increased transcription by activating RNA polymerase II which in turn, results in transcription of messenger RNA (mRNA).

2.5. Specific and Ubiquitous Transcription Factors

Many transcription factors have now been identified and a large proportion of the genome appears to code for these proteins. Many transcription factors are cell specific and are responsible for the selective expression of genes that characterize a particular cell in terms of its structural characteristics, differentiation or function. One example of a specific transcription factor is nuclear factor of activated T cells (NF-AT) which regulates the expression of the lymphocyte proliferative factor interleukin-2 (IL-2) in T lymphocytes. Many transcription factors, such as AP-1 and nuclear factor κB (NF-κB), are ubiquitous and regulate large sets of genes, so that a coordinated cellular response is produced. There may also be important interactions between transcription factors, so that it is necessary to have coincident activation of several transcription factors in order to have maximal gene expression. For example, IL-8 is regulated by NF-κB and C/EBPβ (or nuclear factor of IL-6). C/EBPβ binding alone has little effect on IL-6 transcription but markedly enhances the effect of NF-κB binding, resulting in maximal gene expression [9]. This means that IL-8 will be maximally transcribed only when both transcription factors are activated simultaneously by coincident activating signals. These sorts of interaction explain how transcription factors that are ubiquitous may regulate particular genes in certain types of cell.

3. Nuclear Factor-κB (NF-κB)

NF-κB is a ubiquitous transcription factor that appears to be of particular importance in inflammatory and immune responses. There is increasing evidence that NF-κB plays a pivotal role in orchestrating the inflammatory response and acts as an amplifying and perpetuating mechanism [10]. NF-κB was first identified as a regulator of immunoglobulin κ light chain gene expression in murine B lymphocytes [11], but has subsequently been identified in most cell types. NF-κB binds to the κB DNA sequence 5'-GGGACTTTCC-3'. Several different NF-κB proteins have been characterized and belong to the Rel family of proteins, which share a region of about 300 amino acids known as the Rel homology domain and containing the DNA-binding elements [12, 13]. The activated form of NF-κB is a heterodimer, which usually consists of two subunits, p65 (RelA) and p50, although other forms such as Rel, RelB, v-Rel, p52, p105 (NF-κB1) and p100 (NF-κB2) may also occur. The p50 may be constitutively bound to DNA but requires p65 for transactivation activity. Rel proteins were identified even in invertebrates, such as *Drosophila* sp., where they play an important role in both development and primitive inflammatory responses. Targeted disruption of the genes coding for p65 or p50 in mice ("knock-outs") results in severe immune deficiency which is lethal in the case of p65 [14, 15].

3.1. Activation of NF-κB

In unstimulated cells. NF-κB is localized to the cytoplasm because of binding to inhibitory proteins (IκB), of which several isoforms exist (IκB-α, IκB-β, IκB-γ, IκB-δ, IκB-ε), the most abundant being IκB-α [16, 17]. When the cell is appropriately stimulated, specific IκB kinases phosphorylate IκB, leading to the rapid addition of ubiquitin residues (ubiquitination) which make it a substrate for the proteasome, a multifunctional cellular protease [18, 19] (Figure 3). A specific IκB-α kinase complex (IKK) has now been identified and contains at least two interacting subunits [20]. Several signal transduction pathways are involved in the activation of NF-κB and enzymes from the mitogen-activated protein (MAP) kinase pathways may interact at various points in the activation of NF-κB [21]. A newly described kinase, NF-κB-inducing kinase (NIK), is a MAP3K-related enzyme involved in the activation of IKK by tumour nectoris factor-α (TNF-α) and IL-1β [22]. A key enzyme in the stress-activated MAP kinase pathway, which leads to the activation of c-Jun N-terminal kinase, is MEKK1, which also activates the IκB-α kinase complex, indicating that mechanisms that activate JNK and AP-1 may also activate NF-κB [23].

Degradation of IκB uncovers nuclear localization signals on p65 and p50, so it is rapidly transported into the nucleus where it binds to specific

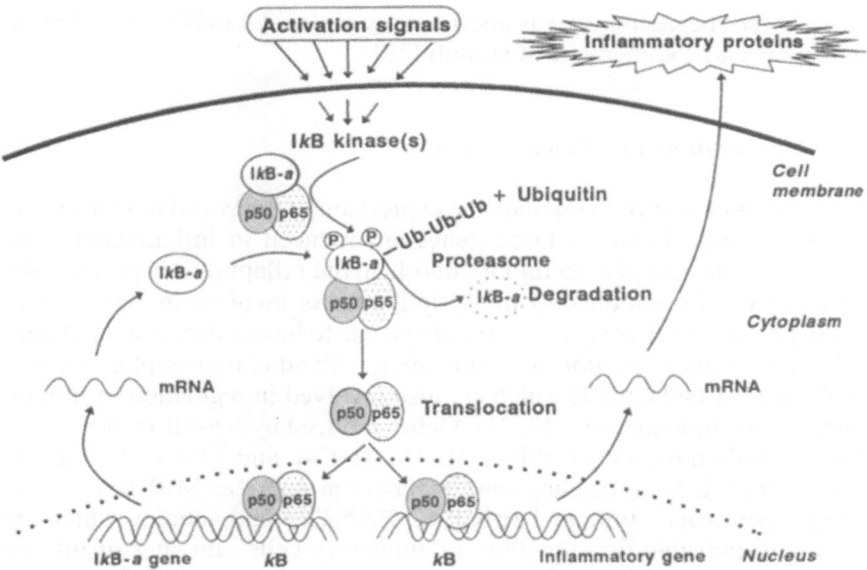

Figure 3. Activation of nuclear factor-κB (NF-κB) involves phosphorylation of the inhibitory protein IκB by specific kinase(s), with subsequent ubiquitination and proteolytic degradation by the proteasome. The free NF-κB then translocates to the nucleus, where it binds to κB sites in the promoter regions of inflammatory genes. Activation of the IκB-α gene results in increased synthesis of IκB-α to terminate the activation of NF-κB.

κB recognition elements in the promoter regions of target genes. The IκB-α gene (MAD-3) itself has several κB sequences in its promoter region, so that NF-κB induces the synthesis of IκB-α, which enters the nucleus to bind NF-κB and induce its export to the cytoplasm, thus terminating activation [24]. Newly synthesized IκB-α interacts with and binds to NF-κB heterodimers within the cytoplasm and to NF-κB bound to κB sites within the nucleus [25]. Targeted disruption of the IκB-α gene results in prolonged activation of NF-κB and animals die of inflammation [26]. By contrast, IκB-β is not induced by NF-κB, so NF-κB is likely to be activated for a more prolonged period in cell types in which IκB-β predominates [27].

Many stimuli activate NF-κB, including cytokines IL-1β, TNF-α, IL-2 and granulocyte-macrophage colony-stimulating factor (GM-CSF) [12], oxidative stress (particularly hydrogen peroxide) [28], viruses (such as rhinovirus and adenovirus) [29], phorbol esters, lipopolysaccharide, and B- and T-lymphocyte activation. Several signal transduction pathways may be involved in this activation, but all of these stimuli appear to act via rapidly activated protein kinases that lead to IκB phosphorylation. The activation of these protein kinases may be blocked by antioxidants, such as pyrrolidine dithiocarbamate (PDTC) and N-acetylcysteine, suggesting that reactive oxygen species may act as intermediary molecules in NF-κB activation in response to a wide range of stimuli [30].

3.2. Inflammatory and Immune Genes

NF-κB is now known to regulate the expression of many inflammatory and immune genes. Many of these genes are induced in inflammatory and structural cells and play an important role in the inflammatory process. Although NF-κB is not the only transcription factor involved in regulation of the expression of these genes, it often appears to have a decisive regulatory role. NF-κB often functions in cooperation with other transcription factors, such as AP-1 and C/EBP, which are also involved in regulation of inflammatory and immune genes [9, 31]. Genes induced by NF-κB include those for the inflammatory cytokines IL-1β, TNF-α and GM-CSF, and the chemokines IL-8, macrophage inflammatory protein-1α (MIP-1α), macrophage chemotactic protein-1 (MCP-1), RANTES and eotaxin, which are largely responsible for attracting inflammatory cells into sites of inflammation [12, 32–35]. NF-κB also regulates the expression of inflammatory enzymes, including the inducible form of nitric oxide synthase (iNOS), which produces large amounts of NO [36], and inducible cyclo-oxygenase (COX-2), which produces prostanoids [37, 38]. NF-κB also plays an important role in regulating expression of adhesion molecules, such as E-selectin, vascular cell adhesion molecule-1 (VCAM-1) and intercellular adhesion molcule-1 (ICAM-1), which are expressed on endothelial and epithelial cells at inflammatory sites and play a key role in the initial recruitment of inflammatory cells [39, 40]. This suggests that activation of NF-κB leads to the coordinated induction of multiple genes that are expressed in inflammatory and immune responses.

Products of genes that are regulated by NF-κB also cause its activation. Thus the proinflammatory cytokines IL-1β and TNF-α both activate and are activated by NF-κB; this may result in a positive regulatory loop which may be important in amplifying and perpetuating the inflammatory response at the local site (Figure 4).

NF-κB also plays a complex role in apoptosis. Inhibition of NF-κB increases apoptosis in response to TNF-α in several cell types, including lymphocytes, suggesting that NF-κB counteracts apoptosis [41, 42].

3.3. Role in Inflammatory Lung Diseases

NF-κB may be activated by many of the stimuli that exacerbate asthmatic inflammation. In experimental animals allergen exposure in sensitized animals activates NF-κB in the lung [43] with concomitant expression of iNOS and chemokines [44]. In animal studies *in vivo* activation of T lym-

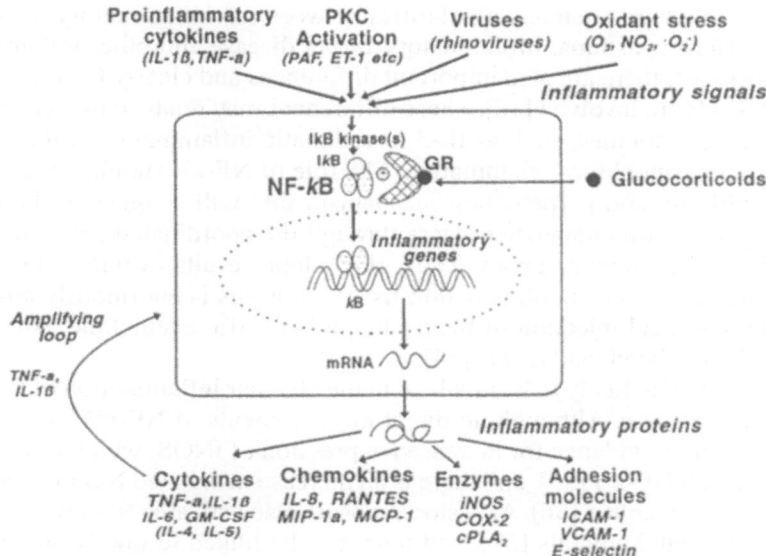

Figure 4. NF-κB may be activated by a variety of inflammatory signals, resulting in the co-ordinated expression of multiple inflammatory genes, including cytokines, chemokines, enzymes and adhesion molecules. The cytokines IL-1β and TNF-α both activate and are regulated by NF-κB and may act as an amplifying feed-forward loop. The actions of NF-κB are inhibited by glucocorticoids by binding to activated glucocorticoid receptors (GR).

phocytes with CD3 antibodies results in marked activation of NF-κB [45]. Oxidants activate NF-κB in a human epithelial line, resulting in increased expression of iNOS [46], and exposure of animals to the oxidant ozone results in NF-κB expression in lung [47]. Exposure of human peripheral blood mononuclear cells, epithelial cells and lung tissue to proinflammatory cytokines results in marked activation of NF-κB which may be prolonged [48–50]. Virus infections are common triggers of acute severe exacerbations of asthma and are thought to initiate a prolonged inflammatory response. Thus experimental rhinovirus infection results in activation of NF-κB and IL-6 secretion in nasal epithelial cells [29]. Viruses may activate NF-κB through mechanisms that involve generation of reactive oxygen intermediates [28]. There is also evidence for activation of NF-κB in biopsies of patients with asthma and in inflammatory cells in the sputum [51].

Many of the inflammatory and immunoregulatory genes (cytokines, enzymes, adhesion molecules) expressed in asthma are regulated predominantly by NF-κB. One such gene that has been studied extensively is iNOS which is expressed in airway epithelial cells and macrophages in asthma [52]. This increased iNOS expression is reflected by increased amounts of NO in exhaled air of asthmatic patients [53].

Although there are many similarities between the inflammatory responses in arthritis, asthma, inflammatory bowel disease and other inflammatory diseases, there are also important differences and clearly factors other
than NF-κB are involved [10]. These differences may relate to the secretion
of specific cytokines, such as IL-5 in asthmatic inflammation which promotes an eosinophilic inflammation. The role of NF-κB should be seen as
an amplifying and perpetuating mechanism that will exaggerate the dis-
ease-specific inflammatory process through the coordinated activation of
multiple inflammatory genes. Thus, IL-5 alone results in relatively little
accumulation of eosinophils within tissues, but this is enormously amplified by the local injection of the eosinophil-specific chemokine, eotaxin,
which is regulated via NF-κB [54].

NF-κB is also likely to be involved in the alveolar inflammation of fibrosing lung disease. Although no direct measurements of NF-κB have been
made, there is evidence for increased expression of iNOS, which is largely
regulated by NF-κB [55], and there is an increase in exhaled NO in patients
with active alveolitis [56]. Asbestos exposure also activates NF-κB in lungs
of experimental animals [57], and thus may be linked to the fibrotic process.

NF-κB is also likely to be involved in ARDS [58]. Endotoxin is a potent
activator of NF-κB in lungs and alveolar macrophages of experimental animals and this may underlie the neutrophil response in the lungs [59]. The
antioxidant N-acetylcysteine inhibits this endotoxin-mediated NF-κB
activation and the neutrophilic response. NF-κB activation is likely to
underlie the increased expression of iNOS in the lungs of rats exposed to
endotoxin [60]. Alveolar macrophages from patients with ARDS have
increased activation of NF-κB compared with patients with other severe
diseases [61]. This would be consistent with reports of increased IL-8 in
bronchoalveolar lavage fluid of patients with ARDS [62].

4. Activator Protein-1 (AP-1)

AP-1 is a heterodimer of Fos and Jun oncoproteins, which is a member of
the basic leucine zipper (bZIP) transcription family, characterized by a
basic leucine-rich area that is involved with dimerization with other transcription factors (Figure 5). AP-1 was originally described by binding to the
TPA (tetradecanoylphorbol-13-acetate) response element (TRE: 5'-TGAC/
GTCA-3') and is responsible for the transcriptional activation of various
genes that were activated by phorbol esters (such as TPA, also known as
phorbol mysistate acetate or PMA) via activation of protein kinase C
(PKC) [63]. It is now apparent that AP-1 is a collection of related transcription factors belonging to the Fos (c-Fos, FosB, Fra1, Fra2) and Jun
(c-Jun, JunB, JunD) families which dimerize in various combinations
through their leucine zipper region. Fos/Jun heterodimers bind with the

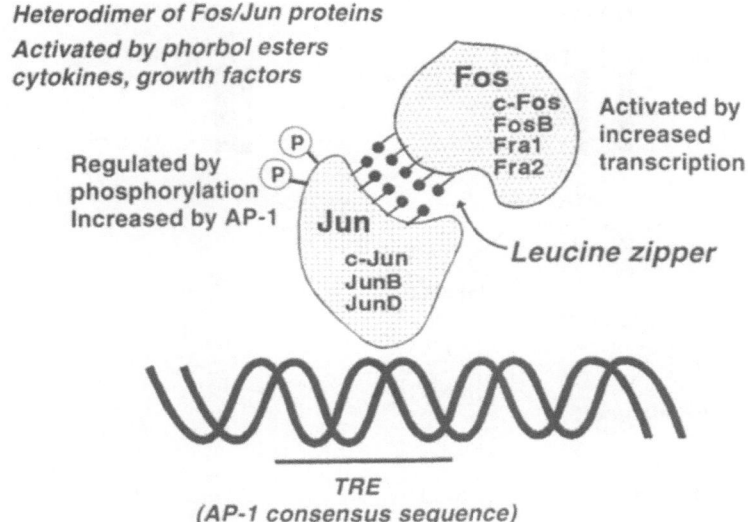

Figure 5. AP-1 is a heterodimer of Fos and Jun proteins.

greatest affinity and are the predominant form of AP-1 in most cells, whereas Jun/Jun homodimers bind with low affinity. AP-1 proteins may also form functionally distinct dimeric complexes with members of the related bZIP family of ATF/CREB transcription factors.

AP-1 may be activated via PKC and by various cytokines, including TNF-α and IL-1β via several types of protein tyrosine kinase (PTK) and mitogen-activated protein (MAP) kinase, which themselves activate a cascade of intracellular kinases [64, 65]. Both TNF-α and IL-1β activate TNF-associated factors (TRAF), which subsequently activate MAP kinases [21]. Recent studies suggest that there may be interactions between the AP-1 activating pathways and NF-κB pathways, in that TRAF2 (activated by TNF-α) and TRAF-6 (activated by IL-1β) may both activate NIK and then IKK [21] (Figure 6).

We have demonstrated the activation of AP-1 in human lung after stimulation with PMA, TNF-α and IL-1β [50, 66], and in peripheral blood mononuclear cells after activation with PMA [48]. Certain signals rapidly increase the transcription of the *fos* gene, resulting in increased synthesis of Fos protein. Other signals lead to activation of kinases that phosphorylate c-Jun, resulting in increased activation. Several specific c-Jun N-terminal kinases (JNK) are now recognized, and may play an important role in the regulation of cellular responsiveness to cytokine signals [65, 67, 68]. Conversely a Jun phosphatase counteracts the activation of AP-1, and a deficiency of this enzyme might lead to amplification of chronic inflammation.

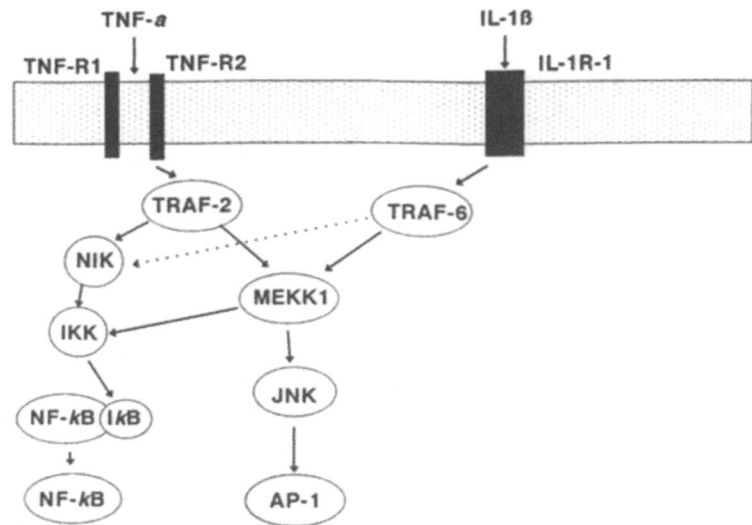

Figure 6. Interaction between AP-1 and NF-κB activating pathways: TNF-α binding to TNF-receptor-2 (TNF-R2) activates TNF-associated factor-2 (TRAF-2) which then activates NF-κB-inducing kinase (NIK); this in turn, leads to activation of NF-κB via activation of the IκB kinase complex (IKK). TRAF-2 also activates a MAP kinase enzyme, MEKK1, which leads to activation of Jun N-terminal kinase (JNK) and activation of AP-1. Similarly, IL-1β binds to the IL-1 receptor (IL-1R-1), leading to activation of TRAF-6, which also activates NIK and MEKK1, resulting in parallel activation of AP-1 and NF-κB.

The role of AP-1 in other inflammatory lung diseases has not been investigated. Endotoxin activates AP-1, so that it is likely to be involved with NF-κB in the regulation of inflammatory genes in this condition. For example, endotoxin induces haem oxygenase-1 via AP-1 activation [69].

There is evidence for increased expression of c-Fos in epithelial cells in asthmatic airways [70], and many of the stimuli relevant to asthma that activate NF-κB will also activate AP-1. AP-1, like NF-κB, regulates many of the inflammatory and immune genes that are over-expressed in asthma. Indeed many of these genes require the simultaneous activation of both transcription factors that work together cooperatively.

The recognition that AP-1 may interact with other transcription factors indicates that cross-talk between different signal transduction pathways is possible [71]. The activated glucocorticoid receptor (GR) directly interacts with activated AP-1, and this may be an important action of steroids to inhibit cytokine-mediated inflammatory responses (see below). AP-1 also interacts with cell-specific transcription factors, such as nuclear factor of activated T cells (NF-AT) (see below).

5. CAAT/Enhancer-Binding Proteins

C/EBP are transcription factors important in IL-1, IL-6 and lipopolysaccharide (LPS)-dependent signal transduction and bind to a consensus sequence ATTGCGCAAT, which includes the CAAT box. These transcription factors are members of the bZIP class of transcription factors and include C/EBPα, C/EBPβ (formerly called nuclear factor for IL-6), C/EBPγ and C/EBPδ [72]. These transcription factors are activated by pathways that involve PKC and regulate the expression of several inflammatory and immune genes. They often cooperate positivelly with other transcription factors, particularly other bZIP proteins, such as AP-1, ATF and CREB, but also with NF-κB. Thus, in the regulation of IL-8 gene expression there is a marked enhancement of transcription when C/EBPβ is activated together with NF-κB, whereas C/EBPβ activation alone has little effect [9]. Splice isoforms of these transcription factors, which appear to have blocking effects on transcription, have been identified.

The role of C/EBP in asthma has not yet been defined, but it is likely that activation of this transcription factor by inflammatory signals is an important amplifying mechanism for the expression of inflammatory genes, such as iNOS, COX-2 and certain chemokines, which have C/EBPβ recognition sequences in their promoter regions. Many of the effects of IL-6 are mediated through activation of C/EBPβ and this cytokine is produced in increased amounts from macrophages of asthmatic patients [73] and is further enhanced by allergen exposure via low-affinity immunoglobulin E (IgE) receptors (FcεRII) [74]. Rhinovirus infection markedly increases the concentrations of IL-6 in induced sputum and levels remain elevated for several days [75].

6. JAK/STAT Family

Several cytokines, including interferons, activate specific cytosolic tyrosine kinases known as Janus kinases (JAK) [76, 77] (Figure 7). Members of the JAK family include JAK1, JAK2, JAK3, TyK1 and TyK2 and may be differentially activated by different cytokines. Thus IL-2 activates JAK1 and JAK3, IL-6 activates JAK1, JAK2 and JAK3, whereas IL-5 activates only JAK2. JAKs are constitutively associated with the cytoplasmic domains of cytokine receptors and become activated upon ligand-induced receptor homo- or heterodimerization. JAKs then phosphorylate tyrosine residues on the cytoplasmic domains of cytokine receptors, which create docking domains for a family of transcription factors known as signal transducers and activators of transcription (STATs) [72]. Phosphorylation of the SH2 domain of STATs results in the formation of homo- or heterodimers which migrate to the nucleus, where they bind to response elements on promoter sequences to regulate the transcription of specific genes. An increasing number of STAT proteins have now been identified and, again,

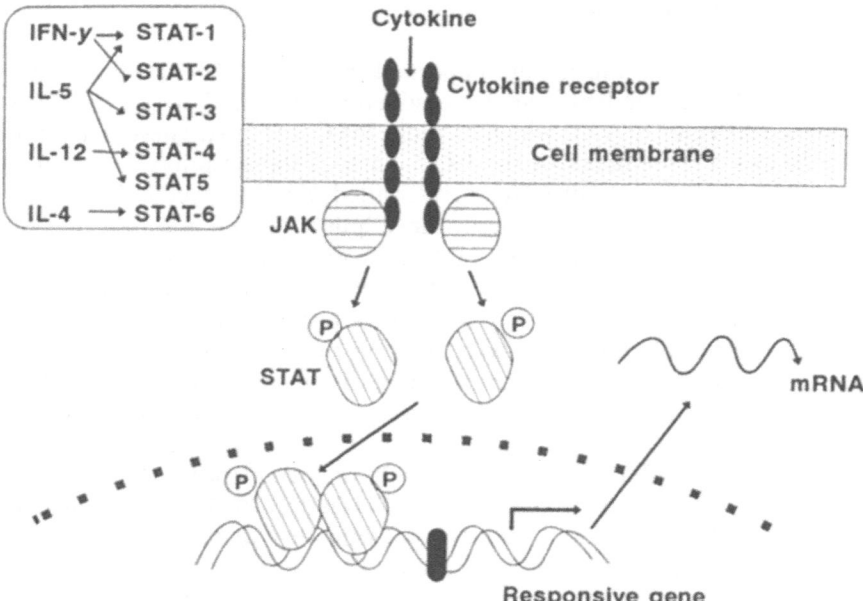

Figure 7. JAK-STAT pathways: cytokine binding to its receptor results in activation of Janus kinases (JAK) which phosphorylate intracellular domains of the receptor, resulting in phosphorylation of signal transduction-activated transcription factors (STATs). Activated STATs dimerize and translocate to the nucleus where they bind to recognition elements on certain genes.

there is specificity with particular cytokines. Thus INF-γ activates STAT1 only, whereas IFN-α activates STAT1 and STAT2 to form a STAT1/STAT2 heterodimer; these, in turn bind to IFN-γ activation sequences (GAS). STATs affect transcription by interacting with the co-activator molecules CBP and p300 [78, 79].

There is specificity in JAK-STAT pathways. Thus IL-6 activates STAT3, whereas IL-4 activates STAT6 [80, 81]. STAT6 therefore provides a novel target for blocking the effects of IL-4 as a potential treatment for allergic asthma. STAT6 knock-out mice have no response to IL-4, fail to produce IgE on allergen sensitization and do not develop Th2 cells in response to IL-4, indicating the critical role of STAT6 in allergic responses [82]. By contrast IL-12 signals via activation of STAT4 [83]. STAT4 knock-out mice have no response to IL-12 and have a propensity to develop Th2 lymphocytes [84]. IL-5 appears to activate several STATs, including STAT1, STAT3 and STAT5α [85–87]. STAT5, originally identified as a mediator of the growth effects of prolactin, also mediates the effects of GM-CSF [87].

Recently, inhibitors of STATs have been identified which are themselves regulated through JAK-STAT pathways and therefore provide a mechanism for switching of cytokine-triggered cellular signalling [88, 89].

7. Cyclic AMP Response Element-Binding Protein

Increased concentrations of cAMP also result in the activation or inhibition of gene transcription; cAMP activates protein kinase A, which phosphorylates the transcription factor CREB, which in turn binds to a CRE in the promoter region of certain genes [90]. CREB is a member of large family of CRE-binding proteins, including members of the activating transcription factor (ATF) family. CREB itself binds to CBP which acts as a co-activator molecule that binds to the TATA box and initiates transcription [91]. CREB may be counteracted by another transcription factor called CRE modulator (CREM) which may block the effects of CREB on CRE (although some splice variants appear to increase CRE binding). CREB appears to be important in the regulation of β_2-adrenoceptor expression [92]. It is activated by relatively high concentrations of β_2-agonists in lung [93] and may play a role in the down-regulation of β_2-receptors after chronic exposure to β_2-agonists [94, 95]. CREB also regulates the expression of several immune and inflammatory genes, including GM-CSF and IL-5.

CREB interacts directly with other transcription factors, allowing crosstalk between different signalling pathways. Thus CREB has a negative effect on AP-1 [96] and GR [97]. High concentrations of β-agonists inhibit the binding of GR to DNA [93, 98]. This may interfere with the anti-inflammatory effects of steroids and may account for the deleterious effects of high-dose inhaled β-agonists in some patients with asthma [99].

8. CREB-Binding Protein

Recent evidence suggests that several transcription factors interact with large co-activator molecules, such as CBP and the related p300, which bind to the basal transcription factor apparatus [100]. Several transcription factors have now been shown to bind directly to CBP, including AP-1, NF-κB and STATs [79, 101–103]. As binding sites on this molecule may be limited, this could result in competition between transcription factors for the limited binding sites available, so that there is an indirect rather than a direct protein–protein interaction (Figure 8). CBP also interacts with nuclear hormone receptors, such as glucocorticoid receptor (GR) and retinoic acid. These nuclear hormone receptors may interact with CBP and the basal transcriptional apparatus through binding to other nuclear co-activator proteins, including steroid receptor co-activator-1 (SRC-1) [104, 105], transcription factor intermediary factor-2 (TIF2) or glucocorticoid receptor-interacting protein-1 (GRIP-1 for the GR) [106]. A newly described nuclear protein called p300/CBP co-integrator-associated protein (p/CIP) appears to be particularly important in the binding of several nuclear receptors to CBP/p300 [107]. These nuclear activator proteins associate with nuclear receptors via a common sequence LXXLL (where L is lysine and X is any amino acid) [108].

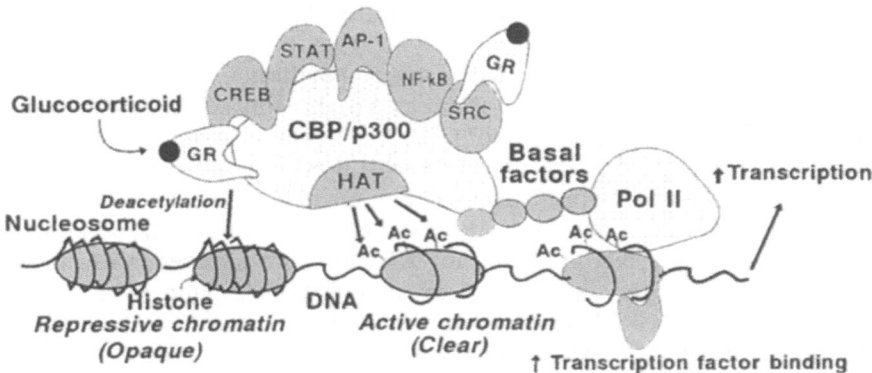

Figure 8. Co-activator molecules: transcription factors, such as STATs, AP-1 and NF-κB, bind to co-activator molecules, such as CREB-binding protein (CBP) or p300, which have intrinsic histone acetyltransferase (HAT) activity, resulting in acetylation (Ac) of histone proteins around which DNA is wound in the chromosome. This leads to unwinding of DNA and so allows increased binding of transcription factors, resulting in increased gene transcription. Glucocorticoid receptors (GR), after activation by corticosteroids, bind to a steroid receptor co-activator which is bound to CBP. This results in deacetylation of histone, with increased coiling of DNA around histone, thus preventing transcription factor binding leading to gene repression.

DNA is wound around histone proteins to form nucleosomes and the chromatin fibre in chromosomes. It has long been recognized at a microscopic level that chromatin may become dense or opaque as a result of the winding or unwinding of DNA around the histone core. CBP and p300 have histone acetylation activity which is activated by the binding of transcription factors, such as AP-1 and NF-κB [109]. Acetylation of histone residues results in unwinding of DNA coiled around the histone core, thus opening up the chromatin structure; this allows transcription factors to bind more readily, thereby increasing transcription (Figure 8). Repression of genes reverses this process by histone deacetylation [110]. The process of deacetylation involves the binding of hormone or vitamin receptors to co-repressor molecules, such as nuclear receptor co-repressor (N-CoR) which forms a complex with another repressor molecule Sin3 and a histone deacetylase [111, 112]. Deacetylation of histone increases the winding of DNA round histone residues, resulting in dense chromatin structure and reduced access of transcription factors to their binding sites, thereby leading to repressed transcription of inflammatory genes.

9. Glucocorticoid Receptors (GRs)

Glucocorticoid receptors are members of the nuclear receptor superfamily which includes other steroids (oestrogen, progesterone), and receptors for vitamins (vitamins A and D) and thyroid hormone. GRs are transcription factors that regulate the transcription of several steroid-responsive target genes [113]. They are expressed in most types of cell, and in human lung there is a high level of expression in airway epithelium and the endothelium of bronchial vessels [114]. The inactive GR is bound to a protein complex which includes two molecules of 90-kDa heat shock protein (hsp90) and an immunophilin; these act as molecular chaperones, protecting the nuclear localization site. Glucocorticoids bind to GRs in the cytoplasm, resulting in dissociation of these molecules and rapid nuclear localization and DNA binding. GRs form homodimers to interact with glucocorticoid response elements (GRE: GGTACAnnnTGTTCT), resulting in increased gene transcription [115]. Recently, it has become apparent that steroid receptors bound to DNA may interact with CBP to enhance transcription and the adenovirus protein E1A, which inactivates CBP, interfere with the action of steroids [104]. Steroids interact with CBP through binding of their ligand-activated GRs to p/CIP and other nuclear proteins [107].

Relatively few genes have GREs. One well-studied example is the human β_2-adrenoceptor gene which has at least three GREs [92]. Cortico-steroids increase transcription of β_2-receptors in animal and human lung and this may prevent tolerance to the effects of β_2-agonists by compen-sating for their down-regulation [95, 116]. Corticosteroids also increase the transcription of several anti-inflammatory proteins, including lipocortin-1, secretory leukoprotease inhibitor, CC-10 and IL-1 receptor antagonist, and these effects are presumably also mediated via GREs in the promoter regions of these genes [117]. Corticosteroids have also been reported to increase the expression of IκB-α in lymphocytes and thus to inhibit NF-κB [45, 118], but this has not been seen in other cell types [119–121]. The IkB-α gene does not appear to have any GRE consensus sequence so any efect of corticosteroids is probably mediated via other transcription factors.

9.1. Interaction With Other Transcription factors

The major anti-inflammatory effects of corticosteroids are through repres-sion of inflammatory and immune genes, and it was believed that this was likely to be mediated through negative GREs resulting in gene repression. However, none of the inflammatory and immune genes that are switched off by steroids in asthma appears to have negative GREs in their promoter sequences, suggesting that there must be some less direct inhibitory mechanism. The inhibitory effect of corticosteroids appears to result largely from a protein–protein interaction between activated GRs and transcrip-tion factors, such as AP-1, NF-κB and C/EBP, which mediate the expres-sion of these inflammatory genes [122] (Figure 9). Direct protein–protein interactions have been demonstrated between GRs and AP-1 [6, 71], and between the p65 component of NF-κB [48, 123, 124] and some STAT pro-teins, such as STAT5 [125], suggesting that corticosteroids block the

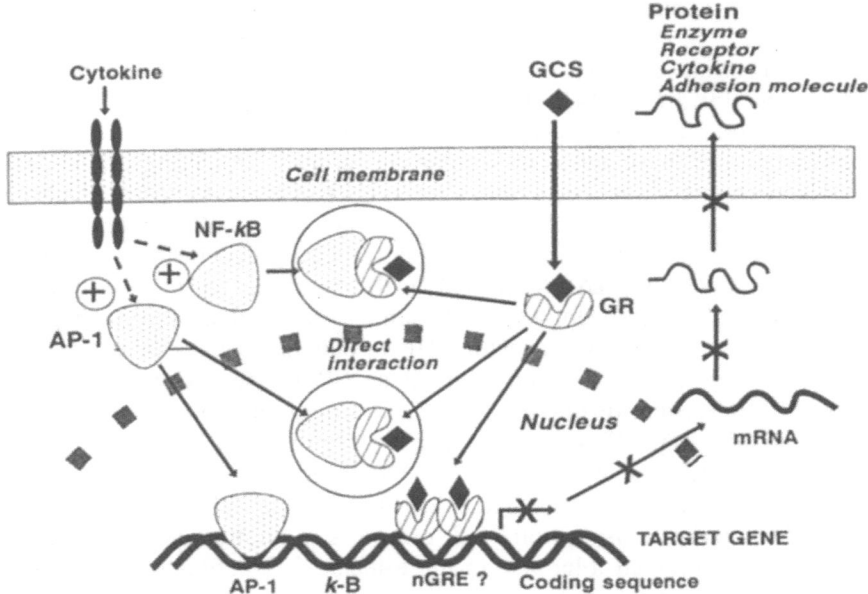

Figure 9. Mechanism of gene repression by corticosteroids. There is little evidence that gluco-corticoid receptors (GR) interact with negative glucocorticoid response elements (nGRE). Direct interaction between the transcription factors activator protein-1 (AP-1) and nuclear factor-κB (NF-κB) and the GR may result in mutual repression. In this way steroids may counteract the chronic inflammatory effects of cytokines and other stimuli that activate these transcription factors.

binding or activation of these transcription factors and thus suppress activated inflammatory genes.

There has recently been increasing evidence that corticosteroids may have effects on the chromatin structure of DNA. The repressive action of steroids may be a result of competition between GRs and the binding sites on CBP for other transcription factors, including AP-1, NF-κB and STATs [79, 101–103]. Activated GRs may bind to several transcription co-repressor molecules which associate with proteins that have histone deacetylase activity, resulting in deacetylation of histone, increased winding of DNA round histone residues, reduced access of transcription factors to their binding sites, and therefore repression of inflammatory genes [110] (see Figure 8).

A good example is the inhibitory effect of steroids on iNOS expression; iNOS is largely regulated via NF-κB [36] and the inhibitory effect of glucocorticoids on induction of iNOS appears to result from a direct interaction of GRs and the p65 component of NF-κB [126]. This results in reduced iNOS expression in asthmatic airways [127] and a reduction in exhaled nitric oxide [128]. Similarly, the eosinophil chemotactic cytokine RANTES, which is up-regulated in asthmatic airways, is inhibited by corticosteroids [129–131]. This is probably the result of an interaction of GRs with NF-κB and AP-1, which are important determinants of RANTES expression [33].

The effect of steroid receptor activation is to interfere with the activation of CBP, which regulates acetylation of the histone around which DNA is coiled. The net effect results in deacetylation of histone residues and thus tighter coiling of DNA, excluding transcription factors such as NF-κB and AP-1 from binding to DNA [102].

9.2. Steroid-Resistant Inflammation

A small proportion of asthmatic patients are steroid resistant and fail to respond to even high doses of oral steroids [132–134]. Similar resistance is seen in other chronic inflammatory diseases, such as inflammatory bowel disease and rheumatoid arthritis, but it has been studied most carefully in patients with asthma. This defect is also seen in mononuclear cells and T lymphocytes isolated from these patients. A reduction in the number or affinity of GRs cannot account for the profound loss of steroid responsiveness, but we have found a marked impairment of GRE binding after exposure of mononuclear cells to steroids *in vitro* [135]. This is associated with a marked reduction in the number of activated GRs available for binding. In the same patients there is a reduced inhibitory effect of corticosteroids on AP-1 activation, but not on NF-κB or CREB activation [136]. Furthermore, there is an increase in the baseline activity of AP-1 and activation of AP-1 with phorbol esters shows a greatly exaggerated expression of c-Fos as a result of increased gene transcription [137]. This appears to be caused by excessive activation of JNK at baseline and in response to TNF-α [138]. The increased activation of AP-1 may result in sequestration of GRs so that no receptors are available for inhibiting NF-κB, C/EBP, etc., resulting in steroid resistance. This resistance will be seen at the site of inflammation where cytokines are produced, i.e. in the airways of asthmatic patients, but not at non-inflamed sites. This may explain why patients with steroid-resistant asthma are not resistant to the endocrine and metabolic effects of steroids, and why they develop steroid side effects [139]. Whether this abnormality is inherited is not yet certain, although there is often a positive family history of asthma in patients with steroid-resistant asthma, indicating that genetic factors may be important.

10. Nuclear Factor of Activated T Cells

The nuclear factor of activated T cells (NF-AT) is a good example of a cell-specific transcription factor, because it is predominantly found in T lymphocytes, although it is also found in other cells such as mast cells. NF-

AT is of key importance in the regulation of the expression of IL-2 and probably other T cell-derived cytokines, such as IL-4 and IL-5. Activation of T cells results in activation of the phosphatase calcineurin, which in turn, activates a preformed cytoplasmic NF-AT (NF-ATp) (Figure 10). Calcineurin binds tightly to NF-ATp and is transported into the nucleus where it continues to dephosphorylate NF-AT, counteracting an NF-AT kinase [140]. At least three other forms of NF-AT have now been identified (NF-ATc, NF-AT3 and NF-AT4) and these are differentially expressed in different tissues, although all have a Rel-like domain [141]. AP-1 forms a transcriptional complex with NF-AT (and is the nuclear NF-AT previously identified) by interacting with the Rel domain to increase IL-2 gene expression [142–144]. This may be inhibited by cyclosporin A and tacrolimus (FK 506) which both inhibit calcineurin, or by steroids which inhibit AP-1 directly. This predicts that there is a synergistic interaction between cyclosporin A and steroid in inhibiting cytokine gene expression in T cells, which has recently been confirmed in studies of lymphocyte proliferation and transcription factor suppression [145].

NF-ATp is important for the regulation of IL-4 and IL-5 genes [146]. NF-AT cooperates with AP-1 in the expression of IL-4 in mice [147] and

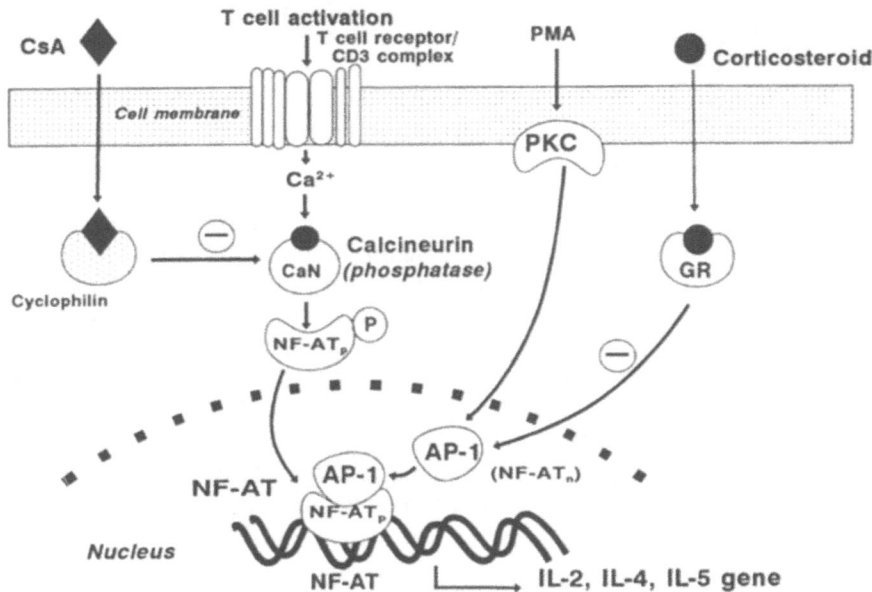

Figure 10. Nuclear factor of activated T cells regulates expression of IL-2, IL-4 and IL-5. It is made up of a cytoplasmic component (NF-AT) and AP-1. Cyclosporin inhibits NF-AT by inhibiting the activity of calcineurin (CaN) which is needed for activation of NF-AT, whereas steroids inhibit by blocking the AP-1 component. This predicts a synergy between these two drugs.

knockout of the NF-ATp gene results in defective IL-4 production [148]. Recently, an additional transcription factor called NF-AT-interacting protein (NIP-45) has been described which appears to be involved in the activation of NF-AT and the proto-oncogene c-*Maf* to activate IL-4 transcription [149]. NF-AT is also implicated in the transcription of IL-5 in T lymphocytes and mast cells, acting in concert with another transcription factor GATA [150, 151]. Corticosteroids potently inhibit IL-5 gene transcription and this may be via inhibitory effects on AP-1 which interacts with NF-ATp [152].

11. Therapeutic Implications

The increased understanding of transcription factors has given new insights into the pathophysiology of inflammatory diseases, such as asthma, but has also opened up an opportunity for the development of new anti-inflammatory treatments. Several new therapies, based on interaction with specific transcription factors or their activation pathways, are now being developed for the treatment of chronic inflammatory diseases and several drugs already in clinical use (corticosteroids, retinoic acid, cyclosporin A) work via transcription factors [153]. One concern about this approach is the specificity of such drugs, but it is clear that transcription factors have selective effects on the expression of certain genes and this may make it possible to be more selective. In addition, there are cell-specific transcription factors that may be targeted for inhibition, which could provide selectivity of drug action. One such example is NF-AT, blocked by cyclosporin A and tacrolimus, which has a restricted cellular distribution. In asthma it may be possible to target drugs to the airways by inhalation, e.g. with inhaled corticosteroids to avoid any systemic effects.

11.1. New Steroids

The recognition that most of the anti-inflammatory effects of steroids are mediated by repression of transcription factors (transrepression), whereas the endocrine and metabolic effects of steroids are likely to be mediated via GRE binding (transactivation), has led to a search for novel corticosteroids that selectively transrepress, thus reducing the risk of systemic side effects. As corticosteroids bind to the same GR, this seems at first to be an unlikely possibility, but although GRE binding involved a GR homodimer, interaction with transcription factors AP-1 and NF-κB involves only a single GR. A separation of transactivation and transrepression has been demonstrated using reporter gene constructs in transfected cells and selective mutations of GRs [154]. Furthermore, some steroids, such as the antagonist RU486, have a greater transrepression than transactivation effect.

Indeed, the topical steroids used in asthma therapy today, such as fluticasone propionate and budesonide, appear to have more potent transrepression than transactivation effects, which may account for their selection as potent anti-inflammatory agents [155]. Recently, a novel class of steroids has been described in which there is potent transrepression with relatively little transactivation. These "dissociated" steroids, including RU24858 and RU40066, have anti-inflammatory effects *in vivo* [156]. This suggests that the development of steroids with a greater margin of safety is possible and may predict the development of oral steroids which could be safe to use in asthma and other inflammatory diseases.

11.2. NF-κB Inhibitors

As NF-κB may play a pivotal role in inflammatory diseases, this has suggested that specific NF-κB inhibitors might be beneficial and could avoid some of the metabolic effects seen with inhaled steroids [10]. There has therefore been interest in NF-κB inhibitors in asthma therapy [157]. Antioxidants have the ability to block activation of NF-κB in response to a wide variety of stimuli, and drugs, such as pyrrolidine dithiocarbamate, have proved useful for *in vitro* studies, but are too toxic for *in vivo* development [28]. Spin-trap antioxidants may be more effective because they work at an intracellular level [158]. However, antioxidants do not block all of the effects of NF-κB and this may require the development of novel drugs.

Some naturally occurring NF-κB inhibitors have already been identified. Thus gliotoxin, derived from *Aspergillus* sp., is a potent NF-κB inhibitor which appears to be relatively specific [159]. The anti-inflammatory cytokine IL-10 also has an inhibitory effect on NF-κB, via an effect on IκB-α [160], and is another therapeutic possibility, particularly as there appears to be a deficit in IL-10 secretion in airway macrophages from asthmatic patients which correlates with increased secretion of proinflammatory cytokines and chemokines [161].

Novel approaches to inhibition of NF-κB would be to develop specific inhibitors of IκB kinases involved in the initial activation of NF-κB or to block the signal transduction pathways leading to activation of IκB kinases. Now that IκB kinases have been identified, it may be possible to screen and design specific inhibitors. It may also be possible to inhibit the activity of the enzymes responsible for its degradation of the IκB complex, although the proteasome has many other important functions and its inhibition is likely to produce severe side effects. Recently, it has been possible to block NF-κB function by targeting of a specific enzyme (ubiquitin ligase) involved in conjugation of ubiquitin [162]. It may be more difficult to develop drugs to inhibit the components of NF-κB itself directly, but antisense oligonucleotides have been shown to be effective inhibitors *in vitro* and stable cell permeable phosphorothioate oligonucleotides are a therapeutic possibility in the future. Recently, adenovirus-mediated gene transfer of IκB-α has been reported to inhibit endothelial cell activation [163].

However, it may be unwise to block NF-κB for prolonged periods, because it plays such a critical role in immune and host defence responses. Targeted disruption ("knock-out") of p65 is lethal because of developmental abnormalities [14], whereas lack of p50 results in immune deficiencies and increased susceptibility to infection [15]. Topical application of NF-κB inhibitors of inhalation may prove to be safe, however.

11.3. Drug Interactions

One of the most important implications of research on transcription factors is that multiple and complex interactions between these proteins are possible and that this leads to cross-talk between different signal transduction pathways. This might be exploited therapeutically by the combination of drugs that act on different transcription factors or pathways which may work together cooperatively. For example, NF-AT has a cytoplasmic component (NF-ATp) which is blocked by cyclosporin and tacrolimus, and a nuclear component AP-1, which is blocked by corticosteroids (see Figure 10). Combining steroids and cyclosporin may therefore have a synergistic inhibitory effect on the expression of genes such as those for IL-2, IL-4 and IL-5. This has indeed been demonstrated for IL-2 in human T cells, where a combination of both drugs has a much greater suppressive effect than either drug alone [145]. This suggests that a dose of cyclosporin A that is too low to give nephrotoxic side effects may be combined with an inhaled steroids, so that this synergistic interaction is confined to the airways.

Another interaction that may be exploited therapeutically is that between retinoic acid and steroids. Retinoic acid (vitamin A) binds to retinoic acid receptors which, like GRs, bind to CBP. There appears to be a synergistic interaction between steroids and retinoic acid in repression of transcription factors, such as NF-κB and AP-1, presumably because of competition for binding sites on CBP. A synergistic interaction between retinoic acid and steroids has been demonstrated in suppression of GM-CSF release from cultured epithelial cells, suggesting that retinoic acid may potentiate the anti-inflammatory effects of steroids [164]. Novel retinoic acid derivatives activate a subtype of retinoic acid receptor (RXR) which interacts with these transcription factors, so that it may be possible to develop more selective retinoids for this purpose [165].

References

1 Hunter T, Karin M (1992) The regulation of transcription by phosphorylation. *Cell* 70: 375–387
2 Karin M, Smeal T (1993) Control of transcription factors by signal transduction pathways: the beginning of the end. *Trends Biochem Sci* 17: 418–422
3 Adcock IM, Barnes PJ (1996) Transcription factors. In: RG Crystal, JB West, WR Weibel, PJ Barnes (eds): *The Lung: Scientific foundations.* Lippincott-Raven, Philadelphia, 255–276
4 Latchman DS (1996) Transcription-factor mutations and disease. *N Engl J Med* 334: 28–33
5 Papavassilou AG (1995) Transcription factors. *N Engl J Med* 332: 45–47
6 Pfahl M (1993) Nuclear receptor/AP-1 interaction. *Endocr Rev* 14: 651–658
7 Tjian R, Maniatis T (1994) Transcriptional activation: a complex puzzle with few easy pieces. *Cell* 77: 5–8
8 Lalli E, Sassone-Corsi P (1994) Signal transduction and gene regulation: the nuclear response to cAMP. *J Biol Chem* 269: 17359–17362
9 Stein B, Baldwin AS (1993) Distinct mechanisms for the regulation of the interleukin-8 gene involve synergism and cooperativity between C/EBP and NF-κB. *Mol Cell Biol* 13: 7191–7198
10 Barnes PJ, Karin M (1997) Nuclear factor-κB: a pivotal transcription factor in chronic inflammatory diseases. *N Engl J Med* 336: 1066–1071
11 Sen R, Baltimore D (1986) Multiple nuclear factors interact with the immunoglobulin enhancer sequences. *Cell* 46: 705–716
12 Siebenlist U, Franzuso G, Brown R (1994) Structure, regulation and function of NF-κB. *Annu Rev Cell Biol* 10: 405–455
13 Baeuerle PA, Henkel T (1994) Function and activation of NF-κB in the immune system. *Annu Rev Immunol* 12: 141–179
14 Beg AA, Sha WC, Bronson RT, Ghosh S, Baltimore D (1995) Embroyonic lethality and liver degeneration in mice lacking the RelA component of NF-κB. *Nature* 376: 167–170
15 Sha WC, Liou HC, Tuomanen EI, Baltimore D (1995) Targeted disruption of the p50 subunit of NF-κB leads to multifocal defects in immune responses. *Cell* 80: 321–330
16 Baldwin AS (1996) The NF-κB and IκB proteins: new discoveries and insights. *Annu Rev Immunol* 14: 649–681
17 Baeuerle PA, Baltimore D (1996) NF-κB: ten years on. *Cell* 87: 13–20
18 DiDonato J, Mercurio F, Rosette C, Wu-Li J, Suyang H, Ghosh S, Karin M (1996) Mapping of the inducible IκB phosphorylation sites that signal its ubiquitination and degradation. *Mol Cell Biol* 16: 1295–1304
19 Chen ZJ, Parent L, Maniatis T (1996) Site-specific phosphorylation of IκBα by a novel ubiquitination-dependent protein kinase activity. *Cell* 84: 853–862
20 Zandi E, Rothwarf DM, Delhase M, Hayakawa M, Karin M (1997) The IκB kinase complex (IKK) contains two kinase subunits, IKKα and IKKβ, necessary for IκB phosphorylation and NF-κB activation. *Cell* 91: 243–252
21 Eder J (1997) Tumour necrosis factor α and interleukin 1 signalling: do MAPKK kinases connect it all? *Trends Pharmacol Sci* 18: 319–322
22 Malinin NL, Boldin MP, Kovalenko AV, Wallach D (1997) MAP3K-related kinase is involved in NF-κB induction by TNF, CD95 and IL-1. *Nature* 385: 540–544
23 Lee FS, Hagler J, Chen ZJ, Maniatis T (1997) Activation of the IκB-α kinase complex by MEKK1, a kinase of the JNK pathway. *Cell* 88: 213–222
24 Arenzana-Seisdedos F, Thomson J, Rodriguez MS, Bachelerie F, Thomas D, Hay RT (1995) Inducible nuclear expression of newly synthesized IκB-α negatively regulates DNA binding and transcriptional activity of NF-κB. *Mol Cell Biol* 15: 2689–2696
25 Adcock IM, Barnes PJ (1996) Tumour necrosis factor alpha causes retention of activated glucocorticoid receptor within the cytoplasm of A549 cells. *Biochem Biophys Res Commun* 225: 1127–1132
26 Klement JF, Rice NR, Car BD et al. (1996) IκB-α deficiency results in a sustained NF-κB response and severe widespread dermatitis in mice. *Mol Cell Biol* 16: 2341–2349
27 Thomspon JE, Phillips RJ, Erdjument-Bromage H, Tempst P, Ghosh S (1995) IκB-β regulates the persistent response in a biphasic activation of NF-κB. *Cell* 80: 573–582

28 Schreck R, Rieber P, Baeuerle PA (1991) Reactive oxygen intermediates as apparently widely used messengers in the activation of the NF-κB transcription factor and HIV-1. *EMBO J* 10: 2247–2258

29 Zhu Z, Tang W, Ray A et al. (1996) Rhinovirus stimulation of interleukin-6 *in vivo* and *in vitro*. Evidence for nuclear factor κB-dependent transcription activation. *J Clin Invest* 97: 421–430

30 Schreck R, Meier B, Männel DN, Dröge W, Baeuerle PA (1991) Dithiocarbamates as potent inhibitors of nuclear factor κB activation in intact cells. *J Exp Med* 175: 1181

31 Stein B, Baldwin AS, Ballard DW, Greene WC, Angel P, Herrlich P (1993) Cross-coupling of the NF-κB p65 and Fos/Jun transcription factors produces potential biological function. *EMBO J* 12: 3879–3891

32 Mukaido N, Morita M, Ishikawa Y, Rice N, Okamoto S, Kasahara T, Matsushima K (1994) Novel mechanisms of glucocorticoid-mediated gene repression: NF-κB is target for glucocorticoid-mediated IL-8 gene expression. *J Biol Chem* 269: 13289–13295

33 Nelson PJ, Kim HT, Manning WC, Goralski TJ, Krensky AM (1993) Genomic organisation and transcriptional regulation of the RANTES chemokine gene. *J Immunol* 151: 2601–2612

34 Ueda A, Okuda K, Shira A et al. (1994) NF-κB and Sp1 regulate transcription of the human monocyte chemoattractant protein-1 gene. *J Immunol* 153: 2052–2063

35 Lilly CM, Nakamura H, Kesselman H et al. (1997) Expression of eotaxin by human lung epithelial cells: induction by cytokines and inhibition by glucocorticoids. *J Clin Invest* 99: 1767–1773

36 Xie Q, Kashiwarbara Y, Nathan C (1994) Role of transcription factor NF-κB/Rel in induction of nitric oxide synthase. *J Biol Chem* 269: 4705–4708

37 Yamamoto K, Arakawa T, Ueda N, Yamamoto S (1995) Transcriptional roles of nuclear factor κB and nuclear factor-interleukin 6 in the tumor necrosis-α-dependent induction of cyclooxygenase-2 in MC3T3-E1 cells. *J Biol Chem* 270: 31315–31320

38 Newton R, Kuitert LM, Bergmann M, Adcock IM, Barnes PJ (1997) Evidence for involvement of NF-κB in the transcriptional control of COX-2 gene expression by IL-1β. *Biochem Biophys Res Commun* 237: 28–32

39 Iademarco MF, McQuillan JJ, Rosen GD, Dean DC (1995) Characterization of the promoter for vascular adhesion molecule-1 (VCAM-1). *J Biol Chem* 267: 16323–16329

40 Van De Stolpe A, Caldenhoven E, Stade BG, Koenderman L, Raaijmakers JA, Johnson JP, van Der Saag PT (1994) 12-O-Tetradecanoyl phorbol-13-acetate and tumor necrosis factor alpha-mediated induction of intercellular adhesion molecule-1 is inhibited by dexamethasone. Functional analysis of the human intercellular adhesion molecule-1 promoter. *J Biol Chem* 269: 6185–6192

41 Liu ZG, Hsu H, Goeddel DV, Karin M (1996) Dissection of TNF receptor 1 effector functions: JNK activation is not linked to apoptosis while NF-κB activation prevents cell death. *Cell* 87: 565–576

42 Beg AA, Baltimore D (1996) An essential role for NF-κB in preventing TNF-α-induced cell death. *Science* 274: 782–784

43 Liu SF, Haddad E, Adcock IM et al. (1997) Inducible nitric oxide synthase after sensitization and allergen challenge of Brown Norway rat lung. *Br J Pharmacol* 121: 1241–1246

44 Haddad E-B, Liu SF, Salmon M, Robichaud A, Barnes PJ, Chung KF (1995) Expression of inducible nitric oxide synthase mRNA in Brown-Norway rats exposed to ozone: effect of dexamethasone. *Eur J Pharmacol (Environ Toxicol Section)* 293: 287–290

45 Auphan N, DiDonato JA, Rosette C, Helmberg A, Karin M (1995) Immunosuppression by glucocorticoids: inhibition of NF-κB activity through induction of IκB synthesis. *Science* 270: 286–290

46 Adcock IM, Brown CR, Kwon OJ, Barnes PJ (1994) Oxidative stress induces NF-κB DNA binding and inducible NOS mRNA in human epithelial cells. *Biochem Biophys Res Commun* 199: 1518–1524

47 Haddad E-B, Salmon M, Koto H, Barnes PJ, Adcock I, Chung KF (1996) Ozone induction of cytokine-induced neutrophil chemoattractant and nuclear factor-κB in rat lung: inhibition by corticosteroids. *FEBS Lett* 379: 265–268

48 Adcock IM, Brown CR, Gelder CM, Shirasaki H, Peters MJ, Barnes PJ (1995) The effects of glucocorticoids on transcription factor activation in human peripheral blood mononuclear cells. *Am J Physiol* 37: C331–C338

49 Jany B, Betz R, Schreck R (1995) Activation of the transcription factor NF-κB in human tracheobronchial epithelial cells by inflammatory stimuli. *Eur Respir J* 8: 387–391

50 Adock IM, Brown CR, Shirasaki H, Barnes PJ (1994) Effects of dexamethasone on cytokine and phorbol ester stimulated c-Fos and c-Jun DNA binding and gene expression in human lung. *Eur Respir J* 7: 2117–2123

51 Hart L, Krishnan VJ, Adcock IM, Barnes PJ, Chung KF (1998) Activation and localization of transcription factor nuclear factor-κB in asthma. *Am J Respir Crit Care Med, in press*

52 Hamid Q, Springall DR, Riveros-Moreno V et al. (1993) Induction of nitric oxide synthase in asthma. *Lancet* 342: 1510–1513

53 Kharitonov SA, Yates D, Robbins RA, Logan-Sinclair R, Shinebourne E, Barnes PJ (1994) Increased nitric oxide in exhaled air of asthmatic patients. *Lancet* 343: 133–135

54 Collins PD, Marleau S, Griffiths-Johnson DA, Jose PJ, Williams TJ (1995) Cooperation between interleukin-5 and the chemokine eotaxin to induce eosinophil accumulation *in vivo. J Exp Med* 182: 1169–1174

55 Saleh D, Barnes PJ, Giaid A (1997) Increased production of the potent oxidant peroxynitrite in the lungs of patients with pulmonary fibrosis. *Am J Respir Crit Care Med* 155: 1763–1769

56 Paredi P, Kharitonov SA, Maziak W, du Bois RM, Barnes PJ (1997) Exhaled nitric oxide (NO) a possible marker for disease activity in patients with interstitial lung disease. *Eur Respir J* 10 (suppl 25): 158S

57 Simeonova PP, Luster MI (1996) Asbestos induction of nuclear transcription factors and interleukin 8 gene regulation. *Am J Respir Cell Mol Biol* 15: 787–795

58 Blackwell TS, Christman JW (1997) The role of nuclear factor-κB in cytokine gene regulation. *Am J Respir Cell Mol Biol* 17: 3–9

59 Blackwell TS, Blackwell TR, Holden EP, Christman BW, Christman JW (1996) *In vivo* antioxidant treatment suppresses nuclear factor-κB activation and neutrophilic lung inflammation. *J Immunol* 157: 1630–1637

60 Liu S, Adcock IM, Old RW, Barnes PJ, Evans TW (1993) Lipopolysaccharide treatment *in vivo* induces widespread expression of inducible nitric oxide synthase mRNA. *Biochem Biophys Res Commun* 196: 1208–1213

61 Schwartz MD, Moore EE, Moore FA, Shenkar R, Moine P, Haenel JB, Abraham E (1996) Nuclear factor-κB is activated in alveolar macrophages from patients with acute respiratory distress syndrome. *Crit Care Med* 24: 1285–1292

62 Donnelly SC, Strieter RM, Kunkel SL et al. (1993) Interleukin-8 and development of adult respiratory distress syndrome in at-risk patient groups. *Lancet* 341: 643–647

63 Hai T, Curran T (1991) Cross-family dimerization of transcription factors Fos/Jun and ATF/CREB alters DNA binding specificity. *Proc Natl Acad Sci USA* 88: 1–5

64 Karin M (1995) The regulation of AP-1 activity by mitogen-activated protein kinases. *J Biol Chem* 270: 16483–16486

65 Karin M, Liu Zg, Zandi E (1997) AP-1 function and regulation. *Curr Opin Cell Biol* 9: 240–246

66 Adcock IM, Shirasaki H, Gelder CM, Peters MJ, Brown CR, Barnes PJ (1994) The effects of glucocorticoids on phorbol ester and cytokine stimulated transcription factor activation in human lung. *Life Sci* 55: 1147–1153

67 Kyriakis JM, Bangrjee P, Nikolakaki E et al. (1994) The stress-activated protein kinase subfamily of c-Jun kinases. *Nature* 369: 156–160

68 Westwick JK, Weitzel C, Minden A, Karin M, Brenner DA (1994) Tumor necrosis factor alpha stimulates AP-1 activity through prolonged activation of the c-Jun kinase. *J Biol Chem* 269: 26396–26401

69 Camhi SL, Alam J, Otterbein L, Sylvester SL, Choi AM (1995) Induction of heme oxygenase-1 gene expression by lipopolysaccharide is mediated by AP-1 activation. *Am J Respir Cell Mol Biol* 13: 387–398

70 Demoly P, Basset-Seguin N, Chanez P et al. (1992) c-*Fos* proto-oncogene expression in bronchial biopsies of asthmatics. *Am J Respir Cell Mol Biol* 7: 128–133

71 Ponta H, Cato ACB, Herrlick P (1992) Interference of specific transcription factors. *Biochim Biophys Acta* 1129: 255–261

72 Kishimoto T, Taga T, Akira S (1994) Cytokine signal transduction. *Cell* 76: 253–262

73 Gosset P, Tsicopoulos A, Wallaert B, Vannimenus C, Joseph M, Tonnel AB, Capron A (1991) Increased secretion by tumor necrosis factor α and interleukin 6 by alveolar macro-

phages consecutive to the development of the late asthmatic reaction. *J Allergy Clin Immunol* 88: 561–571

74 Gosset P, Tsicopoulos A, Wallaert B, Vannimenus C, Joseph M, Tonnel AB, Capron A (1992) Tumor necrosis factor α and interleukin-6 production by human mononuclear phagocytes from allergic asthmatics after IgE-dependent stimulation. *Am Rev Respir Dis* 146: 768–774

75 Grunberg K, Smits HH, Timers MC et al. (1997) Experimental rhinovirus 16 infection. Effects on cell differentials and soluble markers in sputum in asthmatic subjects. *Am J Respir Crit Care Med* 156: 609–616

76 Darnell JE, Kerr IM, Stark GR (1994) Jak-STAT pathways and transcriptional activation in response to IFNs and other extracellular signalling proteins. *Science* 264: 1415–1421

77 Ihle JN, Witthuhn BA, Quelle FW, Yamamoto K, Thienfeloer WC, Kreider B, Silvennoinev O (1994) Signalling by the cytokine receptor superfamily: JAKs and STATs. *Trends Biochem Sci* 19: 222–225

78 Battacharya S, Eckner R, Grossman S, Oldread E, Arany Z, D'Andrea A, Livingston DM (1996) Cooperation of Stat 2 and p300/CBP in signaling induced by interferon-alpha. *Nature* 383: 344–347

79 Zhang JJ, Vinkemeier U, Gu W, Chakravarti D, Horvath CM, Darnell JE (1996) Two contact regions between STAT1 and CBP/p300 in interferon-γ signalling. *Proc Natl Acad Sci USA* 93: 15092–15096

80 Hou J, Schindler U, Henzel WJ, Ho TC, Brasseur M, McKnight SL (1994) An interleukin-4-induced transcription factor: IL-4 stat. *Science* 265: 1701–1706

81 Takeda K, Tanaka T, Shi W et al. (1996) Essential role for Stat6 in IL-4 signaling. *Nature* 380: 627–630

82 Kaplan MH, Schindler U, Smiley ST, Grusby MJ (1996) Stat6 is required for mediating responses to IL-4 and for the development of Th2 cells. *Immunity* 4: 313–319

83 Bacon CM, Petricoin EF, Ortaldo JR, Rees SC, Larner AC, Johnston JA, O'Shea JJ (1995) IL-12 induces tyrosine phosphorylation and activation of STAT-4 in human lymphocytes. *Proc Natl Acad Sci USA* 92: 7303–7311

84 Kaplan MH, Sun Y, Hoey T, Grusby MJ (1996) Impaired IL-12 responses and enhanced development of Th2 cells in Stat4-deficient mice. *Nature* 382: 174–177

85 Pazdrak K, Stafford S, Alam R (1995) The activation of the Jak-STAT 1 signalling pathway by IL-5 in eosinophils. *J Immunol* 155: 397–402

86 van der Bruggen T, Caldenhoven E, Kanters D, Coffer P, Raaijmakers JA, Lammers JW, Koenderman L (1995) Interleukin-5 signaling in human eosinophils involves JAK2 tyrosine kinase and Stat1α. *Blood* 85: 1442–1448

87 Mui ALF, Wakao H, O'Farrell AM, Miyajima A (1995) Interleukin-3, granulocyte-macrophage colony stimulating factor and interleukin-5 transduce signals through two STAT5 homologs. *EMBO J* 14: 1166–1175

88 Naka T, Narazaki M, Hirata M et al. (1997) Structure and function of a new STAT-induced STAT inhibitor. *Nature* 387: 924–929

89 Starr R, Willson TA, Viney EM et al. (1997) A family of cytokine-inducible inhibitors of signalling. *Nature* 387: 917–921

90 Yamamoto KK, Gonzalez GA, Biggs WH, Montminy MR (1988) Phosphorylation-induced binding and transcriptional efficacy of nuclear factor CREB. *Nature* 334: 494–498

91 Chrivia JC, Kwok RPS, Lamb N, Hagiwara M, Montminy MR, Goodman RH (1993) Phosphorylated CREB specifically binds to the nuclear factor CBP. *Nature* 365: 855–859

92 Collins S, Altschmied J, Herbsman O, Caron MG, Mellon PL, Lefkowitz RJ (1990) A cAMP element in the β₂-adrenerigc receptor gene confers autoregulation by cAMP. *J Biol Chem* 265: 19930–19935

93 Peters MJ, Adcock IM, Brown CR, Barnes PJ (1995) β-Adrenoceptor agonists interfere with glucocorticoid receptor DNA binding in rat lung. *Eur J Pharmacol (Mol Pharmacol Section)* 289: 275–281

94 Nishikawa M, Mak JCW, Shirasaki H, Barnes PJ (1993) Differential down-regulation of pulmonary β₁- and β₂-adrenoceptor messenger RNA with prolonged *in vivo* infusion of isoprenaline. *Eur J Pharmacol (Mol Pharmacol Section)* 247: 131–138

95 Mak JCW, Nishikawa M, Shirasaki H, Miyayasu K, Barnes PJ (1995) Protective effects of a glucocorticoid on down-regulation of pulmonary β₂-adrenergic receptors *in vivo*. *J Clin Invest* 96: 99–106

96 Masquilier D, Sassone-Corsi P (1992) Transcriptional cross talk: nuclear factors CREM and CREB bind to AP-1 sites and inhibit activation by Jun. *J Biol Chem* 267: 22460–22466

97 Imai F, Minger JN, Mitchell JA, Yamamoto KR, Granner DK (1993) Glucocorticoid receptor – cAMP response element-binding protein interaction and the response of the phosphoenolpyruvate carboxykinase gene to glucocorticoids. *J Biol Chem* 268: 5353–5356

98 Stevens DA, Barnes PJ, Adcock IM (1995) β-Agonists inhibit DNA binding of glucocorticoid receptors in human pulmonary and bronchial epithelial cells. *Am J Resp Crit Care Med* 151: A195

99 Adcock IM, Stevens DA, Barnes PJ (1996) Interactions between steroids and β_2-agonists. *Eur Respir J* 9: 160–168

100 Janknecht R, Hunter T (1996) A growing coactivator network *Nature* 383: 22–23

101 Arias J, Alberts AS, Brindle P et al. (1994) Activation of cAMP and mitogen responsive genes relies on a common nuclear factor. *Nature* 370: 226–229

102 Kamei Y, Xu L, Heinzel T et al. (1996) A CBP integrator complex mediates transcriptional activation and AP-1 inhibition by nuclear receptors. *Cell* 85: 403–414

103 Perkins ND, Felzien LK, Betts JC, Leung K, Beach DH, Nabel GJ (1997) Regulation of NF-κB by cyclin-dependent kinases associated with the p300 coactivator. *Science* 275: 523–526

104 Smith CL, Onate SA, Tsai MJ, O'Malley BW (1996) CREB binding protein acts synergistically with steroid receptor coactivator-1 to enhance steroid receptor-dependent transcription. *Proc Natl Acad Sci USA* 93: 8884–8888

105 Yao PM, Buhler JM, D'Ortho MP, Lebargy F, Delclaux C, Harf A, Lafuma C (1996) Expression of matrix metalloproteinase gelatinases A and B by cultured epithelial cells from human bronchial explants. *J Biol Chem* 271: 15580–15589

106 Hong H, Kohli K, Garabedian MJ, Stallcup MR (1997) GRIP1, a transcriptional coactivator for the AF-2 transactivation domain of steroid, thyroid, retinoid, and vitamin D receptors. *Mol Cell Biol* 17: 2735–2744

107 Torchia J, Rose DW, Inostroza J, Kamei Y, Westin S, Glass CK, Rosenfeld MG (1997) The transcriptional co-activator p/CIP binds CBP and mediates nuclear receptor function. *Nature* 387: 677–684

108 Heery DM, Kalkhoven E, Hoare S, Parker MG (1997) A signature motif in transcriptional co-activators mediates binding to nuclear receptors. *Nature* 387: 733–736

109 Ogryzko VV, Schlitz RL, Russanova V, Howard BH, Nakatani Y (1996) The transcriptional coactivators p300 and CBP are histone acetyltransferases. *Cell* 87: 953–959

110 Wolffe AP (1997) Sinful repression. *Nature* 387: 16–17

111 Nagy L, Kao HY, Chakravarti D et al. (1997) Nuclear receptor repression mediated by a complex containing SMRT, mSin3A, and histone deacetylase. *Cell* 89: 373–380

112 Heinzel T, Lavinsky RM, Mullen TM et al. (1997) A complex containing N-CoR, mSin3 and histone deacetylase mediates transcriptional repression. *Nature* 387: 43–48

113 Beato M, Herrlich P, Schutz G (1995) Steroid hormone receptors: many actors in search of a plot. *Cell* 83: 851–857

114 Adcock IM, Gilbey T, Gelder CM, Chung KF, Barnes PJ (1996) Glucocorticoid receptor localization in normal human lung and asthmatic lung. *Am J Respir Crit Care Med* 154: 771–782

115 Truss M, Beato M (1993) Steroid hormone receptors: interaction with deoxyribonucleic acid and transcription factors. *Endocr Rev* 14: 459–479

116 Mak JCW, Grandordy B, Barnes PJ (1994) High affinity [³H]formoterol binding sites in lung: characterization and autoradiographic mapping. *Eur J Pharmacol (Mol Section)* 269: 35–41

117 Barnes PJ (1996) Mechanism of action of glucocorticoids in asthma. *Am J Respir Crit Care Med* 154: S21–S27

118 Scheinman RI, Cogswell PC, Lofquist AK, Baldwin AS (1995) Role of transcriptional activation of IκB-α in mediating immunosuppression by glucocorticoids. *Science* 270: 283–286

119 Brostjan C, Anrather J, Csizmadia V, Stoka D, Soares M, Bach FH, Winkler H (1996) Glucocorticoid-mediated repression of NF-κB activity in endothelial cells does not involve induction of IκB α synthesis. *J Biol Chem* 271: 19612–19616

120 Newton R, Hart LA, Adcock IM, Barnes PJ (1997) Effect of glucocorticoids on IL-1β-induced NF-κB binding and expression in type II alveolar cells – no evidence for down-regulation by IκB. *Am J Respir Crit Care Med* 155: A699

121 Heck S, Bender K, Kullmann M, Gottlicher M, Herrlich P, Cato AC (1997) IκB α-independent downregulation of NF-κB activity by glucocorticoid receptor. *EMBO J* 16: 4698–4707

122 Barnes PJ, Adcock IM (1993) Anti-inflammatory actions of steroids: molecular mechanisms. *Trends Pharmacol Sci* 14: 436–441

123 Ray A, Prefontaine KE (1994) Physical association and functional antagonism between the p65 subunit of transcription factor NF-κB and the glucocorticoid receptor. *Proc Natl Acad Sci USA* 91: 752–756

124 Caldenhoven E, Liden J, Wissink S et al. (1995) Negative cross-talk between RelA and the glucocorticoid receptor: a possible mechanism for the antiinflammatory action of gluco-corticoids. *Mol Endocrinol* 9: 401–412

125 Stocklin E, Wisler M, Gouilleux F, Groner B (1996) Functional interactions between Stat5 and the glucocorticoid receptor. *Nature* 383: 726–728

126 Kleinert H, Euchenhofer C, Ihrig Biedert I, Forstermann U (1996) Glucocorticoids inhibit the induction of nitric oxide synthase II by down-regulating cytokine-induced activity of transcription factor nuclear factor-kappa B. *Mol Pharmacol* 49: 15–21

127 Giaid A, Saleh D, Lim S, Barnes PJ, Ernst P (1998) Formation of peroxynitrite in asthmatic airways. *Am J Respir Crit Care Med* 157: A870

128 Kharitonov SA, Yates D, Barnes PJ (1995) Increased nitric oxide in exhaled air of normal human subjects with upper respiratory tract infections. *Eur Respir J* 8: 295–297

129 Kwon OJ, Jose PJ, Robbins RA, Schall TJ, Williams TJ, Barnes PJ (1995) Glucocorticoids inhibition of RANTES expression in human lung epithelial cells. *Am J Respir Cell Mol Med* 12: 488–496

130 Berkman N, Robichaud A, Krishnan VL, Barnes PJ, Chung KF (1996) Expression of RANTES in human airway epithelial cells: effect of corticosteroids and interleukins-4, 10 and 13. *Immunology* 87: 599–603

131 Wang H, Devalia JL, Xia C, Sapsford RJ, Davies RJ (1996) Expression of RANTES by human bronchial epithelial cells *in vitro* and *in vivo* and the effect of corticosteroids. *Am J Respir Cell Mol Biol* 14: 27–35

132 Barnes PJ, Adcock IM (1995) Steroid-resistant asthma. *Q J Med* 88: 455–468

133 Barnes PJ, Greening AP, Crompton GK (1995) Glucocorticoid resistance in asthma. *Am J Respir Crit Care Med* 152: 125S–140S

134 Szefler SJ, Leung DY (1997) Glucocorticoid-resistant asthma: pathogenesis and clinical implications for management. *Eur Respir J* 10: 1640–1647

135 Adcock IM, Lane SJ, Brown CA, Peters MJ, Lee TH, Barnes PJ (1995) Differences in binding of glucocorticoid receptor to DNA in steroid-resistant asthma. *J Immunol* 154: 3000–3005

136 Adcock IM, Lane SJ, Brown CA, Lee TH, Barnes PJ (1995) Abnormal glucocorticoid receptor/AP-1 interaction in steroid resistant asthma. *J Exp Med* 182: 1951–1958

137 Adcock IM, Lane SJ, Barnes PJ, Lee TH (1996) Enhanced phorbol ester-induced c-Fos transcription and translation in steroid-resistant asthma. *Am J Respir Crit Care Med* 153: A682

138 Adcock IM, Brady H, Lim S, Karin M, Barnes PJ (1997) Increased JUN kinase activity in peripheral blood monocytes from steroid-resistant asthmatic subjects. *Am J Respir Crit Care Med* 155: A288

139 Lane SJ, Atkinson BA, Swimanathan R, Lee TH (1996) Hypothalamic–pituitary axis in corticosteroid-resistant asthma. *Am J Respir Crit Care Med* 153: 1510–1514

140 Shibasaki F, Price ER, Milan D, McKeon F (1996) Role of kinases and the phosphatase calcineurin in the nuclear shuttling of transcription factor NF-AT4. *Nature* 382: 370–373

141 Hoey T, Sun YL, Williamson K, Yu X (1995) Isolation of two new members of the NF-AT gene family and functional characterization of the NF-AT proteins. *Immunity* 2: 461–472

142 Jain J, McCaffrey PG, Valge Archer VE, Rao A (1992) Nuclear factor of activated T cells contains Fos and Jun. *Nature* 356: 801–804

143 Northrop JP, Ullman KS, Crabtree GR (1993) Characterization of the nuclear and cyto-plasmic components of the lymphoid-specific nuclear factor of activated T cells (NF-AT). *J Biol Chem* 268: 2917–2923

144 Palmer JBD, Cuss FMC, Mulderry PK et al. (1987) Calcitonin gene-related peptide is localized to human airway nerves and potently constricts human airway smooth muscle. *Br J Pharmacol* 91: 95–101

145 Wright LC, Cammisuli S, Baboulene L, Fozzard J, Adcock IM, Barnes PJ (1995) Cyclosporin A and glucocorticoids interact synergistically in T lymphocytes: implications for asthma therapy. *Am J Resp Crit Care Med* 151: A675

146 Lee HJ, Matsuda I, Naito Y, Yokota T, Arai N, Arai K (1994) Signals and nuclear factors that regulate the expression of interleukin-4 and interleukin-5 genes in helper T cells. *J Allergy Clin Immunol* 94: 594–604

147 Hodge MR, Rooney JW, Glimcher LH (1995) The proximal promoter of the IL-4 gene is composed of multiple essential regulatory sites that bind at least two distinct factors. *J Immunol* 154: 6397–6405

148 Hodge MR, Ranger AM, Charles de la Brousse F, Hoey T, Grusby MJ, Glimcher LH (1996) Hyperproliferation and dysregulation of IL-4 expression in NF-ATp-deficient mice. *Immunity* 4: 397–405

149 Hodge MR, Chun HJ, Rengarajan J, Alt A, Lieberson R, Glimcher LH (1996) NF-AT-driven interleukin-4 transcription potentiated by NIP45. *Science* 274: 1903–1905

150 Lee HJ, Masuda ES, Arai N, Arai K, Yokota T (1995) Definition of *cis*-regulatory elements of the mouse interleukin-5 gene promoter. Involvement of nuclear factor of activated T cell-related factors in interleukin-5 expression. *J Biol Chem* 270: 17541–17550

151 Prieschl EE, Gouilleux Gruart V, Walker C, Harrer NE, Baumruker T (1995) A nuclear factor of activated T cell-like transcription factor in mast cells is involved in IL-5 gene regulation after IgE plus antigen stimulation. *J Immunol* 154: 6112–6119

152 Mori A, Kaminuma O, Suko M et al. (1997) Two distinct pathways of interleukin-5 synthesis in allergen-specific human T cell clones are suppressed by glucocorticoids. *Blood* 89: 2891–2900

153 Manning AM (1996) Transcription factors: a new frontier in drug discovery. *Drug Devel Ther* 1: 151–160

154 Heck S, Kullmann M, Grast A, Ponta H, Rahmsdorf HJ, Herrlich P, Cato ACB (1994) A distinct modulating domain in glucocorticoid receptor monomers in the repression of activity of the transcription factor AP-1. *EMBO J* 13: 4087–4095

155 Adcock IM, Barnes PJ (1996) Ligand-induced differentiation of glucocorticoid receptor (GR) transrepression and transactivation. *Am J Respir Crit Care Med* 153: A243

156 Vayssière BM, Dupont S, Choquart A et al. (1997) Synthetic glucocorticoids that dissociate transactivation and AP-1 transrepresson exhibit antiinflammatory activity *in vivo*. *Mol Endocrinol* 11: 1245–1255

157 Barnes PJ, Adcock IM (1997) NF-κB: a pivotal role in asthma and a new target for therapy. *Trends Pharmacol Sci* 18: 46–50

158 Miyajima T, Kotake Y (1995) Spin trapping agent, phenyl *N*-tert-butyl nitrone, inhibits induction of nitric oxide synthase in endotoxin-induced shock in mice. *Biochem Biophys Res Commun* 215: 114–121

159 Pahl HL, Krauss B, Schultze-Osthoff K et al. (1996) The immunosuppressive fungal metabolite gliotoxin specifically inhibits transcription factor NF-κB. *J Exp Med* 183: 1829–1840

160 Wang P, Wu P, Siegel MI, Egan RW, Billah MM (1995) Interleukin(IL)-10 inhibits nuclear factor kappa B activation in human monocytes. IL-10 and IL-4 suppress cytokine synthesis by different mechanisms. *J Biol Chem* 270: 9558–9563

161 John M, Lim S, Seybold J, Robichaud A, O'Connor B, Barnes PJ, Chung KF (1997) Inhaled corticosteroids increase IL-10 but reduce MIP-1α, GM-CSF and IFN-γ release from alveolar macrophages in asthma. *Am J Respir Crit Care Med*

162 Yaron A, Gonen H, Alkalay I et al. (1997) Inhibition of NF-κB cellular function via specific targeting of the IκB-ubiquitin ligase. *EMBO J* 16: 6486–6494

163 Wrighton CJ, Hofer-Warbinek R, Moll T, Eytner R, Bach FH, de Martin R (1996) Inhibition of endothelial cell activation by adenovirus-mediated expression of IκB-α, an inhibitor of transcription factor NF-κB. *J Exp Med* 183: 1013–1022

164 Wallace J, Adcock IM, Barnes PJ (1996) Retinoic acid potentiates the inhibitory effects of dexamethasone on AP-1 DNA binding in epithelial cells. *Am J Respir Crit Care Med* 153: A209

165 Rowe A (1997) Retinoid X receptors. *Int J Biochem Cell Biol* 29: 275–278

Molecular Biology of the Lung
Vol. 2: Asthma and Cancer
ed. by R. A. Stockley
© 1999 Birkhäuser Verlag Basel/Switzerland

CHAPTER 4
Regulation of the Cytokine Gene Cluster on Chromosome 5q

David J. Cousins, Dontcho Z. Staynov and Tak H. Lee

Department of Respiratory Medicine and Allergy, GKT Medical School, Kings College, Guy's Hospital, London, UK

1   Introduction
2   Involvement of IL-4, IL-5, IL-13 and GM-CSF in Asthma
3   Regulation of the Chromosome 5 Gene Cluster in T Cells
3.1 GM-CSF Gene Regulation
3.2 IL-4 Gene Regulation
3.3 IL-3 Gene Regulation
3.4 IL-5 Gene Regulation
4   Conclusions
     References

1. Introduction

The role of cytokines in the inflammatory processes observed in asthma and atopy has become an area of intense research in recent years. This research has demonstrated that a large number of cytokine genes are overexpressed by inflammatory cells, including T lymphocytes, in patients with atopic disease. CD4$^+$ T-helper lymphocytes have been divided into subsets based upon the cytokine genes that they express on activation [1]. T-helper (Th)1 cells express interleukin (IL)-2 and interferon-γ (IFN-γ) but not IL-4 or IL-5, whereas Th2 cells express IL-4, IL-5, IL-10 and IL-13, but not IL-2 or IFN-γ. Both cell types express IL-3 and granulocyte-macrophage colony-stimulating factor (GM-CSF). A third subset of cells termed Th0 has also been identified which express all of the aforementioned cytokines. These T cell subsets were originally identified in the mouse and a similar, though not identical, pattern of cytokine expression has since been observed in human T cells [2]. The cytokine genes encoding IL-3, IL-4, IL-5, IL-13 and GM-CSF are located in close proximity on human chromosome 5q with a similar gene cluster found on mouse chromosome 11q. This chapter looks at the evidence for the overexpression of a Th2-like cytokine profile in asthma, focusing on the gene cluster on chromosome 5q, and the mechanisms by which these genes are regulated in T cells.

2. Involvement of IL-4, IL-5, IL-13 and GM-CSF in Asthma

Several research groups have studied the expression of these cytokines in asthma by T cell cloning, immunohistochemistry and *in situ* hybridization. Allergen-specific CD4+ T cell clones derived from bronchial biopsy specimens taken from patients with grass pollen-induced asthma displayed a Th2-like phenotype [3]. Bronchoalveolar lavage (BAL) samples from patients with atopic asthma contain increased levels of IL-4, IL-5 and GM-CSF in the lavage fluid [4–6]. Interestingly, the levels of IL-5 correlated with the extent of eosinophil infiltrate in the BAL suggesting that IL-5 may be responsible for the eosinophilia characteristic of atopic asthma [4]. More recently, it has been shown that lung eosinophilia is abolished in a mouse asthma model using IL-5 knock-out mice [7]. Using *in situ* hybridization and immunohistochemistry Robinson et al. confirmed that a predominantly Th2-like T cell population exists in the BAL from patients with atopic asthma with an increase in T cells positive for IL-4, IL-5 and GM-CSF messenger RNA (mRNA) [8]. It is also interesting to note that treatment with corticosteroids, which alleviates the symptoms of asthma, causes a decrease in the numbers of BAL cells positive for IL-4 and IL-5 mRNA [9].

Several studies have demonstrated increased mRNA and protein production of IL-4, IL-5, GM-CSF and IL-13 in bronchial biopsies from patients with atopic asthma and rhinitis [10–16]. Interestingly, the source of these cytokines in biopsy specimens was not exclusively T cells with mast cells [12, 17–19]; eosinophils [15, 18, 20] and epithelial cells [12, 14, 21, 22] also expressing these genes. However, Kay et al. have reported that the predominant cell type (70%) transcribing IL-4 and IL-5 mRNA in patients with atopic asthma and rhinitis is CD3+ T cells with the remaining cells being eosinophils and mast cells [13].

Using a genetic approach several studies have demonstrated linkage of markers on human chromosome 5 to a gene regulating total serum IgE levels in atopic patients [23–26]; particularly close linkage was observed to the IL-4 gene in some of these studies [23, 25]. Bronchial hyperresponsiveness has also been linked to chromosome 5q [27] and has been shown to be co-inherited with total IgE levels [28, 29]. This information suggests that a defect in the regulated expression of these genes may be a factor in atopic disease and asthma, emphasizing the importance of understanding the mechanisms by which expression of this gene cluster is controlled.

3. Regulation of the Chromosome 5 Gene Cluster in T Cells

GM-CSF, IL-3, IL-4, IL-5 and IL-13 are located in a small segment (5q23–31) on the long arm of human chromosome 5 in close proximity to interferon regulatory factor 1 (IRF-1) and several other as yet unidentified genes [25]. The gene order is: IL-13, IL-4, IL-5, IL-3, GM-CSF (Figure 1).

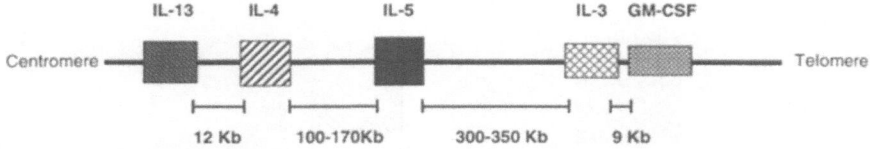

Figure 1. Map of cytokine gene cluster on human chromosome 5q.

This suggests a common origin via gene duplication and/or some common regulatory mechanisms for expression of these genes; however, it is still unclear exactly which mechanisms are involved. Over the last few years a large body of work has been published involving the dissection of the proximal promoters of these genes in both murine and human T cells. Historically, the GM-CSF promoter has been most intensively studied followed by IL-4 and IL-3; more recently work on the IL-5 promoter has been published (see below). There is no information currently available on the IL-13 promoter. Overall this work has indicated that elements identified in one species are not necessarily present (or active) in the other.

3.1. GM-CSF Gene Regulation

Several groups have reported *cis*-acting elements in the promoter of GM-CSF which are active in T cells (Figure 2). The most proximal to the transcription start site is the conserved lymphokine element 0 (CLE0) [30–33]; this region is required for PMA/A23187 induction of GM-CSF. The CLE0 has been shown to bind several factors: nuclear factor of activated T cells (NF-ATp), activator protein-1 (AP-1), Ets1 and Elf1 [34–39]. All of these transcription factors are required for IL-2 activation [40]. Interestingly the CLE0 element is very highly conserved in several genes, notably IL-4, IL-5 and G-CSF. The proteins NF-AT and AP-1 can bind to the CLE0 elements from IL-5 and IL-4 (poorly), but not G-CSF which is not produced by T cells [32]. This suggests that the CLE0 element plays a role in the coordinate induction of these cytokines in T cells. Adjacent to the CLE0 element in the promoter is a more recently characterized region known as PEBP2 [41]. This element binds transcription factors of the polyoma virus enhancer-binding protein 2 (PEBP2) family (also known as core-binding factor or CBF) [42]. Different members of the PEBP2 family have different effects upon transcription of GM-CSF and the activity of this element is dependent upon the relative ratios of these proteins in the nucleus. This region also appears to bind the transcription factor YY-1 which represses the promoter [43]. To date the role of this element in the regulation of GM-CSF remains unclear.

Upstream of these elements are two regions: the CLE1 and CLE2/GC box [44–46]. The CLE1 motif is required for the induction of GM-CSF

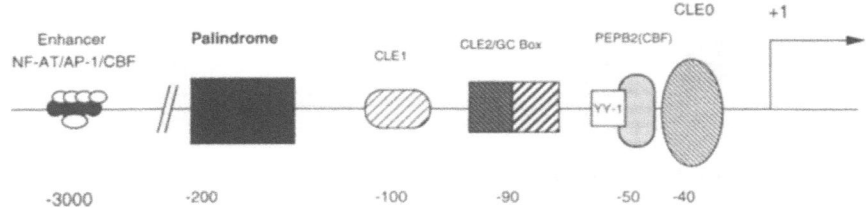

Figure 2. Regulatory elements of the GM-CSF promoter (see text).

transcription by the $p40^X$-transactivating protein (from HTLV-I) but has no effect on PMA/A23187 induction. The CLE2/GC box motif is required for efficient activation by PMA/A23187 or $p40^X$. It contains two protein-binding motifs, the GM2 sequence GGTAGTTCCC, which binds the PMA/A23187 inducible factor nuclear factor of GM-CSF2, and CCGCCC which binds the constitutive factors A_1, A_2 and B [47]. NF-GM2 appears to be nuclear factor-κB (NF-κB) [39, 48, 49], and purified A_1 was identified as the transcription factor Sp1 [47, 50]. The human GM2 sequence is identical to that of the mouse, but the GC box has a C to T mutation (CCGCCT). This may be important because a mutation from C to A abolishes binding of all three constitutive factors and also causes loss of transcriptional inducibility, suggesting that Sp1 may not be involved in the regulation of human GM-CSF [47, 50]. It is interesting to note that they have reported that this element is also involved in the regulation of IL-3 [51].

We have reported a novel regulatory element in the promoter of the human GM-CSF gene upstream of these elements [52]. It contains two symmetrically nested inverted repeats (−192 CTTGGAAAGGTTCATT AATGAAAACCCCCAAG −161 base-pairs). In transfection assays using the human GM-CSF promoter, this element has a strong positive effect on the expression of a reporter gene by the human T cell line Jurkat J6 upon stimulation with phorbol dibutyrate (PDBu) and ionomycin or anti-CD3. In DNA band-retardation assays, this sequence produces six specific bands which invole one or other of the inverted repeats. We have also shown that a DNA−protein complex can be formed involving both repeats and probably more than one protein. The external inverted repeat contains a core sequence CTTGG...CCAAG which is also present in the promoters of several other T cell-expressed human cytokine genes, including IL-4 and IL-5 (labelled palindrome in Figure 3 and 5). However, the palindromic elements in these genes are larger than the core sequence, suggesting that some of the interacting proteins may be different for different genes and may represent a family of novel transcription factors. As this element is present in the promoters of all human Th2-like genes it may contribute to the coordinated expression of this group of cytokines. Although this element is present in the mouse and human promoters of the GM-CSF gene,

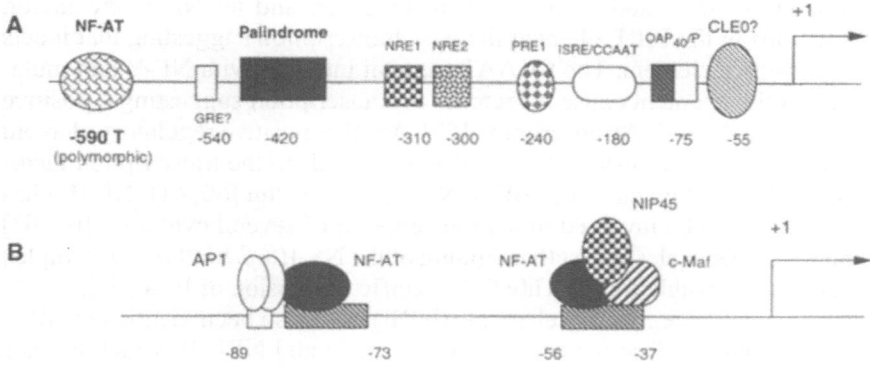

Figure 3. (A) Regulatory elements of the human IL-4 promoter. (B) Regulatory elements of the murine IL-4 promoter (see text).

which is expressed by all T cells, it is only present in the promoters of human and not mouse IL-4, IL-5 and IL-13 genes which are expressed by Th2-like cells. This suggests that there may be differences in the way in which these genes are regulated in human and mouse T cells.

By performing DNase I hypersensitive site mapping Cockerill et al. have identified an enhancer element 3 kilobases upstream of the GM-CSF gene [53]. It contains four binding sites for the transcription factors AP-1, NF-AT [54] and CBF [42]. They suggest that this enhancer is required for complete regulated activation of both GM-CSF and IL-3 in T cells.

3.2. IL-4 Gene Regulation

The human IL-4 promoter differs considerably from the promoters of IL-3, IL-5 and GM-CSF (Figure 3A). It contains a putative glucocorticoid response element (AGAACA) and only a short fragment of the CLE0 element present in IL-5 and GM-CSF is conserved. Studies on the human IL-4 promoter have identified several cis-acting regions, the most proximal of which is the positive (P) sequence [55]. This region is required for activation of IL-4 in the T cell line Jurkat and binds a factor NF(P) that appears to be very closely related to NF-κB, NF-AT [56] and also NF-Y [57], a factor required for expression of major histocompatibility class (MHC) II genes. Immediately adjacent to the P sequence is an element known as octamer-associated protein 40 (OAP$_{40}$) which is also involved in activation of IL-4 transcription. Song et al. have shown that a polymorphism at this site can cause overexpression of IL-4 in T cells, although no relationship is shown between this polymorphism and atopy or asthma [58].

Two elements adjacent to each other have been reported, an interferon stimulatory response element (ISRE) and a CCAAT motif. The ISRE element is associated with IRF-2, a repressor, and an NF-1 like factor. Mutations in the ISRE element increase transcription suggesting that it acts as a negative element. The CCAAT element interacts with NF-Y and mutations in this element cause a decrease in transcription suggesting a positive role for NF-Y in IL-4 transcription [57]. Another positive regulatory element (PRE-1) is located distally [59]; this region binds to the transcription factor NF-IL6β (also known as C/EBPδ), NF-ATc/p and Jun [60, 61]. NF-IL6 has been shown to be involved in the transcription of several cytokines [62, 63] and Li-Weber et al. suggest that binding of the NF-IL6β/Jun/NF-AT complex may be responsible for the Th0/Th2-specific expression of IL-4 [61].

Two negative regulatory elements (NRE) have also been identified: NRE-I, which binds a T cell-specific factor (Neg-1) and NRE-II, which binds a ubiquitous protein (Neg-2) [64]. In Jurkat cells, which are activated with phorbol myristate acetate (PMA)/ionomycin, the two NREs act in tandem to down-regulate the PRE-1 [59]. Unfortunately, all of these studies have been performed using the Jurkat cell line which constitutively transcribes IL-4 and only shows limited up-regulation of IL-4 upon activation. This is a very different situation to that of a normal human T cell and therefore the activities of all of these elements will have to be validated in more suitable cells. Recently, a polymorphism has been identified in the human IL-4 promoter distal to all of these elements at position −590 relative to the open reading frame [65]. The mutation from C to T appears to be associated with an increase in total serum IgE and an increase in IL-4 promoter activity.

It is becoming increasingly clear that NF-AT plays an important role in the control of transcription of these genes; NF-ATp knock-out mice display a profound defect in IL-4 transcription and also decreased transcription of GM-CSF [66]. Analysis of the murine IL-4 promoter, in which the precise role of NF-AT has been more clearly defined (Figure 3B), has revealed at least two proximal binding sites for NF-AT. At the more distal site it binds cooperatively with AP-1 to activate the promoter and at the proximal site it acts synergistically with the protein c-Maf to activate the promoter, even in non-T cells [67, 68]. The protein c-Maf appears to be Th2 cell specific and may therefore be crucial to the expression of Th2-specific cytokines. The same group have recently described a novel protein termed NIP45 (for NF-AT interacting protein) which also appears to act synergistically at this point with both NF-AT and c-Maf [69]. A very recent paper by Zheng and Flavell indicates that GATA-3 is also Th2 specific and required for murine IL-4 expression; however, the exact location of the GATA-3 binding site is not reported [70].

3.3. IL-3 Gene Regulation

The IL-3 promoter has also been shown to contain multiple elements using transient transfection assays as shown in Figure 4. The most proximal of

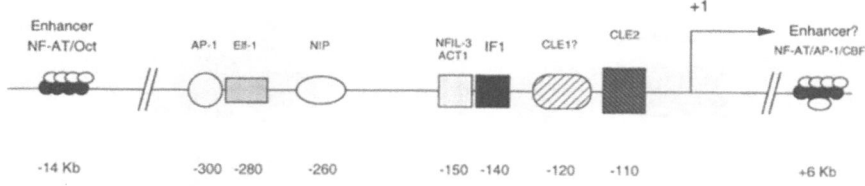

Figure 4. Regulatory elements of the IL-3 promoter (see text).

these is a region homologous to CLE2 of the GM-CSF promoter, and appears to be required for basal level expression of IL-3 and may bind AP-2 and Sp1 [71,72]. Distal to this is a site known as IF-1 (*in vivo* footprint-1) which appears to be necessary but not sufficient for inducible expression of IL-3 in T cells; the factors that bind at this site are as yet uncharacterized [73]. Adjacent to this site is a region known as ACT1 (NFIL-3) which is an activating region and contains binding sites for AP-1 and Oct proteins [71, 74, 75]. Further upstream around −260 bp is a negative domain known as NIP which is involved in restricting IL-3 expression to T cells [75]. Adjacent to this site are Elf-1 and AP-1 binding sites which are also required for inducible T cell-restricted expression of IL-3 [71, 74−76]. A recent report by Duncliffe et al. has identified an enhancer element 14 kb upstream of IL-3 which appears to be T cell specific, involving NF-AT and Oct proteins in activation of IL-3 expression [77]. The same group has also suggested that the GM-CSF enhancer may also play a role in IL-3 activation [42, 53, 54, 78].

3.4. IL-5 Gene Regulation

The data available on the transcriptional regulation of human IL-5 is limited as a result of the lack of a suitable cell line for use in transient transfection assays. However, several papers have recently been published which have used transfection assays to identify regulatory elements in the mouse IL-5 promoter (Figure 5) [79−88]. The most proximal of these is the IL-5 CLE0 which has been shown to be required for functional activation [80−82, 84, 88]. It has also been shown that this region apparently binds NF-AT and Oct1, upon activation through different signalling pathways to those that activate GM-CSF [81, 84, 89]. Adjacent to this is a region IL-5C which is also required for transcription and appears to bind octamer and GATA transcription factors [80, 86, 88, 90]. Upstream of this region is the IL-5P element, mutation of this resulted in the loss of 80% of promoter activity" and it appears to be an NF-AT-binding element [80, 87, 91]. In a recent paper Stranick et al. have identified a negative regulatory region known as RE-III; the factors that bind to this region are not yet characterized [92].

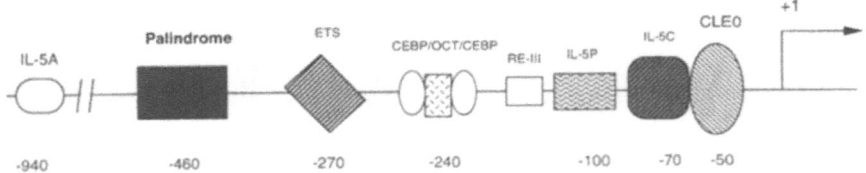

Figure 5. Regulatory elements of the IL-5 promoter (see text).

Using DNase I footprinting we have identified elements of the human IL-5 promoter that bind nuclear proteins derived from allergen-specific human T cell clones [83]. This method has identified several regions that interact with transcription factors. The most proximal of these is an octamer site flanked by two NF-IL6 sites between -227 and -251 bp. Deletion of this region has shown that it is a positive element [85]. Distal to this, an ETS site was also identified and it is different to the consensus sequence for the ets1 factor found in an activated T cells, which is a negative regulator of IL-2 expression [92]. The region furthest from the transcription start site is IL-5A which has homology to NF-1-binding elements. Mutations in this region caused a 40% loss of promoter activity when activated with PMA and Bt_2cAMP [80]. However, mutation of the NF-1 site actually causes constitutive transcription, suggesting that NF-1 may act as a negative regulator of IL-5 transcription [82].

4. Conclusions

Overall the results detailed above show that the transcriptional regulation of IL-3, IL-4, IL-5 and GM-CSF is a very complex process involving interactions between different cis-acting elements and transcription factors. It is clear that the coordinated control of expression of this gene cluster in T cells is only beginning to be elucidated. It is important to note that NF-AT appears to be required for the efficient activation of all of these genes in T cells. This is interesting because it is also essential for the activation of IL-2 [93], a Th1 cytokine. The NF-AT complex is a family of related proteins (NF-AT1–4) [94]; it will be interesting to identify the role of each NF-AT family member in the coordinated expression of these cytokines, especially in the light of the results from the NF-ATp knockout mouse showing that IL-2 is expressed normally [66]. Similarly elucidation of the functions of the palindromic elements that we have recently described and identification of the factors that bind to them will be central to the mechanisms that control the expression of these cytokines.

References

1 Mosmann TR, Coffman RL (1989) T_{h1} and T_{h2} cells: Different patterns of lymphokine secretion lead to different functional properties. *Annu Rev Immunol* 7: 145–173
2 Romagnani S (1991) Human Th1 and Th2 subsets: doubt no more. *Immunol Today* 12: 256–257
3 Del Prete GF, De Carli M, D'Elios MM, Maestrelli P, Ricci M, Fabbri L, Romagnani S (1993) Allergen exposure induces the activation of allergen-specific Th2 cells in the airway mucosa of patients with allergic respiratory disorders. *Eur J Immunol* 23: 1445–1449
4 Walker C, Bode E, Boer L, Hansel TT, Blaser K, Virchow J-C (1991) Allergic and non-allergic asthmatics have distinct patterns of T cell activation and cytokine production in peripheral blood and bronchoalveolar lavage. *Am Rev Respir Dis* 146: 109–115
5 Walker C, Bauer W, Braun RK, Menz G, Braun P, Schwarz F, Hansel TT, Villiger B (1994) Activated T cells and cytokines in bronchoalveolar lavages from patients with various lung diseases associated with eosinophilia. *Am J Respir Crit Care Med* 150: 1038–1048
6 Howell CJ, Pujol J-L, Crea AEG, Davidson R, Gearing AJH, Godard PH, Lee TH (1989) Identification of an alveolar macrophage-derived activity in bronchial asthme that enhances leukotriene C4 generation by human eosinophils stimulated by ionophore A23187 as a granulocyte-macrophage colony-stimulating factor. *Am Rev Respir Dis* 149: 1340–1347
7 Foster PS, Hogan SP, Ramsay AJ, Matthaei KI, Young IG (1996) Interleukin 5 deficiency abolishes eosinophilia, airways hyperreactivity and lung damage in a mouse asthma model. *J Exp Md* 183: 195–201
8 Robinson DS, Hamid Q, Ying S, Tsicopoulos A, Barkans J, Bentley AM, Corrigan C, Durham R, Kay AB (1992) Predominant T_{h2}-like bronchoalveolar T lymphocyte population in atopic asthma. *N Engl J Med* 326: 298–304
9 Robinson D, Hamid Q, Ying S, Bentley A, Assoufi B, Durham S, Kay AB (1993) Prednisolone treatment in asthma in associated with modulation of bronchoalveolar lavage cell interleukin 4, interleukin 5 and interferon-γ cytokine gene expression. *Am Rev Respir Dis* 148: 401–406
10 Durham SR, Ying S, Varney VA, Jacobson MR, Sudderick RM, Mackay IS, Kay AB, Hamid QA (1992) Cytokine messenger RNA expression for IL-3, IL-4, IL-5 and granulocyte/macrophage colony-stimulating factor in the nasal mucosa after local allergen provocation: relationship to tissue eosinophilia. *J Immunol* 148: 2390–2394
11 Hamid Q, Azzawi M, Ying S, Moqbel R, Wardlaw AJ, Corrigan CJ, Bradley B, Durham SR, Collins JV, Jeffery PK et al. (1991) Expression of mRNA for Interleukin-5 in Mucosal Bronchial Biopsies from Asthma. *J Clin Invest* 87: 1541–1546
12 Ackerman V, Marini M, Vittori E, Bellini A, Vassali G, Mattoli S (1994) Detection of cytokines and their cell sources in bronchial biopsy specimens from asthmatic patients; Relationship to atopic status, symptoms, and level of airway hyperresponsiveness. *Chest* 105: 687–696
13 Ying S, Humbert M, Barkans J, Corrigan CJ, Pfister R, Menz G, Larche M, Robinson DS, Durham SR, Kay AB (1997) Expression of IL-4 and IL-5 mRNA and protein product by CD4+ and CD8+ T cells, eosinophils, and mast cells in bronchial biopsies obtained from atopic and nonatopic (intrinsic) asthmatics. *J Immunol* 158: 3539–3544
14 Sousa AR, Poston RN, Lane SJ, Nakhosteen JA, Lee TH (1993) Detection of GM-CSF in asthmatic bronchial epithelium and decrease by inhaled corticosteroids. *Am Rev Respir Dis* 147: 1557–1561
15 Nonaka M, Nonaka R, Woolley K, Adelroth E, Miura K, O'Byrne P, Dolovich J, Jordana M (1995) Localization of interleukin-4 in eosinophils in nasal polyps and asthmatic bronchial mucosa. *J Allergy Clin Immunol* 95: 220
16 Humbert M, Durham SR, Kimmitt P, Powell N, Assoufi B, Pfister R, Menz G, Kay AB, Corrigan CJ (1997) Elevated expression of messenger RNA encoding IL-13 in the bronchial mucosa of atopic and nonatopic subjects with asthma. *J Allergy Clin Immunol* 99: 657–665
17 Bradding P, Feather IH, Howarth PH, Mueller R, Roberts JA, Britten K, Bews JPA, Hunt TC, Okayama Y, Heusser CH et al. (1992) Interleukin 4 is localized to and released by human mast cells. *J Exp Med* 176: 1381–1386
18 Bradding P, Feather IH, Wilson S, Bardin PG, Heusser CH, Holgate ST, Howarth PH (1993) Immunolocalization of cytokines in the nasal mucosa of normal and perennial rhinitic sujects. *J Immunol* 151: 3853–3865
19 Bradding P, Roberts JA, Britten K, Montefort S, Djukanovic R, Mueller R, Heusser CH, Howarth PH, Holgate ST (1994) Interleukin-4, -5, and -6 and tumor necrosis factor-α in

normal and asthmatic airways: evidence for the human mast cell as a source of these cytokines. *Am J Respir Cell Mol Biol* 10: 471–480

20 Broide DH, Paine MM, Firestein GS (1992) Eosinophils express interleukin-5 and granulocyte macrophage-colony-stimulating factor mRNA at sites of allergic inflammation in Asthmatics. *J Clin Invest* 90: 1414–1424

21 Marini M, Vittori E, Hollemborg J, Mattoli S (1992) Expression of the potent inflammatory cytokines, granulocyte-macrophage colony-stimulating factor and interleukin-6 and interleukin-8, in bronchial epithelial cells of patients with asthma. *J Allergy Clin Immunol* 89: 1001–1009

22 Cromwell O, Hamid Q, Corrigan CJ, Barkans J, Meng Q, Collins PD, Kay AB (1992) Expression and generation of interleukin-8, IL-6 and granulocyte-macrophage colony-stimulating factor by bronchial epithelial cells and enhancement by IL-1β and tumour necrosis factor-α. *Immunology* 77: 330–337

23 Marsh DB, Neely JD, Breazeale DR, Ghosh B, Friedhoff LR, Ehrlich-Kautzky E, Schou C, Krishnaswamy G, Beaty TH (1994) Linkage analysis of IL-4 and other chromosome 5q31.1 markers and total serum IrE concentrations. *Science* 264: 1152–1156

24 Meyers DA, Postma DS, Panhuysen CIM, Xu J, Amelung PJ, Levitt RC, Bleecker ER (1994) Evidence for a locus regulating total serum IgE levels mapping to chromosome 5. *Genomics* 23: 464–470

25 Marsh DG, Neely JD, Breazeale DR, Ghosh B, Friedhoff LR, Schou C, Beaty TH (1995) Total serum IgE levels and chromosome 5q. *Clin Exp Allergy* 25: 79–83

26 Xu J, Levitt RC, Panhuysen CIM, Postma DS, Taylor EW, Amelung PJ, Holroyd KJ, Bleecker ER, Meyers DA (1995) Evidence for two unlinked loci regulating total serum IgE levels. *Am J Hum Genet* 57: 425–430

27 Levitt RC, Eleff SM, Zhang L-Y, Kleeberger SR, Ewart SL (1995) Linkage homology for bronchial hyperresponsiveness between DNA markers on human chromosome 5q31–33 and mouse chromosome 13. *Clin Exp Allergy* 25: 61–63

28 Bleeker ER, Amelung PJ, Levitt RC, Postma DS, Meyers DA (1995) Evidence for linkage of total serum IgE and bronchial hyperresponsiveness to chromosom 5q: a major regulatory locus important in asthma. *Clin Exp Allergy* 25: 84–88

29 Postma DS, Bleecker ER, Amelung PJ, Holroyd KJ, Xu JF, Panhuysen CIM, Meyers DA, Levitt RC (1995) Genetic susceptibility to asthma-Bronchial hyperresponsiveness coinherited with a major gene for atopy. *N Engl J Med* 333: 894–900

30 Chan JY, Slamon DJ, Nimer SD, Golde DW, Gasson JC (1986) Regulation of expression of human granulocyte-macrophage colony stimulating factor. *Proc Natl Acad Sci USA* 83: 8669–8673

31 Nimer SD, Morita EA, Martis MJ, Wachsman W, Gasson J (1988) Characterization of the human granulocyte-macrophage colony-stimulating factor promoter region by genetic analysis: Correlation with DNase I footprinting. *Mol Cell Biol* 8: 1979–1984

32 Miyatake S, Shlomai J, Arai K-I, Arai N (1991) Characterization of the mouse granulocyte-macrophage colony-stimulating factor (GM-CSF) gene promoter: Nuclear factors that interact with an element shared by three lymphokine genes – those for GM-CSF, Interleukin-4 (IL-4) and IL-5. *Mol Cell Biol* 11: 5894–5901

33 Heike T, Miyatake S, Yoshida M, Arai K, Arai N (1989) Bovine papilloma virus encoded E2 protein activates lymphokine genes through DNA elements distinct from the consensus motif, in the long control region of its own genome. *EMBO J* 8: 1411–1417

34 Tokumitsu H, Masuda ES, Tsuboi A, Arai K-I, Arai N (1993) Purification of the 120 kDa component of the human nuclear factor of activated T cells (NF-AT). *Biochem Biophys Res Commun* 196: 737–744

35 Masuda ES, Tokumitsu H, Tsuboi A, Shlomai J, Hung P, Arai K-I, Arai N (1993) The granulocyte-macrophage colony stimulating factor promoter cis-acting element CLE0 mediates induction signals in T cells and is recognized by factors related to AP1 and NFAT. *Mol Cell Biol* 13: 7399–7407

36 Thomas RS, Tymms MJ, Seth A, Shannon MF, Kola I (1995) ETS1 transactivates the human GM-CSF promoter in Jurkat T cells stimulated with PMA and ionomycin. *Oncogene* 11: 2135–2143

37 Fraser JK, Tran S, Nimer SD, Gasson JC (1994) Characterization of nuclear factors that bind to a critical positive regulatory element of the human granulocyte-macrophage colony-stimulating factor promoter. *Blood* 84: 2523–2530

38 Wang C-Y, Bassuk AG, Boise LH, Thompson CB, Bravo R, Leiden JM (1994) Activation of the granulocyte-macrophage colony-stimulating factor promoter in T cells requires cooperative binding of Elf-1 and AP-1 transcription factors. *Mol Cell Biol* 14: 1153–1159

39 Jenkins F, Cockerill PN, Bohmann D, Shannon MF (1995) Multiple signals are required for function of the human granulocyte-macrophage colony-stimulating factor gene promoter in T cells. *J Immunol* 155: 1240–1251

40 Ullman KS, Northrop JP, Verweij CL, Crabtree GR (1990) Transmission of signals from the T lymphocyte antigen receptor to the genes responsible for cell proliferation and immune function. *Annu Rev Immunol* 8: 421–452

41 Takahashi A, Satake M, Yamaguchi-Iwai Y, Bae S-C, Lu J, Maruyama M, Zhang YW, Oka H, Arai N, Arai K-I, Ito Y (1995) Positive and negative regulation of granulocyte-macrophage colony-stimulating factor promoter activity by *AML1*-related transcription factor, PEBP2. *Blood* 86: 607–616

42 Cockerill PN, Osborne CS, Bert AG, Grotto RJM (1996) Regulation of GM-CSF gene transcription by core-binding factor. *Cell Growth Differentiation* 7: 917–922

43 Jianping Y, Young HA, Ortaldo JR, Ghosh P (1994) Identification of a DNA binding site for the nuclear factor YY1 in the human GM-CSF core promoter. *Nucleic Acids Res* 22: 5672–5678

44 Shannon MF, Gamble JR, Vadas MA (1988) Nuclear proteins interacting with the promoter region of the human granulocyte-macrophage colony-stimulating factor gene. *Proc Natl Acad Sci USA* 85: 674–678

45 Miyatake S, Seiki M, DeWaal Malefijt R, Heike T, Fujisawa J-I, Takebe Y, Nishida J, Shloami J, Yokota T et al. (1988) Activation of T cell-derived lymphokine genes in T cells and fibroblasts: effects of human T cell leukemia virus type 1 p40X protein and bovine papilloma virus encoded E2 protein. *Nucleic Acids Res* 16: 6547–6566

46 Miyatake S, Seiki M, Yoshida M, Arai K-I (1988) T cell activation signals and human T cell leukemia virus type I-encoded p40x protein activate the mouse granulocyte-macrophage colony-stimulating factor gene through a common DNA element. *Mol Cell Biol* 8: 5581–5587

47 Sugimoto K, Tsuboi A, Miyatake S, Arai K, Arai N (1990) Inducible and non-inducible factors co-operatively activate the GM-CSF promoter by interacting with two adjacent DNA motifs. *Int Immunol* 2: 787–794

48 Tsuboi A, Sugimoto K, Yodoi J, Miyastake S, Arai K, Arai N (1991) A nuclear factor NF-GM2 that interacts with a regulatory region of the GM-CSF gene essential for its induction in response to T cell leukemia line Jurkat cells and similarity to NF-κB. *Int Immunol* 3: 807–817

49 Schreck R, Baeuerle PA (1994) NF-κB as inducible transcriptional activator of the granulocyte-macrophage colony-stimulating factor gene. *Mol Cell Biol* 1990; 10: 1281–1286

50 Masuda ES, Yamaguchi-Iwai Y, Tsuboi A, Hung P, Arai K-I, Arai N (1994) The transcription factor Sp1 is required for induction of the murine GM-CSF promoter in T cells. *Biochem Biophys Res Commun* 205: 1518–1525

51 Nishida Y, Yoshida M, Arai K, Yokota T (1991) Definition of a GC-rich motif as regulatory sequence of the human IL-3 gene: coordinate regulation of the IL-3 gene by CLE2/GC box of the GM-CSF gene in T cell activation. *Int Immunol* 3: 245–254

52 Staynov DZ, Cousins DJ, Lee TH (1995) A regulatory element in the promoter of the human granulocyte-macrophage colony-stimulating factor gene that has related sequences in other T cell-expressed cytokine genes. *Proc Natl Acad Sci USA* 92: 3606–3610

53 Cockerill PN, Shannon MF, Bert AG, Ryan GR, Vadas MA (1993) The granulocyte-macrophage colony stimulating factor/interleukin 3 locus is regulated by an inducible cyclosporin A-sensitive enhancer. *Proc Natl Acad Sci USA* 90: 2466–2470

54 Cockerill PN, Bert AG, Jenkins F, Ryan GR, Shannon MF, Vadas MA (1995) Human granulocyte-macrophage colony-stimulating factor enhancer function is associated with cooperative interactions between AP-1 and NFATp/c. *Mol Cell Biol* 15: 2071–2079

55 Abe E, DeWaal Malefyt R, Matsuda I, Arai K, Arai N (1992) An 11-base-pair DNA sequence motif apparently unique to the human interleukin 4 gene confers responsiveness to T cell activation signals. *Proc Natl Acad Sci USA* 89: 2864–2868

56 Matsuda I, Masuda ES, Tsuboi A, Behnam S, Arai N, Arai K-I (1994) Characterization of NF(P), the nuclear factor that interacts with the regulatory P sequence (5'-CGAAAATTT-CC-3') of the human interleukin-4 gene: relationship to NF-κB and NF-AT. *Biochem Biophys Res Commun* 199: 439–446

57 Li-Weber M, Davydov IV, Frafft H, Krammer P (1994) The role of NF-Y and IRF-1 in the regulation of human IL-4 gene expression. *J Immunol* 153: 4122–4133
58 Song Z, Casolaro V, Chen R, Georas SN, Monas D, Ono SJ (1996) Polymorphic nucleotides within the human IL-4 promoter that mediate overexpression of the gene. *J Immunol* 156: 424–429
59 Li-Weber M, Krafft H, Krammer PH (1993) A novel enhancer element in the human IL-4 promoter is suppressed by a position-independent silencer. *J Immunol* 151: 1371–1382
60 Davydov IV, Krammer PH, Li-Weber M (1995) Nuclear factor-IL-6 activates the human IL-4 promoter in T cells. *J Immunol* 155: 5273–5279
61 Li-Weber M, Salgame P, Hu C, Davydov IV, Krammer PH (1997) Differential interaction of nuclear factors with the PRE-I enhancer element of the human IL-4 promoter in different T cell subsets. *J Immunol* 158: 1194–1200
62 Akira S, Isshiki H, Sugita T, Tanabe O, Kinoshita S, Nishio Y, Nakajima T, Hirano T, Kishimoto T (1990) A nuclear factor for IL-6 expression (NF-IL-6) is a member of a C/EBP family. *EMBO J* 9: 1897–1906
63 Kunsch C, Lang RK, Rosen CA, Shannon MF (1994) Synergistic transcriptional activation of the IL-8 gene by NF-κB p65 (RelA) and NF-IL-6. *J Immunol* 153: 153–164
64 Li-Weber M, Eder A, Krafft-Czepa H, Krammer PH (1992) T cell-specific negative regulation of transcription of the human cytokine IL-4. *J Immunol* 148: 1913–1918
65 Rosenwasser LJ, Klemm DJ, Dresback JK, Inamura H, Mascali JJ, Klinnert M, Borish L (1995) Promoter polymorphisms in the chromosome 5 gene cluster in asthma and atopy. *Clin Exp Allergy* 25: 74–78
66 Hodge MR, Ranger AM, de la Brousse FC, Hoey T, Grusby MJ, Glimcher LH (1996) Hyperproliferation and dysregulation of IL-4 expression in NF-ATp-deficient mice. *Immunity* 4: 397–405
67 Ho I-C, Hodge MR, Rooney JW, Glimcher LH (1996) The proto-oncogenen c-*maf* is responsible for tissue-specific expression of interleukin-4. *Cell* 85: 973–983
68 Wenner CA, Szabo SJ, Murphy KM (1997) Identification of IL-4 promoter elements conferring Th2-restricted expression during T helper cell subset development. *J Immunol* 158: 765–773
69 Hodge MR, Chun HJ, Rengarajan J, Alt A, Lieberson R, Glimcher LH (1996) NF-AT-driven Interleukin-4 transcription potentiated by NIP45. *Science* 274: 1903–1905
70 Zheng W-P, Flavell RA (1997) The transcription factor GATA-3 is necessary and sufficient for Th2 cytokine gene expression in CD4 T cells. *Cell* 89: 587–596
71 Park J-H, Kaushansky K, Levitt L (1993) Transcriptional regulation of interleukin 3 (IL-3) in primary human T lymphocytes. Role of AP-1 and octamer-binding proteins in control of IL-3 gene expression. *J Biol Chem* 268: 6299–6308
72 Nishida J, Yoshida M, Arai K-I, Yokota T (1991) Definition of a GC-rich motif as regulatory sequence of the human IL-3 gene: coordinate regulation of the IL-3 gene by CLE2/GC box of the GM-CSF gene in T cell activation. *Int Immunol* 3: 245–254
73 Cameron S, Taylor DS, TePas EC, Speck NA, Mathey-Prevot B (1994) Identification of a critical regulatory site in the human interleukin-3 promoter by *in vivo* footprinting. *Blood* 83: 2851–2859
74 Shoemaker SG, Hroms R, Kaushansky K (1990) Transcriptional regulation of interleukin 3 gene expression in T lymphocytes. *Proc Natl Acad Sci USA* 87: 9650–9654
75 Mathey-Prevot B, Andrews NC, Murphy HS, Kreissman SG, Nathan DG (1990) Positive and negative elements regulate human interleukin 3 expression. *Proc Natl Acad Sci USA* 87: 5046–5050
76 Gottschalk LR, Giannola DM, Emerson SG (1993) Molecular regulation of the human IL-3 gene: Inducible T cell-restricted expression requires intact AP-1 and Elf-1 nuclear protein binding sites. *J Exp Med* 178: 1681–1692
77 Duncliffe KN, Bert AG, Vadas MA, Cockerill PN (1997) A T cell-specific enhancer in the interleukin-3 locus is activated cooperatively by Oct and NFAT elements within a DNase 1-hypersensitive site. *Immunity* 6: 175–185
78 Osborne CS, Vadas MA, Cockerill PN (1995) Transcriptional regulation of mouse granulocyte-macrophage colony-stimulating factor/IL-3 locus. *J Immunol* 155: 226–235
79 Lee HJ, Koyano-Nakagawa N, Naito Y, Nishida J, Arai N, Arai K-I, Yokota T (1993) cAMP Activates the IL-5 promoter synergistically with phorbol ester through the signaling pathway involving protein kinase A in mouse thymoma line EL-4. *J Immunol* 151: 6135–6142

80 Lee HJ, Masuda ES, Arai N, Arai K-I, Yokota T (1995) Definition of *cis*-regulatory elements of the mouse interleukin-5 gene promoter. *J Biol Chem* 270: 17541–17550

81 Naora H, van Leeuwen BH, Bourke PF, Young IG (1994) Functional role and signal-induced modulation of proteins recognizing the conserved TCATTT-containing promoter elements in the murine IL-5 and GM-CSF genes in T lymphocytes. *J Immunol* 153: 3466–3475

82 Bourke PF, van Leeuwen BH, Campbell HD, Young IG (1995) Localization of the inducible enhancer in the mouse interleukin-5 gene that is responsive to T cell receptor stimulation. *Blood* 85: 2069–2077

83 Cousins DJ, Staynov DZ, Lee TH (1994) Transcriptional Regulation of IL-5 gene expression in human T cells. *J Allergy Clin Immunol* 93: 679

84 Karlen S, D'Ercole M, Sanderson CJ (1996) Two pathways can activate the interleukin-5 gene and induce binding to the conserved lymphokine element 0. *Blood* 88: 211–221

85 Gruart-Gouilleux V, Engels P, Sullivan M (1995) Characterization of the human interleukin-5 gene promoter: involvement of octamer binding sites in the gene promoter activity. *Eur J Immunol* 25: 1431–1435

86 Yamagata T, Nishida J, Sakai R, Tanaka T, Honda H, Hirano N, Mano H, Yazaki Y, Hirai H (1995) Of the GATA-binding proteins, only GATA-4 selectively regulates the human interleukin-5 gene promoter in interleukin-5 producing cells which express multiple GATA-binding proteins. *Mol Cell Biol* 15: 3830–3839

87 Stranick KS, Payvandi F, Zambas DN, Umland SP, Egan RW, Billah MM (1995) Transcription of the murine interleukin 5 gene is regulated by multiple promoter elements. *J Biol Chem* 270: 20575–20582

88 Siegel MD, Zhang D-H, Ray P, Ray A (1995) Activation of the interleukin-5 promoter by cAMP in murine EL4 cells requires the GATA-3 and CLE0 elements. *J Biol Chem* 270: 24548–24555

89 Mori A, Suko M, Kaminuma O, Hoshino A, Ohmura T, Miyazawa K, Ito K, Okidaira H (1997) Oct-1 binding element is essential for human IL-5 gene transcription. *J Allergy Clin Immunol* 99: 1952

90 Yamagata T, Mitani K, Ueno H, Kanda Y, Yazaki Y, Hirai H (1997) Triple synergism of human T lymphotropic virus type 1-encoded tax, GATA-binding protein and AP-1 is required for constitutive expression of the interleukin-5 gene in adult T cell leukemia cells. *Mol Cell Biol* 17: 4272–4281

91 Stranick KS, Zambas DN, Uss AS, Egan RW, Billah MM, Umland SP (1997) Identification of transcription factor binding sites important in the regulation of the human interleukin-5 gene. *J Biol Chem* 272: 16453–16465

92 Romano-Spica V, Georgiou P, Suzuki H, Papas TS, Bhat NK (1995) Role of ETS1 in IL-2 gene expression. *J Immunol* 154: 2724–2732

93 Northrop JP, Ho SN, Chen L, Thomas DJ, Timmerman LA, Nolan GP, Admon A, Crabtree GR (1994) NF-AT components define a family of transcription factors targeted in T cell activation. *Nature* 369: 497–502

94 Hoey T, Sun YL, Williamson K, Xu X (1995) Isolation of two new members of the NF-AT gene family and functional characterization of the NF-AT proteins. *Immunity* 2: 461–472

Molecular Biology of the Lung
Vol. 2: Asthma and Cancer
ed. by R. A. Stockley
© 1999 Birkhäuser Verlag Basel/Switzerland

CHAPTER 5
Cytokine Expression in Asthma

C. J. Corrigan

Department of Respiratory Medicine, National Heart and Lung Institute, Imperial College School of Medicine, Charing Cross Hospital, London, UK

1 Introduction
2 T Cells, Cytokines and the Atopic Diathesis
3 T Cells, Cytokines, Chemokines and Eosinophil Recruitment
4 CD4 T Cells, Cytokines and Bronchial Mucosal Inflammation in Asthma
5 Cellular Origins of Cytokines in Asthmatic Inflammation
6 Are Asthmatic CD4 T Cells "Th2 Like"?
7 The Atopic Diathesis and Asthma
8 Conclusion
   References

1. Introduction

Asthma is a disease characterized clinically by reversible obstruction of the airways, or bronchi, and bronchial hyperresponsiveness, which indicates the tendency of the bronchi in asthmatic patients to constrict in response to a wide range of specific and non-specific stimuli. It is now widely accepted that chronic inflammation of the bronchial mucosal lining plays a fundamental role in the genesis of these clinical manifestations. The most striking feature of this inflammation is the intense infiltration of the bronchial mucosa with eosinophils, macrophages and lymphocytes [1]. In this chapter, how cytokine and chemokine products of activated T cells have the propensity to bring about this selective eosinophil accumulation and activation is described. The eosinophil, in turn, appears to be a key cell in producing injury to the bronchial mucosa, which is believed to result in bronchial obstruction and irritability, although the precise mechanisms by which this occurs are not clear.

2. T Cells, Cytokines and the Atopic Diathesis

Cytokines play an important role in the control of switching of antibody isotypes in humans away from immunoglobulin M (IgM) during the evolution of the immune response, and also in regulating the amounts of antibody that are secreted through their growth-regulating effects on B cells. They are thus at least partly responsible for the genesis of the inappropriate synthesis of IgE which characterizes atopy. Cytokines that play a role in this process may be classified as follows:

1. Cytokines that specifically induce IgE switching in B cells. Only the cytokines interleukin 4 (IL-4) and IL-13 have been shown to induce switching to IgE synthesis in human B cells, transcription of which is preceded by the synthesis of non-productive, intermediate splice variants termed "germline" Cε transcripts [2, 3].
2. Cytokines that influence IgE production by B cells through effects other than the induction of switching. Some of these cytokines are generally facilitatory or inhibitory to B cell activation and clonal expansion. Thus the interferons IFN-α, IFN-γ, transforming growth factor β (TGF-β), IL-2, IL-8 and IL-12 inhibit IL-4-induced IgE synthesis, whereas IL-5, IL-6 and tumour necrosis factor α (TNF-α) enhance it [4–10].

Allergen-specific CD4 T cells are activated when processed fragments of allergen are presented to their receptor/CD3 complex by antigen-presenting cells on major histocompatibility complex (MHC) class II molecules. B cells expressing allergen-specific immunoglobulin capture, process and present allergen in this way. In addition to these "cognate" interactions, additional signals are provided to B cells through T cell contact which, along with IL-4/IL-13 are essential for subsequent secretion of allergen-specific IgE. At least two signals are important in this respect:

1. CD40/CD40L ligand interaction: CD40 is a surface glycoprotein express-ed on B cells as well as thymic epithelial and dendritic cells [11]. The importance of this interaction was first inferred when it was discovered that anti-CD40 monoclonal antibodies could replace contact with acti-vated T cells in induction of IgE synthesis [12]. These experiments con-versely suggested the presence of a ligand for CD40 (CD40L) on T cells, which was later cloned [13].
2. CD21/CD23 interaction: CD23 is the low-affinity receptor for IgE pre-sent on many cells including B cells, monocytes and a subset of T cells, whereas CD21, identified as the Epstein-Barr virus and C3 desArg receptor on B cells, is also found on some T cells as well as follicular dendritic cells. It has been shown that triggering of CD21, either with anti-CD21 antibody or with recombinant soluble CD23, increases IL-4-induced IgE production by B cells [14].

In summary, it is clear that many T cell-derived cytokines play an impor-tant role (in the case of IL-4 or IL-13 indispensably so) in the initiation and propagation of IgE synthesis by B cells. Nevertheless, it is not clear how far IL-4 and IL-13 play a role in the *maintenance*, as distinct from the *initiation* of IgE synthesis, because "memory" allergen-specific B cells may be long lived and capable of continued IgE synthesis long after the original "switch" stimulus has been removed.

3. T Cells, Cytokines, Chemokines and Eosinophil Recruitment

A fundamental problem in asthma pathogenesis has been elucidation of the mechanisms leading to the marked and specific infiltration of eosinophils into the asthmatic bronchial mucosa, which is the hallmark of the disease. Cytokines play a prominent role in these mechanisms. Of the cytokines secreted by activated T cells, IL-3, IL-5 and granulocyte-macrophage colony-stimulating factor (GM-CSF) promote maturation, activation and prolonged survival of the eosinophil [15–17]. IL-5 is unique in that, unlike IL-3 and GM-CSF, it acts specifically on eosinophils in terms of activation and terminal differentiation of the eosinophil precursor [18]. IL-5 is probably the most important cytokine regulating eosinophil differentiation *in vivo,* because transgenic mice constitutively expressing the gene for IL-5 (but not the genes for IL-3 and GM-CSF) show a marked, specific expansion of blood and tissue eosinophils [19]. Thus, local expression of cytokines such as IL-5 may partly account for selective eosinophil accumulation in asthmatic inflammation, through selective enhancement of eosinophil differentiation in the bone marrow and survival (and possibly differentiation) in the target organ.

Selective local recruitment of eosinophils from the bronchial mucosal microcirculation may also contribute to this process. Eosinophil migration is initiated by an interaction between receptors on the cell surface with their ligands on the surface of vascular endothelial cells. The β_2-integrins, such as LFA-1 and Mac-1 on the eosinophil surface, mediate firm adhesion of these cells to endothelium by binding to endothelial adhesion molecules such as intercellular adhesion molecule-1 (ICAM-1) and vascular cell adhesion molecule-1 (VCAM-1) [20, 21]. IL-5 selectively enhances eosinophil adhesion to unstimulated endothelial cells 22], probably by selective upmodulation of the expression of integrins on eosinophils. Furthermore, eosinophils, but not neutrophils, express the β_1-integrin VLA-4, a ligand for VCAM-1 on the surface of stimulated endothelial cells [23]. The expression of VCAM-1 on endothelial cells is increased by exposure to IL-4 and IL-13, which enhances VLA-4/VCAM-1-dependent adherence of eosinophils, but not neutrophils, to endothelium [24]. Thus, local secretion of cytokines such as IL-4, IL-5 and IL-13 may selectively enhance eosinophil adhesion to vascular endothelium, although it is not clear how far these cytokines play a role in effecting eosinophil endothelial transmigration.

Finally, "chemotactic cytokines" or chemokines are important in the mechanism of selective eosinophil recruitment to sites of inflammation. The β-chemokines, particularly RANTES, macrophage chemotactic factor-3 (MCP-3) and, to a lesser extent, macrophage inflammatory protein-1α (MIP-1α), are powerful and relatively selective chemoattractants for eosinophils and basophils *in vitro* [25], whereas a novel β-chemokine termed eotaxin [26] appears to be exquisitely eosinophil specific. Injection of eotaxin into the skin of experimental guinea-pigs produced a rapid and selective accumulation of eosinophils, an effect that was interestingly not seen with eosinophil-active cytokines such as IL-5 [27, 28]. These observations support the hypothesis that β-chemokines act in concert with cytokines such as IL-5 in asthmatic inflammation, with IL-5 enhancing eosinophil release from the bone marrow and local endothelial adhesion, and β-chemokines causing selective tissue sequestration. In summary, the important role of cytokines and chemokines in bringing about selective accumulation of eosinophils in the asthmatic bronchial mucosa is self-evident.

4. CD4 T Cells, Cytokines and Bronchial Mucosal Inflammation in Asthma

Bronchial mucosal inflammation has been extensively studied in people with mild asthma using the techniques of bronchoalveolar lavage (BAL) and bronchial biopsy. In addition, examination of bronchial luminal inflammatory cells in sputum (typically induced by inhalation of hyper-tonic saline) is gaining popularity as an investigative tool. Such techniques have consistently demonstrated elevated numbers of eosinophils and activated (CD25+) T cells in the bronchial mucosa and lumen of people with mild asthma compared with controls [29–32].

The present clinical classification of asthma (intrinsic, extrinsic and occupational) implies possible variability in its pathogenesis, but such distinctions are not apparent in histopthological terms. Thus, immunocyto-chemical studies [29, 33–35] comparing bronchial biopsies from people with extrinsic, intrinsic and occupational asthma showed marked similari-ties in terms of their inflammatory cell infiltrate. These observations suggest that bronchial inflammation, at least in terms of overall inflamma-tory cell numbers, in patients with asthma has similar characteristics regardless of the nature of identifiable provoking agents.

Immunocytochemical studies of bronchial biopsies taken from people with asthma [29, 30, 33–35] have shown that the numbers of activated (CD25+) T cells correlate both with the numbers of locally activated eosin-ophils and with disease severity. Studies on the peripheral blood of adults and children with asthma have shown elevated numbers of activated T cells, the numbers of wich correlate with disease severity and the numbers of peripheral blood eosinophils, and a reduction in the extent of this activation after glucocorticoid therapy [36–39]. Similarly, elevated serum concentra-tions of IL-5 and IL-5 mRNA copy numbers in peripheral blood T cells have been demonstrated in people with asthma compared with controls, with a reduction in association with glucocorticoid therapy [38, 40, 41]. Peripheral blood T cells from patients with asthma who are clinically resistant to glucocorticoid therapy were shown to express activation markers *in vivo* [42] and to be refractory to the inhibitory effects of gluco-corticoids *in vitro* [43, 44]. These studies suggest that glucocorticoids exert their anti-asthma effect at least partly by inhibiting the release of cytokines from activated T cells.

Measurement of cytokines *in vivo* is problematic because of their low concentrations and unquantifiable degree of metabolism, clearance and dilution. One alternative to the direct measurement of cytokines is the detection of their mRNA using the technique of *in situ* hybridization with cytokine-specific cRNA probes or riboprobes. Although this is not a strictly quantitative technique, and with the proviso that mRNA synthesis does not necessarily equate with secretion of the corresponding protein, it does have the advantage the it can localize the secretion of cytokines within cells and tissues. Using this technique, it was demonstrated that IL-5 mRNA was elaborated by cells in bronchial biopsies from a majority of patients with mild asthma but not from normal controls [45] (Figure 1). The amount of mRNA correlated broadly with the numbers of activated T cells and eosinophils in biopsies from the same subjects.

It was shown [46] that significantly elevated percentages of BAL cells expressed mRNA encoding IL-2, IL-3, IL-4, IL-5 and GM-CSF, but not IFN-γ, in patients with mild atopic asthma compared with non-atopic

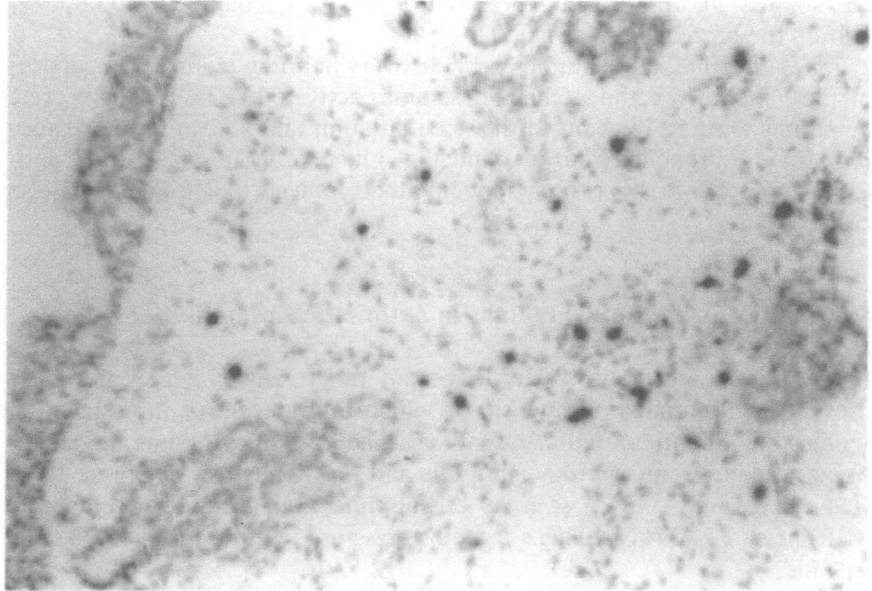

Figure 1. Bronchial biopsy section from an atopic asthmatic individual incubated with a radio-labelled IL-5 antisense riboprobe, washed stringently, then dipped in photographic emulsion, exposed and developed. Discrete clumps of silver grains are visible over those cells that have hybridized with the radioactive probe and thus express IL-5 mRNA.

normal controls, and that the majority (>90%) of the cells expressing IL-5 and IL-4 mRNA were T cells. Over a broad range of asthma severity, the percentages of BAL fluid cells from patients with atopic asthma expressing mRNA encoding IL-5, IL-4, IL-3 and GM-CSF, but not IL-2 and IFN-γ, could be correlated with the severity of asthma symptoms and bronchial hyperresponsiveness [47]. Elevated percentages of peripheral blood CD4, but not CD8, T cells from patients with exacerbation of asthma expressed mRNA encoding IL-3, IL-4, IL-5 and GM-CSF, but not IL-2 and IFN-γ, compared with controls [48]. Elevated spontaneous secretion of IL-3, IL-5 and GM-CSF was also demonstrable in these patients using an eosinophil survival-prolonging assay. Again, the percentages of CD4 T cells expressing mRNA encoding IL-3, IL-5 and GM-CSF, as well as spontaneous secretion of these cytokines by the CD4 T cells, were reduced in association with glucocorticoid therapy and clinical improvement. In a double-blind, parallel group study, therapy of people with mild atopic asthma with oral prednisolone, but not placebo, resulted in clinical improvement associated with a reduction in the percentages of BAL fluid cells expressing IL-5 and IL-4 and an increase in those expressing IFN-γ [49]. These changes were not seen in asthma patients who were clinically resistant to glucocorticoid therapy [50]. Conversely, artificial exacerbation of asthma by allergen bronchial challenge of patients with sensitized atopic asthma was associated with increased numbers of activated T cells and eosinophils, and increased expression of mRNA encoding IL-5 and GM-CSF in the bronchial mucosa [51].

Taken together, these studies provide overwhelming evidence in support of the general hypothesis that, in asthma, activated CD4 T cells secrete cytokines that are relevant to the accumulation and activation of eosinophils in the bronchial mucosa, and that glucocorticoids exert their anti-asthma effect at least partly by reducing the synthesis of cytokines by these cells.

5. Cellular Origins of Cytokines in Asthmatic Inflammation

In addition to T cells, it is clear that many other cells which are normally present in the bronchial mucosa, or which migrate into it in association with asthmatic inflammation, are potential sources of cytokines and chemokines. For example, both eosinophils and mast cells can elaborate IL-4, IL-5, IL-6 and TNF-α whereas eosinophils in addition can elaborate MIP-1α and RANTES. These proteins are stored within intracytoplasmic granules.

The relative contributions of all these cells to cytokine expression in the asthmatic bronchial mucosa *in vivo* is difficult to assess using currently available techniques, and the data obtained are probably dependent to some extent on the particular technique employed. Detection of cytokine mRNA synthesis (as above) by inflammatory cells is arguably mostly physiological because it implies *de novo* synthesis of the corresponding protein, although it does not necessarily imply translation and release of that protein. Using immunocytochemistry to identify cellular phenotypes with sequential *in situ* hybridization, it was shown that T cells were the predominant cells expressing IL-4 and IL-5 mRNA in the bronchial mucosa and BAL fluid of patients with atopic asthma, with smaller but significant contributions from mast cells and eosinophils [52]. In contrast, direct staining of intracellular cytokine protein in bronchial biopsies from similar patients using specific monoclonal antibodies, with identification of the phenotypes of positively stained cells in thin serial sections, suggested that mast cells were the principal source of IL-4 and IL-5 protein, whereas T cell staining was undetectable [53]. These observations suggest the possibilities that secretion and storage of cytokine proteins in leukocytes may not be synchronous with transcription of their mRNA, and that T cells may secrete cytokines rapidly, without storage, after synthesis such that intracytoplasmic cytokines are not detectable by immunocytochemistry.

Using a third technique [54], in which cytokine protein expression in BAL T cells was assessed by flow cytometry after treatment with monensin (an inhibitor of cellular protein export) and staining with specific monoclonal antibodies, it was concluded that elevated percentages of these cells expressed IFN-γ, a Th1 (T helper) cytokine, in patients with asthma compared with controls, whereas IL-4 and IL-5 staining was barely detectable. This technique, however, necessitated *ex vivo* stimulation of the T cells with phorbol ester and ionomycin, powerful polyclonal T cell stimulators, which may have distorted the pattern of cytokine expression *in vivo*. In contrast, CD4 T cell lines propagated from BAL fluid cells from patients with asthma secreted readily measurable quantities of these cytokines which were elevated, on a per cell basis, compared with lines derived from controls [55]. In summary, it is clear that no single technique currently available to assess cytokine expression and release by inflammatory cells *in vivo* is definitive. Further clarification of the relative contributions of these cells to cytokine release *in vivo* must await further studies.

6. Are Asthmatic CD4 T Cells "Th2 Like"?

The nature of immune responses initiated by activated CD4 T cells is at least partly dependent on the "selection" or preferential activation of particular subsets of these cells secreting defined patterns of cytokines. Studies of cytokine secretion by mouse CD4 T cell clones revealed that these could be divided into two basic functional subsets termed Th1 and Th2. Th1 T cells were characterized by the predominant secretion of IL-2, IFN-γ and TNF-β, whereas Th2 cells predominantly secreted IL-4, IL-5, IL-6 and IL-10. Other cytokines, such as TNF-α, IL-3 and GM-CSF, were produced by both Th1 and Th2 T cells [56, 57]. These differing patterns of cytokine secretion by CD4 T cells result in distinct effector functions. Broadly speaking, Th1 cells participate in delayed-type hypersensitivity (DTH) reactions, whereas Th2 cells, by their pattern of secretion of B cell co-stimulatory cytokines, enhance the synthesis of immunoglobulin, including IgE, thus promoting "humoral" immune responses. In the centre of this spectrum, T cell clones secreting cytokines characteristic of both Th1 and Th2 cells, termed Th0 cells, have also been described [58]. It is still not clear whether these Th0 cells represent distinct functional subsets or precursor cells in the process of differentiating into Th1 or Th2 cells.

Some of the most convincing evidence for a role for Th1 and Th2 cytokines in orchestrating distinct inflammatory responses *in vivo* has come from the studies of cytokine mRNA expression in asthma, as described above. In other studies employing *in situ* hybridization, the cutaneous inflammatory responses to challenge with allergen in atopic subjects and tuberculin in non-atopic subjects were compared [59, 60]. Both types of response (late-phase allergic and DTH) were associated with an influx of activated CD4 T cells, although, whereas mRNA molecules encoding IL-2 and IFN-γ were abundant within the tuberculin reactions, very little mRNA encoding these cytokines was observed in the late-phase allergic reactions. Conversely, mRNA encoding IL-4 and IL-5 was abundant in the late-phase allergic but not the tuberculin reactions. These observations provide direct evidence in support of the hypothesis that Th1 and Th2 CD4 T cell responses can be detected in humans under physiological conditions, and that the antigen specificity of the T cells might be one factor that determines which type of response is initiated. Taken together with the observations described above, they provide a considerable body of evidence for the existence of Th1 and Th2 *patterns* of cytokine secretion *in vivo*, although it cannot be ascertained from such studes whether or not these cytokines originate from the same cells. Support of the existence of *clonal* Th2 differentiation in allergic diseases has been provided by the demonstration that most T cell clones derived from cells within the "target" organ in patients with vernal conjunctivitis or atopic dermatitis show a Th2 profile of cytokine secretion [61, 62]. Some of these clones were allergen specific. On the other hand, it has been suggested [63] that co-expression of IL-4 and IL-5 by cloned T cells *in vitro* may reflect an artefactual effect of T cell activation, and that T cells isolated *ex vivo* rarely co-express IL-4 and IL-5. Furthermore, although studies on T cell clones provide information about patterns of cytokine synthesis, they do not allow comparison of the amount of secretion of cytokines in T cell population *in vivo*. In summary, the proposition that asthmatic inflammation is driven, at least in part, by clonally expanded Th2 T cells, some of which are allergen specific, is a reasonable one, although this remains to be demonstrated clearly, and particular uncertainty arises in the case of non-atopic asthma (see below).

7. The Atopic Diathesis and Asthma

The term "atopy" refers to the predisposition of certain individuals to synthesize, inappropriately, IgE specific for protein components of antigens ("allergens") encountered at mucosal surfaces. This is frequently, but not always, accompanied by generalized, elevated IgE synthesis. As described above, IL-4 secreted by Th2 T cells is strongly implicated in the pathogenesis of atopy, because it is one of only two cytokines that are able to bring about isotype switching to IgE synthesis in the course of allergen-specific B cell antibody responses. Allergen-specific IgE antibodies are commonly detected in the peripheral circulation by skin-prick tests or a radioallergosorbent test (RAST), although it is not clear precisely where these antibodies are made and whether or not putative localized allergen-specific IgE synthesis, for example, in the bronchial mucosa, is always reflected by elevated circulating antibody concentrations. Once formed, allergen-specific IgE may bind to cells with high-affinity (classically mast cells and basophils) or low-affinity (B cells, monocytes and a subset of T cells) IgE receptors, thus sensitizing them for activation when this surface IgE is cross-linked on further allergen exposure. This of course is the basis of "immediate hypersensitivity". IgE-mediated mechanisms have been assumed to play a role in the pathogenesis of asthma in atopic subjects, because natural or experimental exposure of patients with atopic asthma to "extrinsic" allergens to which they are sensitized results in exacerbation of disease – hence the term "extrinsic" asthma. Strictly, however, such observations do not necessarily imply a role for IgE-mediated mechanisms in asthma *pathogenesis*, as distinct from *exacerbation*, because they may simply reflect the release of bronchoconstricting mediators (such as histamine and leukotrienes) from IgE-sensitized cells (such as mast cells) into airways rendered hyperresponsive by eosinophil products. Furthermore, IgE-mediated mechanisms do not inevitably result in asthma, because many highly sensitized atopic individuals never develop the disease.

People with non-atopic asthma, who are not apparently sensitized to environmental allergens, and in whom IgE-mediated mechanisms are assumed not to operate, have been labelled "intrinsic" after an early clinical description [64]. It is now generally accepted that this term is used to describe a group of asthmatic people who are skin-prick test negative to extracts of aeroallergens, and whose serum total IgE concentrations are within the normal range. This clinical distinction between "extrinsic" and "intrinsic" asthma implies corresponding pathogenic distinctions. It has been shown, however, that the numbers and nature of the inflammatory cells infiltrating the bronchial mucosa in people with "extrinsic" and "intrinsic" asthma are remarkably similar [29, 34], and more recently that elevated numbers of these cells in people with both "extrinsic" and "intrinsic" asthma express both IL-4 and IL-5 mRNA and protein and high-affinity IgE receptors compared with non-asthmatic controls matched for atopic status [65, 66]. Does this IL-4 direct IgE synthesis in people with "intrinsic" asthma, and if not, why not? Is IL-4 synthesis in this situation nothing more than a surrogate marker of Th2-type T cell activation with no pathophysiological significance? The answers to these questions are not yet known. Unfortunately, experiments with IL-5 and IL-4 "knock-out" mice used in "models" of asthma have not clarified the relative roles of these cytokines in asthma pathogenesis; on the contrary, they have clouded the picture still further [67, 68]. Nevertheless, the data raise the theoretical possibility that elevated IgE synthesis may occur in the bronchial mucosa of people with "intrinsic" asthma in the presence of cells that are capable of being activated by IgE-mediated mechanisms, even though circulating concentrations of allergen-specific IgE in these patients are not detectably elevated.

To reconcile these observations, it is possible to speculate that asthmatic and atopic subjects have some more fundamental, possibly congenital, defect of mucosal surfaces which permits the local development of both IL-5-mediated eosinophilic inflammation and IL-4-mediated inappropriate IgE synthesis (both T cell driven) under the influence of environmental factors, but that these processes need not occur concurrently or to the same degree. In support of this, studies on genetic susceptibility to asthma and atopy have uncovered distinct loci which are associated with increased risk of development of atopy, on the one hand [69], and bronchial hyperresponsiveness, on the other [70].

In summary, although IgE-mediated mechanisms may clearly be important in allergen-induced, short-term *exacerbations* of asthma in atopic individuals, their role in the *pathogenesis* of chronic disease, in both atopic and non-atopic subjects alike, is less certain. Clearer answers to these questions may become available if and when specific antagonists of key cytokines such as IL-4 and IL-5 become available for clinical use.

8. Conclusion

There now exists considerable support for the hypothesis that asthma represents a specialized form of cell-mediated immunity, in which cytokines and possibly other mediators secreted by activated T cells bring about the specific accumulation and activation of eosinophils in the bronchial mucosa (Figure 2). These cytokines are secreted in the context of a Th2-type pattern and putatively reflect a locally directed T cell response against mucosal antigens, including aeroallergens. The relative roles of T cell-dependent and IgE-mediated mechanisms in the pathogenesis of asthma in various clinical settings remain to be defined, although there is some evidence that IgE-mediated mechanisms may play a role even in so-called "intrinsic" asthma. These observations suggest that strategies directed at inhibition of T cells or antagonism of cytokines that they produce are like-

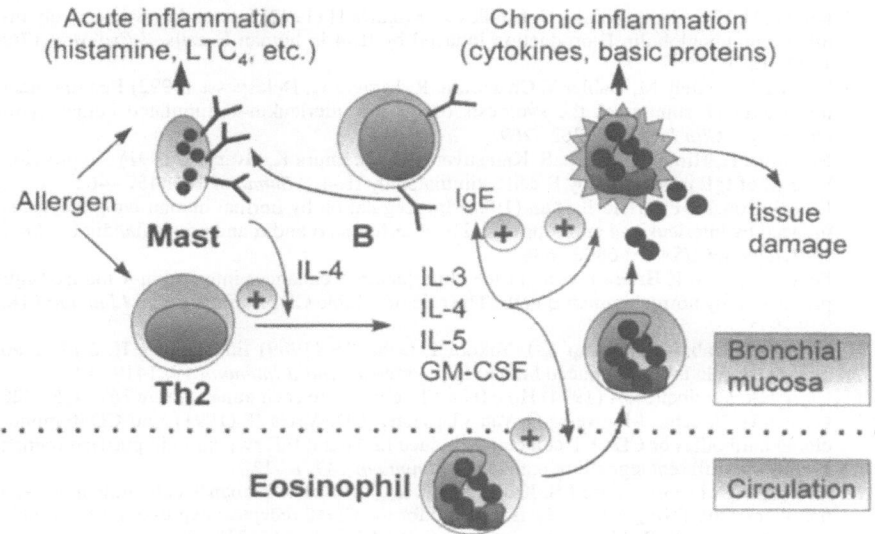

Figure 2. Inflammatory mechanisms in asthma: activation of Th2 CD4+ T cells (Th2) by specific antigen including (although not necessarily exclusively) allergen results in the secretion of cytokines, particularly IL-5, IL-4, IL-3 and GM-CSF, which influence eosinophil survival, differentiation, activation and adherence, and are implicated in orchestrating the specific eosinophil infiltration that characterizes chronic asthmatic inflammation. In parallel, allergens may trigger inflammatory processes, at least in those patients who are atopic, through the cross-linking of surface allergen-specific IgE on mast cells (Mast), resulting in the acute release of mediators such as histamine and leukotrienes with acute exacerbation of inflammation. The relative importance of these processes in asthmatic inflammation in different clinical settings remains to be determined. The two systems are interdependent in the sense that IL-4 derived from Th2 T cells is essential for IgE switching by B cells (B), and thus mast cell sensitization, whereas IL-4 release from IgE-triggered mast cells may further promote Th2 T cell development.

ly to continue to form part of the fundamental basis for future asthma therapy.

References

1 Dunnill MS (1960) The pathology of asthma with special reference to changes in the bronchial mucosa. *J Clin Pathol* 3: 27–33
2 Gauchat J-F, Lebman DA, Coffman RL, Gascan H, De Vries JE (1990) Structure and expression of germline ε transcripts in human B cells induced by IL-4 to switch to IgE production. *J Exp Med* 172: 463–473
3 Punnonen J, Aversa G, Cocks BG et al. (1993) Interleukin-13 induces interleukin-4-independent IgG4 and IgE synthesis and CD23 expression by human B cells. *Proc Natl Acad Sci USA* 90: 3730–3734
4 Gauchat J-F, Aversa G, Gascan H, De Vries JE (1992) Modulation of IL-4 induced germline ε mRNA synthesis in human B cells by tumour necrosis factor-α, anti-CD40 monoclonal antibodies or transforming growth factor-β correlates with levels of IgE production. *Int Immunol* 4: 397–406

5 Kimata H, Yoshida A, Ishioka C, Lindley L, Mikawa H (1992) Interleukin-8 selectively inhibits immunoglobulin E production induced by IL-4 in human B cells. *J Exp Med* 176: 1227–1231

6 Kinawa M, Gately M, Gabler V, Chizzonite R, Fargeas C, Delespesse (1992) Recombinant interleukin-12 suppresses the synthesis of IgE by interleukin-4-stimulated human lymphocytes. *J Clin Invest* 90: 262–269

7 Miyajima H, Hirano T, Hirose S, Karasuyama H, Okamura K, Ovary Z (1991) Suppression by IL-2 of IgE production by B cells stimulated by IL-4. *J Immunol* 146: 457–462

8 Pene J, Rousset F, Briere F et al. (1988) IgE regulation by normal human lymphocytes is induced by interleukin-4 and suppressed by interferons α and α and prostaglandin E_2. *Proc Natl Acad Sci USA* 85: 6880–6884

9 Pene J, Rousset F, Briere F et al. (1988) Interleukin-5 enhances interleukin-4-induced IgE production by normal human B cells. The role of soluble CD23 antigen. *Eur J Immunol* 18: 929–935

10 Vercelli D, Jabara HH, Arai K-I, Yokota T, Geha RS (1989) Endogenous IL-6 plays an obligatory role in IL-4-induced human IgE synthesis. *Eur J Immunol* 19: 1419–1424

11 Clark EA, Leadbetter JA (1994) How B and T cells talk to each other. *Nature* 367: 425–428

12 Gascan H, Gauchat J-F, Aversa G, Van Vlasselaer P, De Vries JE (1991) Anti-CD40 monoclonal antibodies or CD4+ T cell clones induce IgG4 and IgE switching in purified human B cells via different signalling pathways. *J Immunol* 147: 8–13

13 Hollenbaugh D, Grosmaire LS, Kullas CD et al. (1992) The human T cell antigen gp39, a member of the TNF gene family, is a ligand for the CD40 receptor: expression of a soluble form of gp39 with B cell co-stimulatory activity. *EMBO J* 11: 4313–4321

14 Aubry J-P, Pochon S, Graber P, Jansen KU, Bonnefoy J-Y (1992) CD21 is a ligand for CD23 and regulates IgE production. *Nature* 358: 505–507

15 Lopez AF, Williamson DJ, Gamble JR, Begley CG, Harian JM, Klebanoff SJ, Waltersdorph A, Wong G, Clark SC, Vadas MA (1986) Recombinant human granulocyte-macrophage colony stimulating factor stimulates *in vitro* mature human eosinophil and neutrophil function surface receptor expression and survival. *J Clin Invest* 78: 1220–1228

16 Rothenberg ME, Owen WF, Silberstein DS, Woods J, Soberman RJ, Austen KF, Stevens RL (1988) Human eosinophils have prolonged survival, enhanced functional properties and become hypodense when exposed to human interleukin-3. *J Clin Invest* 81: 1986–1992

17 Rothenberg ME, Petersen J, Stevens RL, Silberstein DS, McKenzie DT, Austen KF, Owen WF (1989) IL-5 dependent conversion of normodense human eosinophils to the hypodense phenotype uses 3T3 fibroblasts for enhanced viability, accelerated hypodensity and sustained antibody-dependent cytotoxicity. *J Immunol* 143: 2311–2316

18 Lopez AF, Sanderson CJ, Gamble JR, Campbell HD, Young IG, Vadas MA (1988) Recombinant human interleukin-5 is a selective activator of eosinophil function. *J Exp Med* 167: 219–224

19 Dent LA, Strath M, Mellor AL, Sanderson CJ (1990) Eosinophilia in transgenic mice expressing interleukin-5. *J Exp Med* 172: 1425–1431

20 Bochner BS, Luscinskas FW, Gimbrone MAJ, Newman W, Sterbinsky SA, Derse-Anthony CP, Klunk D, Schleimer RP (1993) Adhesion of human basophils, eosinophils and neutrophils to IL-1 activated human vascular endothelial cells: contributions of endothelial cell adhesion molecules. *J Exp Med* 173: 1553–1557

21 Kyan-Aung U, Haskard DO, Poston RN, Thornhill MH, Lee TH (1991) Endothelial leukocyte adhesion molecule 1 and intercellular adhesion molecule 1 mediate adhesion of eosinophils to endothelial cell *in vitro* and are expressed by endothelium in allergic cutaneous inflammation *in vivo*. *J Immunol* 146: 521–528

22 Walsh GM, Hartnell A, Wardlaw AJ, Moqbel R, Kay AB (1990) IL-5 enhances the *in vitro* adhesion of human eosinophils, but not neutrophils, in a leukocyte integrin (CD11/CD18)-dependent manner. *Immunology* 71: 258–265

23 Walsh GM, Hartnell A, Mermod J-J, Kay AB, Wardlaw AJ (1991) Human eosinophil, but not neutrophil adherence to IL-1 stimulated HUVEC is $\alpha 4\beta 1$ (VLA-4) dependent. *J Immunol* 146: 3419–3423

24 Schleimer RP, Sterbinsky SA, Kaiser J et al. (1992) IL-induces adherence of human eosinophils and basophils but not neutrophils to endothelium: association with expression of VCAM-1. *J Immunol* 148: 1086–1092

25 Baggiolini M, Dahinden CA (1994) CC chemokines in allergic inflammation. *Immunol Today* 15: 127–133

26 Garcia-Zapeda EA, Rothenberg ME, Ownbey RT et al. (1996) Human eotaxin is a specific chemoattractant for eosinophil cells and provides a new mechanism to explain tissue eosinophila. *Nature Med* 2: 449–456

27 Collins PD, Marleau S, Griffits-Johnson DA et al. (1995) Co-operation between interleukin-5 and the chemokine eotaxin to induce eosinophil accumulation *in vivo*. *J Exp Med* 182: 1169–1174

28 Jose PJ, Griffiths-Johnson DA, Collins PD et al. (1994) Eotaxin: a potent eosinophil chemoattractant cytokine detected in a guinea pig model of allergic airways inflammation. *J Exp Med* 179: 881–887

29 Azzawi M, Bradley B, Jeffery PK, Frew AJ, Wardlaw AJ, Knowles G, Assoufi B, Collins JV, Durham SR, Kay AB (1990) Identification of activated T lymphocytes and eosinophils in bronchial biopsies in stable atopic asthma. *Am Rev Respir Dis* 142: 1410–1413

30 Hamid Q, Barkans J, Robinson DS, Durham SR, Kay AB (1992) Co-expression of CD25 and CD3 in atopic allergy and asthma. *Immunology* 75: 659–663

31 Pizzichini MM, Popov TA, Efthimiadis A et al. (1996) Spontaneous and induced sputum to measure indices of airway inflammation in asthma. *Am J Respir Crit Care Med* 154: 866–869

32 Wardlaw AJ, Dunnette S, Gleich GJ, Collins JV, Kay AB (1988) Eosinophils and mast cells in bronchoalveolar lavage in mild asthma: relationship to bronchial hyperreactivity. *Am Rev Respir Dis* 137: 62–69

33 Bradley BL, Azzawi M, Assoufi B, Jacobson M, Collins JV, Irani A, Schwartz LB, Durham SR, Kay AB (1991) Eosinophils, T lymphocytes, mast cells, neutrophils and macrophages in bronchial biopsies from atopic asthmatics: comparison with atopic non-asthma and normal controls and relationship to bronchial hyperresponsiveness. *J Allergy Clin Immunol* 88: 661–674

34 Bentley AM, Menz G, Storz C, Robinson DS, Bradley B, Jeffery PK, Durham SR, Kay AB (1992) Identification of T lymphocytes, macrophages and activated eosinophils in the bronchial mucosa in intrinsic asthma: relationship to symptoms and bronchial responsiveness. *Am Rev Respir Dis* 146: 500–506

35 Bentley AM, Maestrelli P, Saetta M, Fabbri LM, Robinson DS, Bradley BL, Jeffery PK, Durham SR, Kay AB (1992) Activated T lymphocytes and eosinophils in the bronchial mucosa in isocyanate-induced asthma. *J Allergy Clin Immunol* 89: 821–829

36 Corrigan CJ, Hartnell A, Kay AB (1988) T lymphocyte activation in acute severe asthma. *Lancet* i: 1129–1131

37 Corrigan CJ, Kay AB (1990) CD4 T lymphocyte activation in acute severe asthma. Relationship to disease severity and atopic status. *Am Rev Respir Dis* 141: 970–977

38 Corrigan CJ, Haczku A, Gemou-Engesaeth V, Doi S, Kikuchi Y, Takatsu K, Durham SR, Kay AB (1993) CD4 T lymphocyte activation in asthma is accompanied by increased concentrations of interleukin-5: effect of glucocorticoid therapy. *Am Rev Respir Dis* 147: 540–547

39 Gemou-Engesaeth V, Kay AB, Bush A, Corrigan CJ (1994) Activated peripheral blood CD4 and CD8 T lymphocytes in childhood asthma: correlation with eosinophila and disease severity. *Pediatr Allergy Immunol* 5: 170–177

40 Alexander AG, Barkans J, Moqbel R, Barnes NC, Kay AB, Corrigan CJ (1994) Serum interleukin-5 concentrations in atopic and non-atopic patients with glucocorticoid-dependent chronic severe asthma. *Thorax* 49: 1231–1233

41 Doi S, Gemou-Engesaeth V, Kay AB, Corrigan CJ (1994) Polymerase chain reaction quantification of cytokine messenger RNA expression in peripheral blood mononuclear cells of patients with severe asthma: effect of glucocorticoid therapy. *Clin Exp Allergy* 24: 854–687

42 Corrigan CJ, Brown PH, Barnes NC, Tsai J-J, Frew AJ, Kay AB (1991) Glucocorticoid resistance in chronic asthma: peripheral blood T lymphocyte activation and a comparison of the T lymphocyte inhibitory effects of glucocorticoids and cyclosporin A. *Am Rev Respir Dis* 144: 1026–1032

43 Corrigan CJ, Brown PH, Barnes NC, Tsai J-J, Frew AJ, Kay AB (1991) Glucocorticoid resistance in chronic asthma: glucocorticoid pharmacokinetics, glucocorticoid receptor characteristics and inhibition of peripheral blood T cell proliferation by glucocorticoids *in vitro*. *Am Rev Respir Dis* 144: 1016–1025

44 Haczku A, Alexander A, Brown P, Kay AB, Corrigan CJ (1994) The effect of dexamethasone, cyclosporin A and rapamycin on T lymphocyte proliferation *in vitro*: comparison of cells from corticosteroid sensitive and corticosteroid resistant chronic asthmatics. *J Allergy Clin Immunol* 93: 510–519

45 Hamid Q, Azzawi M, Ying S, Moqbel R, Wardlaw AJ, Corrigan CJ, Bradley B, Durham SR, Kay AB (1991) Expression of mRNA for interleukin-5 in mucosal bronchial biopsies from asthma. *J Clin Invest* 87: 1541–1546

46 Robinson DS, Hamid Q, Ying S, Tsicopoulos A, Barkans J, Bentley AM, Corrigan C, Durham SR, Kay AB (1992) Evidence for a predominant "Th2-type" bronchoalveolar lavage T lymphocyte population in atopic asthma. *N Engl J Med* 326: 298–304

47 Robinson DS, Ying S, Bentley AM, Meng Q, North J, Durham SR, Kay AB (1993) Relationships among numbers of bronchoalveolar lavage cells expressing messenger ribonucleic acid for cytokines, asthma symptoms, and airway methacholine responsiveness in atopic asthma. *J Allergy Clin Immunol* 92: 397–403

48 Corrigan CJ, Hamid Q, North J, Barkans J, Moqbel R, Durham SR, Kay AB (1995) Peripheral blood CD4, but not CD8 T lymphocytes in patients with exacerbation of asthma transcribe and translate messenger RNA encoding cytokines which prolong eosinophil survival in the context of a Th2-type pattern: effect of glucocorticoid therapy. *Am J Respir Cell Mol Biol* 12: 567–578

49 Robinson DS, Hamid Q, Ying S, Bentley AM, Assoufi B, North J, Meng Q, Durham SR, Kay AB (1993) Prednisolone treatment in asthma in associated with modulation of bronchoalveolar lavage cell interleukin-4, interleukin-5 and interferon-gamma cytokine gene expression. *Am Rev Respir Dis* 148: 402–406

50 Leung DY, Martin RJ, Szefler SJ et al. (1995) Dysregulation of interleukin-4, interleukin-5 and interferon gamma gene expression in steroid-resistant asthma. *J Exp Med* 181: 33–40

51 Bentley AM, Meng Q, Robinson DS et al. (1993) Increases in activated T lymphocytes, eosinophils and cytokine messenger RNA for IL-5 and GM-CSF in bronchial biopsies after allergen inhalation challenge in atopic asthmatics. *Am J Respir Cell Mol Biol* 8: 35–42

52 Ying S, Durham SR, Corrigan CJ, Hamid Q, Kay AB (1995) Phenotype of cells expressing mRNA for Th2-type (interleukin-4 and interleukin-5) and Th1-type (interleukin-2 and interferon-gamma) cytokines in bronchoalveolar lavage and bronchial biopsies from atopic asthmatics and normal control subjects. *Am J Respir Cell Mol Biol* 12: 477–487

53 Bradding P, Roberts JA, Britten KM et al. (1994) Interleukin-4, -5, -6 and tumour necrosis factor-α in normal and asthmatic airways: evidence for the human mast cell as a source of these cytokines. *Am J Respir Cell Mol Biol* 10: 471–480

54 Krug N, Madden J, Redington AE et al. (1996) T cell cytokine profile evaluated at the single cell level in blood and allergic asthma. *Am J Respir Cell Mol Biol* 14: 319–326

55 Till SJ, Li B, Durham S, Humbert M, Assoufi B, Jeannin P, Huston D, Dickason R, Kay AB, Corrigan CJ (1995) Secretion of the eosinophil-active cytokines IL-5, GM-CSF and IL-3 by bronchoalveolar lavage CD4+ and CD8+ T cell lines in atopic asthmatics and atopic and non-atopic controls. *Eur J Immunol* 25: 2727–2731

56 Mosmann TR, Coffman RL (1989) Th1 and Th2 cells: different patterns of lymphokine secretion lead to different functional properties. *Annu Rev Immunol* 7: 145–173

57 Mosmann TR, Moore KW (1991) The role of IL-10 in cross-regulation of Th1 and Th2 responses. *Immunoparasitol Today* 12: 49–53

58 Firestein GS, Roeder WD, Laxer JA et al. (1989) A new murine CD4+ T cell subset with an unrestricted cytokine profile. *J Immunol* 143: 518–525

59 Kay AB, Ying S, Varney V, Gaga M, Durham SH, Moqbel R, Wardlaw AJ, Hamid Q (1991) Messenger RNA expression of the cytokine gene cluster IL-3, IL-4, IL-5 and GM-CSF in allergen-induced late phase cutaneous reactions in atopic subjects. *J Exp Med* 173: 775–778

60 Tsicopoulos A, Hamid Q, Varney V, Ying S, Moqbel R, Durham SR, Kay AB (1992) Preferential messenger RNA expression of Th1-type cells (IFN-γ+, IL-2+) in classical delayed-type (tuberculin) hypersensitivity reactions in human skin. *J Immunol* 148: 2058–2061

61 Maggi E, Biswas P, Del Prete G et al. (1991) Accumulation of Th2-like helper T cells in the conjunctiva of patients with vernal conjunctivitis. *J Immunol* 146: 1169–1174

62 Van der Heijden FL, Wierenga EA, Bos JD, Kapsenberg ML (1991) High frequency of IL-4 producing CD4+ allergen-specific T lymphocytes in atopic dermatitis lesional skin. *J Invest Dermatol* 97: 389–394

63 Jung T, Schauer U, Rieger C et al. (1995) Interleukin-4 and interleukin-5 are rarely co-expressed by human T cells. *Eur J Immunol* 25: 2413–2416
64 Rackemann FM (1947) A working classification of asthma. *Am J Med* 3: 601–606
65 Humbert M, Durham SR, Ying S, Kimmitt P, Barkans J, Assoufi B, Pfister R, Mewnz G, Robinson DS, Kay AB, Corrigan CJ (1966) IL-4 and IL-5 mRNA and protein in bronchial biopsies from patients with atopic and non-atopic asthma: evidence against "intrinsic" asthma being a distinct immunopathologic entity. *Am J Respir Crit Care Med* 154: 1497–1504
66 Humbert M, Grant JA, Taborda-Barata L et al. (1996) High affinity IgE receptor (FCεRI)-bearing cells in bronchial biopsies from atopic and non-atopic athma. *Am Rev Respir Crit Care Med* 153: 1931–1937
67 Corry DB, Folkesson HG, Warnock ML et al. (1996) Interleukin 4, but not interleukin 5 or eosinophils is required in a murine model of acute airway hyperreactivity. *J Exp Med* 183; 109–117
68 Foster PS, Hogan SP, Ramsay AJ, Matthaei KI, Young IG (1996) Interleukin-5 deficiency abolishes eosinophilia, airways hyperreactivity and lung damage in a mouse asthma model. *J Exp Med* 183: 195–201
69 Shirakawa T, Li A, Dubowitz M, Dekker JW, Shaw AE, Faux JA, Ra C, Cookson WOCM, Hopkin JM (1994) Association between atopy and variants of the β subunit of the high-affinity immunoglobulin E receptor. *Nature Genet* 7: 125–130
70 Postma DS, Bleeker ER, Amelung PJ et al. (1995) Genetic susceptibility to asthma – bronchial hyperresponsiveness coinherited with a major gene for atopy. *N Engl J Med* 333: 894–900

Molecular Biology of the Lung
Vol. 2: Asthma and Cancer
ed. by R. A. Stockley
© 1999 Birkhäuser Verlag Basel/Switzerland

CHAPTER 6
β-Adrenoceptors

Peter J. Barnes and Judith C. W. Mak

Department of Thoracic Medicine, National Heart and Lung Institute, Imperial College School of Medicine, London, UK

1   Introduction
2   β-Adrenoceptor Structure
2.1 Cloning of β-Receptors
2.1.1 Ligand-binding domain
2.1.2 G-protein Coupling Domain
3   Expression of β-Receptor Genes in the Lung
4   Intracellular Mechanisms
4.1 G-Proteins
4.2 Cyclic AMP
4.3 K⁺ channels
4.4 Cyclic AMP Response Element Binding Protein
4.5 Receptor Cross-Talk
5   Regulation of β-Receptors
5.1 Desensitization and Down-Regulation
5.2 Effect of Glucocorticosteroids
5.3 Inflammation
5.4 Asthmatic Airways
6   β₂-Receptors Polymorphisms
     References

1. Introduction

β-Adrenoceptors regulate many aspects of lung function and β-adrenergic agonists have become the most widely used bronchodilators for the treatment of obstructive airway diseases. There have been important advances in our understanding of the molecular structure and regulation of β-adrenoceptors, which have implications for elucidating β-adrenoceptor function in airway disease and the mechanisms of action of β-agonists [1, 2]. At least three β-adrenoceptors are now recognized (Table 1). β_1-Receptors, which are preferentially activated by noradrenaline, are physiologically regulated by sympathetic nerves; β_2-receptors are preferentially regulated by circulating adrenaline; β_3-receptors or "atypical" β-receptors are involved in lipolysis but are increasingly recognized in other functions. β_2-Receptors predominate in lungs and mediate most of the effects of β-agonist on airway function.

Table 1. Human β-adrenoceptor subtypes

Subtype	Agonist potency	Size	Selective agonist	Selective antagonist
β_1	NA > A > I	477	Xamoterol	CGP 20712 Atenolol
β_2	I > A > NA	413	Procaterol Albuterol Salmeterol	ICI 118,551 Butoxamine
β_3	NA > A > I	402	BRL37344	SR58894

NA, noradrenaline; A, adrenaline; I, isoprenaline.

2. β-Adrenoceptor Structure

2.1. Cloning of β-Receptors

Three β-adrenoceptors have now been cloned [3–6] and this has made it possible to elucidate the structure of the receptor protein and the way in which the receptor interacts with β-agonists and intracellular pathways [7]. β-Adrenoceptors have the characteristic structure associated with G-protein-coupled receptors of seven hydrophobic stretches of 20–25 amino acids, which take the form of an α-helix that crosses the cell membrane. The intervening hydrophilic sections are alternately exposed intracellularly and extracellularly with the amino (N) terminus exposed to the outside and the carboxyl (C) terminus within the cytoplasm (Figure 1). The three-dimensional structure of β-receptors is derived by analogy to bacterial rhodopsin, and it has not been possible to confirm this by X-ray crystallography as a result of the difficulty in obtaining sufficient receptor protein. The molecular weight of the cloned receptors predicted from the copy DNA (cDNA) sequence is less than the molecular mass of the wild receptors when assessed by polyacrylamide gel electrophoresis. This discrepancy results from glycosylation of the native receptor, for example, β_2-receptors contain two sites for glycosylation on asparagine (Asn) residues near the amino terminus, and it is estimated that N-glycosylation accounts for 25–30% of the molecular mass of the native receptor. The functional significance of glycosylation is not yet clear; it does not affect receptor affinity for ligand or coupling to G-proteins, but it may be important for the trafficking of the receptor through the cell during down-regulation, or for keeping the receptor correctly orientated in the lipid bilayer. There is a palitylolation site in the third intracellular loop which anchors it to the lipid bilayer.

The three β-receptors so far identified have distinctly different sequences. The human β_1-receptor has only 54% homology with the human β_2-receptor. The human β_2-receptor gene is localized to chromosome 5q and codes for a protein of 413 amino acids. β_3-Receptors have been identified,

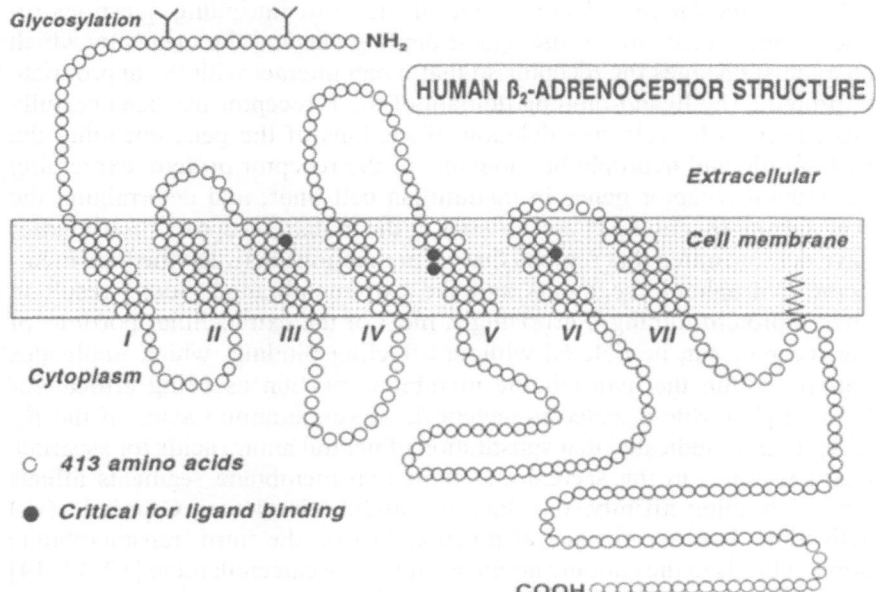

Figure 1. Structure of the human β₂-adrenoceptor: the protein chain is believed to have seven transmembrane α-helices (I–VII). Filled circles indicate the amino acids that are essential for β-agonist binding.

cloned, sequenced and expressed [6]. The β₃-receptor is clearly different from either β₁- or β₂-receptors (about 50% amino acid sequence homology) and appears to correspond to the "atypical" β-receptors described in adipose tissue. β₃-Receptors appear to be important in regulation of metabolic rate and have not yet been detected in lung homogenates [8, 9].

Mutant receptors with substitution of single nucleotide bases at different positions in the sequence (site-directed mutagenesis) have proved to be invaluable in elucidating β-receptor structure and function. Replacement of the cysteine (Cys) residues at positions 106 and 184 in the second and third extracellular domain in the hamster lung β₂-receptor shows that they are important in maintaining the correct three-dimensional shape of the receptor in the cell membrane by the formation of a disulphide link between the two loops. Substitution of either of these Cys residues with isoleucine (Ile) impairs β-receptor ligand-binding affinity [10]. Similarly, substitution of either of the adjacent Cys residues, at positions 190 and 191 on the third cytoplasmic loop of the human β₂-receptor, markedly reduces binding affinity and coupling to adenylate cyclase [11]. It is interesting that the Cys residues on the second and third extracellular loops are highly conserved among receptors and suggests that they may be critical in stabilizing their three-dimensional structure.

2.1.1. Ligand-binding domain: One of the most intriguing questions relates to the elucidation of the ligand-binding site and the means by which
an agonist changes the receptor so that it can interact with the appropriate
G-protein. The ligand-binding domain of the β-receptor has been carfully
characterized by selective deletion of sections of the gene encoding the
hydrophilic and hydrophobic domains of the receptor protein, expressing
the mutant receptor genes in mammilian cell lines, and determining the
binding and functional characteristics of the mutant receptor. These studies
have demonstrated that regions that form junctions between the transmembrane hydrophobic segments and the extramembranous loops result in
altered protein folding. Surprisingly, most of the extracellular portions of
the receptor can be deleted without affecting binding, which implicates
regions within the hydrophobic membrane portion as being critical for
binding [12]. Site-directed mutagenesis of single amino acids of the β_2-
receptor have indicated that substitution of neutral amino acids for aspartate
(Asp) residues in the second and third transmembrane segments affects
agonist binding affinity, but does not affect stimulatory G-protein (G$_s$)
activation. The Asp residue at position 113 on the third transmembrane
domain binds to the cationic amine group of the catecholamine [10, 13, 14]
(Figure 2). Asp 113 is highly conserved between adrenoceptors and between different species. It is of interest that equivalent Asp residues are
conserved in all other adrenergic receptors which all bind ligands with a
charged amine group.

Site-directed mutagenesis of serine (Ser) residues, which may form a
hydrogen bond with the catechol ring, suggests that Ser residues in the fifth
transmembrane helix (Ser 204 and Ser 207) are also important. These
studies indicate that a ligand-binding pocket may fit between the third to

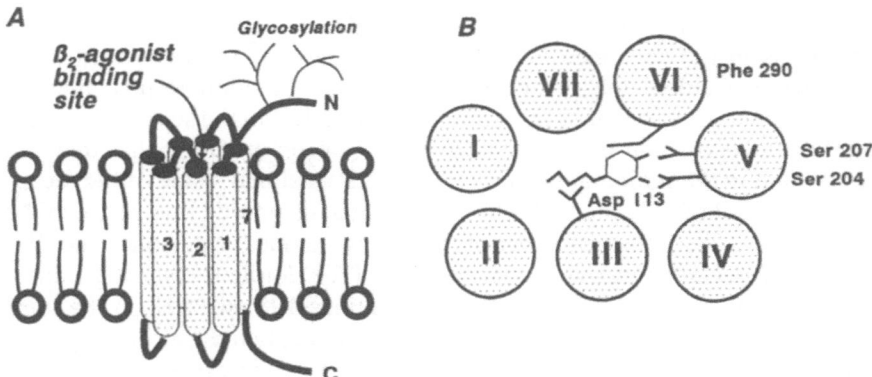

Figure 2. Three-dimensional structure of the β-receptor (A) and plan of the ligand-binding
domain, indicating how the catechol ring of β-agonists associates with critical amino acids in
the transmembrane spanning segments (B).

sixth transmembrane helix [10]. Using the fluorescent β-blocker carazolol, which binds with high affinity to the β_2-receptor, it has been possible with fluorescence spectroscopy to demonstrate in quenching experiments that the ligand-binding site is buried deep (at least 1.1 nm) within the receptor [15].

The reason why β_2-receptors prefer adrenaline (which is more bulky as a result of an additional methyl group) to noradrenaline is not completely understood. Recent studies with chimaric receptors, which are a combination of the sequence of β_1- and β_2-receptors, indicate that the sequences of amino acids in transmembrane helices 4 and 5 are critical and probably determine the shape of the binding pocket [16].

The discovery of long-acting β_2-agonists, such as salmeterol and formoterol, has revealed additional information about the ligand-binding domain. Salmeterol has a long aliphatic side chain that may anchor the catechol end of the molecule of the binding cleft in the β-receptor. Salmeterol displays a characteristic behaviour *in vitro* with a slow onset of action and a very slow recovery even after extensive washing [17]. Addition of a β-adrenergic antagonist reverses the relaxation effect of salmeterol, but when the antagonist is washed out salmeterol "reasserts" its action, indicating that it is still bound to the receptor. Site-directed mutagenesis has demonstrated that residues 149–158 localized at the interface of transmembrane domain 4 and the cytoplasm are critical for the long duration of salmeterol binding [18], suggesting that this region is involved in anchoring the molecule within the binding cleft. By contrast, formoterol appears to have a long duration of action by virtue of its lipophilicity and the drug simply dissolves in the lipid bilayer, which acts as a depot [19].

2.1.2. G-protein Coupling Domain: The intracellular loops located on the inner surface of the plasma membrane interact with the α-subunit of G_s (α_s). Deletion mutagenesis studies, in which stretches of the amino acid sequence are removed, indicate that the third intracellular loop is critical for interaction between β_2-receptors and α_s [20]. This loop contains a sequence of amino acids which includes charged amino acids in the form of an α-helix. Sequences in the fourth intracellular loop also cooperate in activation of α_s. Synthetic peptides derived from the third intracellular loop are capable of activating G_s and substitution of only a single amino acid results in mutant receptors that have constitutive activity and activate G_s [21]. This suggests that, in the unoccupied state, the β_2-receptor is constrained, but binding of a β-agonist may lead to a conformational change which reveals these sequences in the third intracellular loop, resulting in activation of G_s.

3. Expression of β-Receptor Genes in the Lung

β_2-Adrenoceptors are expressed in many cell tyes in the lung and subserve many different cellular functions (Table 2). The presence of β_2-receptor

Table 2. Localization and function of airway β-adrenoceptors

Cell type	Subtype	Function
Smooth muscle	β_2	Relaxation (proximal = distal) Inhibition of proliferation
Epithelium	β_2	Increased ion transport Secretion of inhibitory factor? Increased ciliary beating Increased mucociliary clearance
Submucosal glands	β_1/β_2	Increased secretion (mucus cells)
Clara cells	β_2	Increased secretion
Cholinergic nerves	β_2	Reduced acetylcholine release
Sensory nerves	β_2/β_3	Reduced neuropeptide release Reduced activation?
Bronchial vessels	β_2	Vasodilatation Reduced plasma extravasation
Inflammatory cells		
Mast cells	β_2	Reduced mediator release
Macrophages	β_2	No effect?
Eosinophils	β_2	Reduced mediator release
T lymphocytes	β_2	Reduced cytokine release?

mRNA has been detected in human and rat lung by northern analysis using radiolabelled cDNA (or cRNA) probes [22–24]. Northern blotting shows a single transcript of 2.2 kilobases (kb), as observed in other tissues and cells. β_2-Receptor mRNA has been localized by *in situ* hybridization and corresponds, as expected, to β-receptor-binding sites [22]. However, there are discrepancies between the relative density of mRNA and receptors in certain cells. Thus, in airway smooth muscle there is a very high density of β-receptor mRNA, whereas the density of the β-receptors is relatively low; this suggests either that the rate of receptor synthesis is high, and there is a rapid turnover of receptors, or that the stability of mRNA is high. This may explain why it is difficult to down-regulate β-receptors in airway smooth muscle, and therefore to demonstrate tachyphylaxis to the bronchodilator action of β-agonists. By contrast, in the alveolar walls there is a low level of mRNA but a very high receptor density, which may indicate a low receptor turnover, and this would be consistent with the fact that down-regulation is readily produced in lung parenchyma.

β_1-Receptor mRNA is also detected in animal and human lung tissue, although as expected it is less abundant than β_2-receptor mRNA [24]. β_1-Receptor mRNA is localized to submucosal glands and alveolar walls, as predicted by autoradiographic receptor mapping [25, 26]. β_3-Receptor mRNA has not been detected in human or animal lung by Northern blotting or *in situ* hybridization [8, 24], or by the more sensitive technique of reverse transcription polymerase chain reaction (RT-PCR) [27].

4. Intracellular Mechanisms

4.1. G-Proteins

The intracellular mechanisms involved in mediating the effects of β-agonists are now reasonably well established, although recent studies have challenged the dogma [28]. Occupation of a β-receptor by an agonist results in a conformational change which leads to the activation of the α-subunit of G_s. G_s is made up of three subunits: $α_s$ which interacts with the receptor and binds GTP and β and γ subunits which appear to anchor or stabilize the α-subunit in the membrane, but are also involved in more long-term signalling events. Activation of $α_s$ in turn activates the cell surface-associated enzyme adenylate cyclase, which results in conversion of ATP to cyclic adenosine 3′,5′-monophosphate (cAMP), the second messenger of β-receptor function (Figure 3).

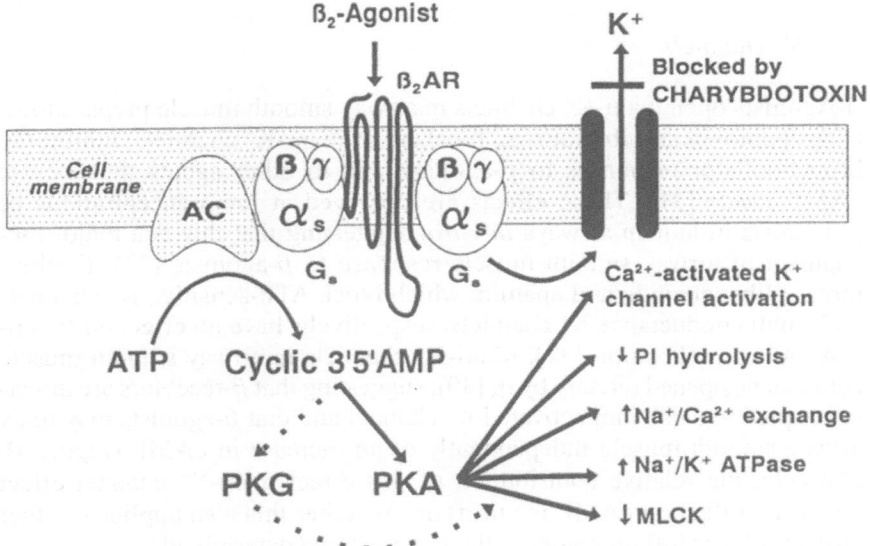

Figure 3. Intracellular mechanisms of $β_2$-receptor activation in airway smooth muscle cells. $β_2$-receptors are coupled to adenylate cyclase (AC) via a stimulatory guanine nucleotide regulatory protein (G_s), consisting of three subunits ($α_s$, $β$, $γ$). A rise in intracellular cAMP activates protein kinase A (PKA) which phosphorylates several proteins that contribute to the relaxant effect of β-agonists. Cyclic AMP may also activate protein kinase G (PKG) which in turn may also phosphorylate several protein targets. β-Receptors may also be coupled directly via G_s to a large conductance calcium-activated K⁺ channel.

4.2. Cyclic AMP

Cyclic AMP activates protein kinase A (PKA), which then phosphorylates
certain key proteins in the cell leading to the characteristic cellular response
[29]. PKA may be physically associated with the cell membrane through
anchoring proteins, so that it is in close proximity to adenylate cyclase. In
airway smooth muscle PKA inhibits myosin light chain phosphorylation,
which inhibits phosphoinositide hydrolysis and promotes Ca^{2+}/Na^+ ex-
change, thus resulting in a fall in intracellular Ca^{2+}. The rise in cAMP also
leads to phosphorylation of a large conductance, calcium-activated potassium (maxi-K^+) channel, which is blocked by the scorpion venom toxins
charybdotoxin and iberiotoxin [30]. There is also evidence that an increase
in cAMP may activate protein kinase G (PKG) and the relaxant effects of
β-agonists in some preparations may be mediated, at least in part, via a
cAMP-induced activation of PKG rather than protein kinase C (PKC) [28].
PKG activation inhibits Ca^{2+} mobilization and this may contribute to the
relaxant effects of β-agonists mediated via PKA and maxi-K^+ channels.

4.3. K^+ channels

β-Agonists open maxi-K^+ channels in airway smooth muscle preparations.
Charybdotoxin and iberiotoxin, blockers of maxi-K^+ channels, inhibit the
bronchodilator responses to β-agonists and to other agents that elevate
cAMP levels [31]. These effects are observed at low concentrations of
β-agonists in human airways *in vitro*, suggesting that this is a major mechanism of airway smooth muscle response to β-agonists [32]. Furthermore, glibenclamide and apamin, which block ATP-sensitive K^+ channels
and small conductance K^+ channels, respectively, have no effect on β-ago-
nist-induced relaxation [32]. Maxi-K^+ channels in airway smooth muscle
cells can be opened directly by α_s [30], suggesting that β-receptors are directly coupled to a calcium activated K^+ channel and that β-agonists may relax
airway smooth muscle independently of an increase in cAMP (Figure 3).
However, the relative contribution of this direct maxi-K^+ channel effect
versus an effect on cAMP is uncertain. Whether this also applies to other
airway cells or inflammatory cells remains to be determined.

4.4. Cyclic AMP Response Element Binding Protein

Cyclic AMP-mediated activation of PKA may lead to the induction of
several genes through a conserved cAMP response element (CRE) on the
promoter sequence of target genes. This effect of cAMP is mediated via a
43-kDa DNA-binding protein CREB (CRE-binding protein), which functions as a transcription factor [33] (Figure 4). CREB is activated by phos-

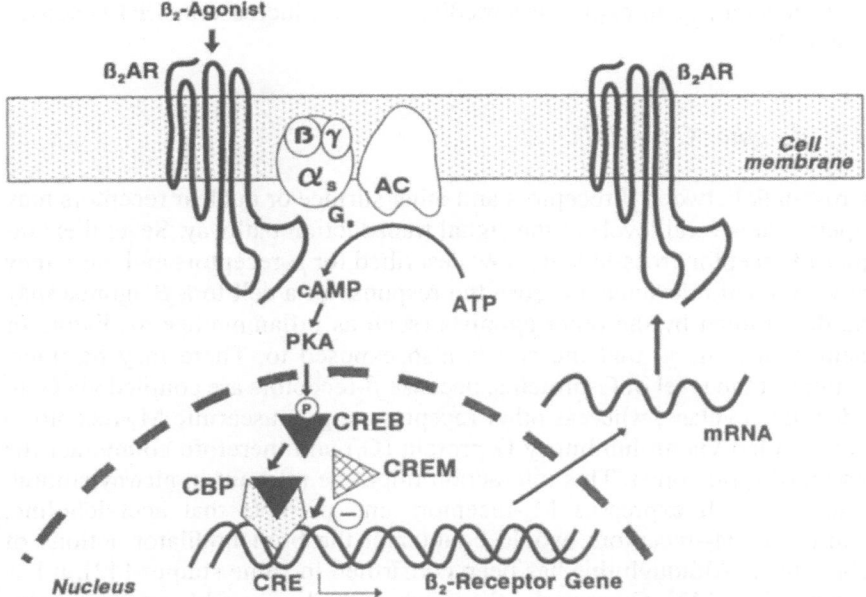

Figure 4. Effect of *β*-agonists on gene transcription: an increase in cAMP activates protein kinase A (PKA), resulting in phosphorylation of cAMP response element-binding protein (CREB) within the nucleus; this binds to a cAMP response element (CRE) in the upstream promoter region of a responsive gene (e.g. the *β*$_2$-receptor gene itself), resulting in increased transcription. Binding of CREB to CRE is facilitated by CREB-binding protein (CBP) and may be blocked by another transcription factor, CRE modulator (CREM).

phorylation (at Ser 133) by the catalytic subunit of PKA which translocates to the nucleus on activation by cAMP. There may be a family of different CREBs that are differentially regulated. The activated phosphophorylated CREB associates with a large CREB-binding protein (CBP), forming a transcriptional activation complex [34]. A transcription factor that also binds to CRE, known as CRE modulator (CREM), exists as three isoforms [35]. CREM usually has opposing effects to CREB, thus blocking the transcriptional actions of CREB. There is evidence that *β*-agonists increase CRE binding in human and rat lung tissue [36–38], although activation of CREB is only seen at relatively high concentration of *β*-agonists (which are needed for an increase in cAMP concentration). The human *β*$_2$-receptor gene has a CRE sequence and CREB increases its expression [39]. Indeed, a CREB may be responsible for the basal expression of *β*$_2$-receptors and may in part determine the *β*-receptor density of different cell types. A CRE sequence has also been described in the promoter region of the human *β*$_1$-receptor gene [40] and there may be multiple CREs in the promoter sequence of the *β*$_3$-receptor gene [41]. Short-term exposure of cells to *β*-agonists results in a transient increase in β_2-receptor gene expression mediated via an increase in CREB activation [39].

4.5. Receptor Cross-Talk

Cross-talk between β-receptors and other surface or nuclear receptors may operate at several levels in the signal transduction pathway. Several examples of receptor cross-talk are now described for β-receptors and these may have clinical relevance, because the response of a cell to a β-agonist may be determined by the other agonists (such as inflammatory mediators or neurotransmitters) that the cell is also exposed to. There may be interactions at the level of G-proteins, because β-receptors are coupled via G_s to adenylate cyclase, whereas other receptors (e.g. muscarinic M_2-receptors) are coupled via an inhibitory G-protein (G_i) and therefore counteract the effect of a β-agonist. This interaction might be relevant in airway smooth muscle which expresses M_2-receptors and predicts that acetylcholine, acting via M_2-receptors, would counteract the bronchodilator actions of β-agonists. Although this has been confirmed in some studies [42], it has not in others [43]. Conversely, β-agonists may decrease M_2-receptor function [44]. Another level of functional antagonism between muscarinic and β-receptors may be at the level of the maxi-K^+ channel, because β-receptors are coupled via G_s to maxi-K^+ channels in airway smooth muscle, whereas M_2-receptors are coupled via G_i to the same channel and would therefore oppose the opening of the channel in response to a β-agonist [45].

Interaction may also occur in signal transduction pathways, because β-agonists inhibit phosphoinositide hydrolysis stimulated via receptors, such as M_3-receptors and histamine receptors, in airway smooth muscle [46]. In turn, muscarinic agonists may activate PKC via stimulation of phosphoinositide hydrolysis, which may result in phosphorylation of both β-receptors and G_s, with resulting down-regulation and uncoupling of surface β-receptors [47]. Such a mechanism has recently been demonstrated in airway smooth muscle [48] (Figure 5).

Complex interactions may also occur within the nucleus between transcription factors activated via different surface receptors. Several interactions have recently been recognized between CREB and other transcription factors, such as activator protein-1 (AP-1) and between the glucocorticoid receptor [49, 50]. This has potentially important clinical implications, because activation of CREB by exposure to β_2-agonists may interfere with the actions of cytokines, such as tumour necrosis factor-α (TNF-α), which activate AP-1, and this would be beneficial in the context of chronic inflammation. On the other hand, CREB also interacts with the glucocorticoid receptor, which may inhibit the anti-inflammatory actions of steroids [37, 51]. The final functional outcome will depend on the net balance between the various interacting forces and will differ from cell to cell.

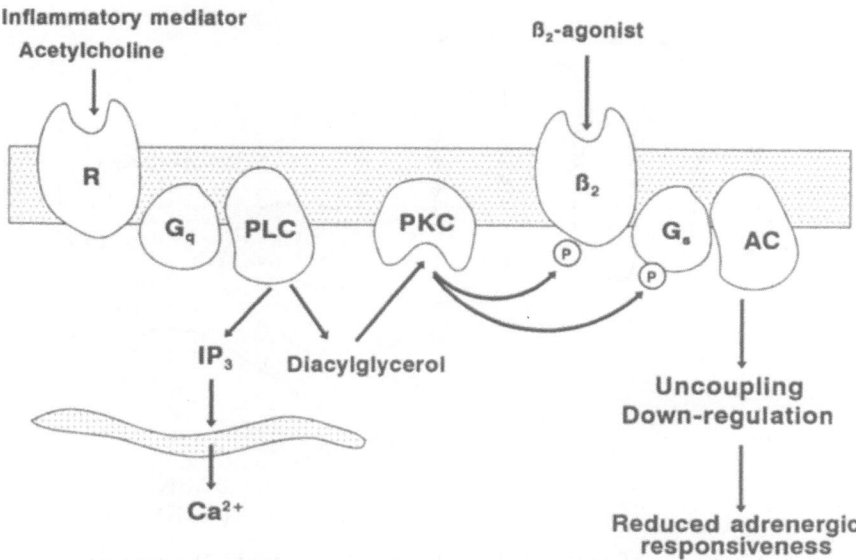

Figure 5. Cross-talk between β_2-receptors and inflammatory mediator and muscarinic receptors. Inflammatory mediators and acetylcholine may activate phosphoinositide hydrolysis, resulting in activation of protein kinase C (PKC), which phosphorylates β_2-receptors and stimulatory G-proteins (G$_s$), resulting in uncoupling and down-regulation of β-receptors.

5. Regulation of β-Receptors

5.1. Desensitization and Down-Regulation

Reduced responsiveness occurs with most cell surface receptors when exposed continuously or repeatedly to an agonist; tachyphylaxis refers to short-term desensitization and tolerance to desensitization after repeated application of an agonist. Several molecular mechanisms are involved in desensitization of β-receptors [52, 53]. Homologous desensitization refers to reduced responsiveness to β-agonists, whereas heterologous desensitization refers to desensitization to other agonists and usually involves cAMP.

In the short term, homologous desensitization involves phosphorylation of the receptor, which results in uncoupling from G$_s$. At least two types of serine/threonine (Ser/Thr) kinase are involved, PKA and β-adrenergic receptor kinase (βARK) [54, 55] (Figure 6). βARK is not specific for β-receptors and may be involved in the phosphorylation of other receptors, including muscarinic and tachykinin receptors. Two distinct βARKs are now recognized and are members of a larger G-protein receptor kinase (GRK) family that are specific for agonist-occupied or activated receptors. βARK1 (GRK2) and βARK2 (GRK3) appear to play similar roles in phos-

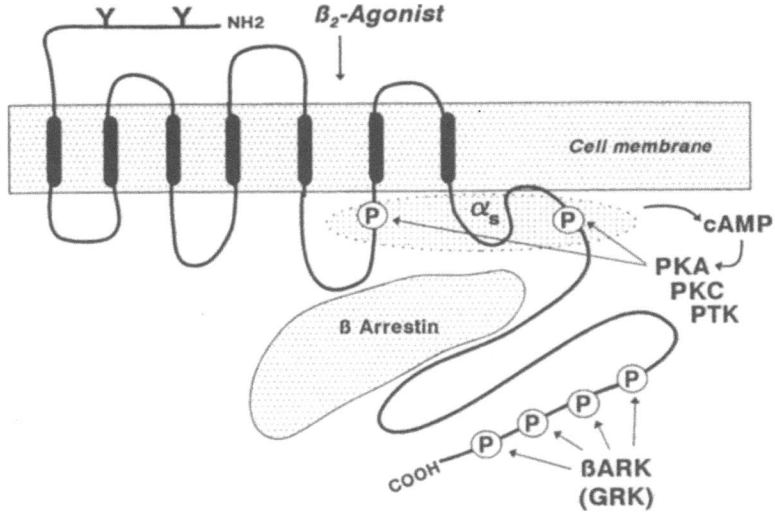

Figure 6. Mechanisms of short-term desensitization of β_2-receptors. The β-receptor is phosphorylated by β-adrenergic receptor kinase (βARK) and other G-protein receptor kinases (GRK) on its carboxyl tail, resulting in increased binding of β-arrestin, which leads to uncoupling and internalization of the receptor. Protein kinase A (PKA), activated by an increase in cAMP, phosphorylates the receptor at other sites on the third intracellular loop. Protein kinase C (PKC) and protein tyrosine kinases (PTK) may also phosphorylate the receptor, resulting in uncoupling.

phorylation of β-receptors and an additional enzyme GRK5 may also be involved. Occupation of β-receptors by a β-agonist activates α_s and the dissociated $\beta\gamma$ units of G_s act as a membrane anchor for βARK which translocates to the cell membrane where it phosphorylates the membrane-bound receptor [56]. The activity of βARK is thus enhanced by $\beta\gamma$ subunits of G-proteins. βARKs have a high degree of specificity because they recognize only agonist-occupied β_2-receptors. The site of phosphorylation of βARK appears to be the Ser/Thr-rich carboxyl tail of the receptor. A co-factor termed "β-arrestin" is necessary for βARK inhibition of receptor function [57, 58]. Phosphorylation of β-receptors by βARK enhances the ability of β-arrestin to bind and thereby to uncouple the receptor from G_s. Overexpression of β-arrestin enhances the desensitization of β-receptors [58].

Heterologous desensitization is seen with stable analogues of cAMP or with forskolin; the reduction in receptor sensitivity is less marked than with β-agonists. Site-directed mutagenesis studies indicate that phosphorylation of the receptor by PK may also enhance the rate of β_2-receptor down-regulation, but that this effect is less marked than that seen with β-agonists. Homologous desensitization thus involves both βARK and a component resulting from PKA-induced phosphorylation. The latter occurs at low concentrations of agonist, whereas higher concentrations are needed for activation of βARK. The site of phosphorylation by PKA is the Ser/Thr residues in the third intracellular loop of the receptor [52, 53]. PKC may also phosphorylate β_2-receptors, resulting in uncoupling [59]. This could be relevant in inflammatory lung diseases, because several inflammatory mediators may activate PKC through stimulation of phosphoinositide hydrolysis [59]. In bovine airway smooth muscle and rabbit airway epithelial cells stimulation of PKC by a phorbol ester results in uncoupling and down-regulation of β_2-receptors [48, 60]. Protein tyrosine kinases (PTKs) may also phosphorylate β-receptors. Thus activation of the insulin receptor, which has intrinsic PTK activity, phosphorylates and desensitizes β_2-receptors [61]. This allows cross-talk between pathways involved in cell growth and β-receptors, and may be relevant in chronic inflammatory diseases of the lung.

Longer-term mechanisms include down-regulation of surface receptor number, a process that involves internalization of the receptor and its subsequent degradation. Surface β-receptors are rapidly internalized (sequestration) after exposure to β_2-agonists and are manifest by a loss of binding of hydrophilic ligands (cell surface receptors) but not lipophilic ligands (total number of receptors). This uncoupled internalized receptor may return to the cell membrane once the β-agonist is removed (resensitization). A highly conserved tyrosine residue at the junction of the seventh transmembrane segment and the fourth intracellular loop (Tyr 326) in the β_2-receptor is required for both sequestration and resensitization [62]. More prolonged exposure to β-agonists results in down-regulation, which involves a permanent loss of receptors from the cell surface; this in turn, involves degradation of the receptors. After down-regulation, responsiveness is only restored by the synthesis of new receptors.

More chronic effects of β-agonists, which are probably of greater relevance to clinical practice, appear to involve changes in β-receptor synthesis. In a cultured hamster cell line, down-regulation of β_2-receptors results in a rapid decline in the steady-state level of β_2-receptor mRNA [63]. Incubation of human lung with salbutamol, and the long-acting β_2-agonists salmeterol and formoterol, results in a reduction in β_2-receptor density and a concomitant decrease in β_2-receptor mRNA [64]. In cultured human airway epithelial cells, incubation with isoprenaline for 24 hours results in reduced expression of surface β_2-receptors as a consequence of reduced stability of β_2-receptor mRNA [65]. This suggests that down-regulation is achieved, in part, either by inhibiting the gene transcription of receptors or by increased post-transcriptional processing of the mRNA in the cell. Using actinomycin D to inhibit transcription, it has been found that β_2-receptor mRNA stability is markedly reduced in these cells after exposure to β-agonists. A specific protein, termed "βARB", that selectively binds to β_2-receptor mRNA is up-regulated by β_2-agonists and may be involved in the reduced stability of mRNA [66, 67]. Short-term exposure to β-agonists may increase β_2-receptor gene transcription through activation of CREB, but with prolonged agonist exposure there may also be inhibition of gene transcription [68].

Molecular mechanisms of down-regulation have recently been investigated in lung tissue after prolonged exposure to β-agonists. After a 7-day infusion of noradrenaline in guinea-pigs, there was a marked reduction in β_2-receptor density in lung parenchyma and this is accompanied by a similar reduction in steady-state β_2-receptor mRNA levels measured by Northern blotting. There is a difference between propensities to down-regulation in different cell types in the lung, as revealed by autoradiography and *in situ* hybridization, which shows a greater reduction in β_2-receptor density and mRNA in the alveolar wall than in airway smooth muscle [69]. This may relate to a greater rate of gene transcription in airway epithelial cells than in lung parenchyma. Similar data are observed in rats after long-term infusion with $(-)$-isoprenaline, with a reduction in β_2- and β_1-receptors [38]. In addition to the reduction in β_2-receptor mRNA, there is also a reduction in the activity of the transcription factor CREB, which may account for the reduced rate of β_2-receptor gene transcription [38]. The mechanisms that lead to reduced CREB activation are not yet understood but may be related to a reduction in cAMP, secondary to uncoupling of the receptor, or possibly to increased activity of CREM (Figure 7).

Less is understood about regulation of β_1-receptors, but in cultured cell lines differential regulation has been reported [70]. After chronic infusion

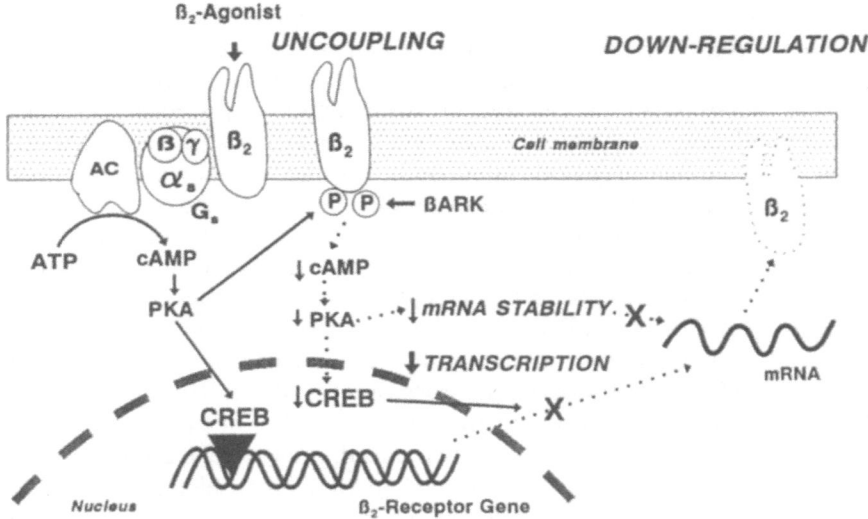

Figure 7. Long-term exposure to β-agonists may result in down-regulation and reduced gene transcription.

of β-agonists in guinea-pigs and rats, there is down-regulation of both β_1- and β_2-receptors and reduced mRNA expression in lung [38, 69]. Although the time course of reduction in β_1- and β_2-receptors is similar, there is a more rapid reduction in β_1-receptor mRNA.

There are marked differences between different cell types in their propensity to down-regulation. It has proved surprisingly difficult to demonstrate desensitization of the bronchodilator effect of β-agonists in asthmatic patients, although a small effect has been observed in normal subjects [71]. This is consistent with the resistance of airway smooth muscle to down-regulation, possibly because of the high level of β_2-receptor gene expression [38, 69]. Alternatively, it may be the result of the high density of "spare receptors", so that even marked reduction in β-receptor density may not be accompanied by a reduced relaxation response. Long-acting inhaled β_2-agonists may be more likely to induce tolerance, but several long-term studies of both salmeterol and formoterol have failed to show significant loss of bronchodilator response [72]. Recent studies with formoterol have demonstrated some loss of bronchodilator response after $1-2$ weeks of administration in asthmatic patients, if the studies are preceded by a wash-out period with anticholinergic drugs substituted for β-agonists [73, 74]. Recently it has been suggested that resistance to desensitization in airway smooth muscle cells may be caused by a very low level of expression of βARK in these cells [75].

Other effects of β-agonists on airway function do not appear to be as resistant to desensitization, presumably because tolerance is more easily produced in other cell types. Recent *in vivo* studies in human using positron emission tomography with a positron-emitting β-blocker (S-[^{11}C]CGP12177) have demonstrated an apparent reduction in pulmonary β-receptor density after 2 weeks of treatment with an inhaled or oral β_2-agonist [76]. Inhaled β_2-agonists have a much greater protective effect against AMP-induced bronchoconstriction than against methacholine-induced constriction, suggesting that there is some extra protective effect on mast cell mediator release [77]. After one week of regular inhaled β_2-agonist (terbutaline 500 μg four times daily) in patients with mild asthma, there is no evidence for tachyphylaxis of the bronchodilator response to terbutaline, a slight reduction in protection against methacholine and a marked reduction in protective effect against AMP, suggesting more marked desensitization of β_2-receptors on mast cells than on airway smooth muscle [78]. This is consistent with a much greater expression of βARK in mast cells than in airway smooth muscle cells [75]. Direct measurement of airway β-receptors has recently been made after inhaled β-agonists in normal subjects and demonstrates substantial down-regulation and uncoupling of β_2-receptors in epithelial cells and macrophages in normal subjects [79]. Desensitization of β_2-receptors on airway epithelial cells was also seen in asthmatic patients after treatment with an inhaled β_2-agonist [80].

5.2. Effect of Glucocorticosteroids

Glucocorticoids increase the transcription of several genes, including the β_2-receptor gene. The human β_2-receptor gene has several glucocorticoid response element consensus sequences (GREs) in its 5′-non-coding, coding and 3′-non-coding regions [81, 82]. The GREs in the 5′-non-coding region are obligatory for glucocorticoid responsiveness [83]. β-Adrenoceptor expression is increased by glucocorticoids in several cell types, including pulmonary cells. Glucocorticoids also prevent desensitization of β-receptors and restore down-reguled receptors to normal levels. In subjects taking a regular oral β_2-agonist, there is a down-regulation of β_2-receptor in lymphocytes; the receptors are restored to normal 16 h after a single dose (100 µg) of prednisone [84]. Similar changes are reported in asthmatic patients after a single dose of intravenous glucocorticoid, although this was not associated with any increase in bronchodilator responsiveness to an inhaled β_2-agonist [85]. Steroids increase the density of β_2-receptors in rat lung and prevent the desensitization and down-regulation of β-receptors on human leukocytes [86]. Corticosteroids increase the steady-state level of β_2-receptor mRNA in cultures hamster smooth muscle cells from the vas deferens without any increase in mRNA stability, thus indicating that steroids may increase β-receptor density by increasing the rate of gene transcription [87], (Figure 8). This is confirmed by an increased transcription rate in these cells

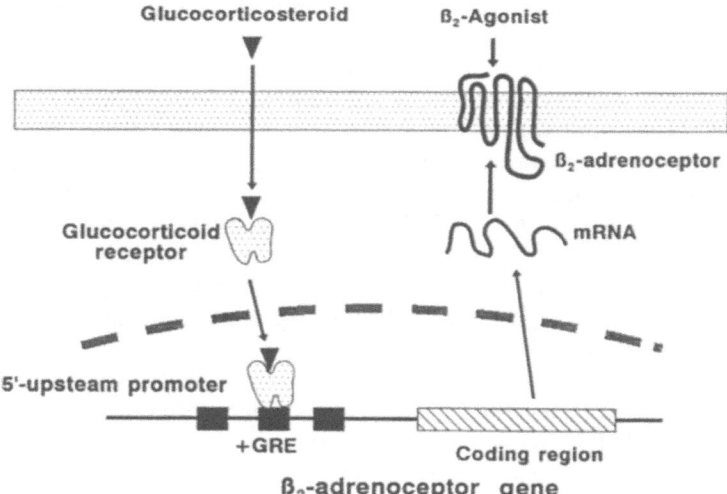

Figure 8. Effect of glucocorticoids on β_2-receptor gene transcription. Glucocorticoids bind to glucocorticoid receptors (GR) which translocate to the nucleus and bind to glucocorticoid response elements (GRE) on the upstream promoter region of the β_2-receptor gene; this leads to increased gene transcription, with an increase in mRNA and increased expression of the β_2-receptor.

measured by a nuclear run-on assay, which directly measures gene transcription [88]. The increase in mRNA occurs rapidly (within 1 h), preceding the increase in β_2-receptors, and then declines to a steady-state level about twice normal. Similarly steroids increase the gene expression of β_2-receptors in human lung tissue [89]. This is the result of increased transcription, as confirmed by a nuclear run-on assay.

Steroids increase the expression of β-receptors in all cell types, as revealed by autoradiographic mapping studies in rat lung [90]. Furthermore, steroids prevent the down-regulation of β_2-receptors in lung tissue after a prolonged infusion of isoprenaline. This appears to be caused by an increase in gene transcription which counteracts the decrease in transcription resulting from chronic β-agonist exposure. This protective effect of steroids is seen in airway smooth muscle and airway epithelial cells [90]. These studies have not been undertaken at a molecular level in humans, but treatment of the nasal mucosa with topical steroids increases β_2-receptor mRNA [91]. However, inhaled corticosteroids do not appear to prevent the development of tolerance to inhaled long-acting β_2-agonists [92, 93], which may be a result of the fact that the inhaled drug does not reach β_2-receptors in airway smooth muscle in adequate concentrations. By contrast, the tolerance to an inhaled β_2-agonist is rapidly reversed by high-dose parenteral corticosteroids [94].

β_1-Receptors, unlike β_2-receptors, have no GREs in their promoter region and glucocorticoids do not increase β_1-receptor density or mRNA in lung, or prevent homologous down-regulation [90].

5.3. Inflammation

Inflammatory mediators may impair the function of β-receptors [1]. In guinea-pigs phospholipase A_2 causes a reduction and uncoupling of pulmonary β-receptors, suggesting that lipid mediators may influence β-receptor function. Platelet-activating factor (PAF), leukotrienes and 15-lipoxygenase products have all been reported to reduce β-receptor function, although the mechanisms are often ill defined. Activation of inflammatory mediator receptors on airway smooth muscle cells may lead to activation of PKC, which has the capacity to phosphorylate both β-receptors and the α_s, thus resulting in either down-regulation or uncoupling of the receptor [95] (see Figure 5). In vitro studies show that bradykinin reduces the cAMP response to isoprenaline in cultured rabbit epithelial cells and that this effect is mimicked by PKC activation [96].

Cytokines may also influence β-receptor expression. In A549 cells (adenocarcinoma cell line with features of type II pneumocytes) interleukin 1β (IL-1β) and TNF-α increase β_2-receptor density and isoprenaline-induced cAMP increase [97] through an effect on gene transcription [98]. In contrast, IL-1β, IL-2 and granulocyte-macrophage colony-stimulating factors (GM-CSFs) are reported to inhibit isoprenaline-induced cAMP in human peripheral blood mononuclear cells [99], although there was no effect on β-agonist-induced relaxation of guinea-pig trachea under the same conditions. By contrast incubation of guinea-pig trachea with IL-1β and TNF-α for 18 h reduced isoprenaline-induced relaxation [100]. This effect was completely reversed by pertussis toxin, which implicates the involvement of G_i. Proinflammatory cytokines may increase the expression of α_i resulting in inhibition of adenylate cyclase and functional antagonism of β-agonists. Similarly, in a cultured human airway epithelial cell line (BEAS-2B), IL-1β decreased the cAMP response to isoprenaline, but paradoxically increased β_2-receptor mRNA, and this may reflect uncoupling and interruption of a negative regulation of gene expression [101]. *In vitro* IL-1β and TNF-α cause uncoupling of β_2-receptors in airway smooth muscle, and this may be a consequence of an increase in the inhibitory coupling protein G_i [102]. Similar results are obtained *in vivo* in rats exposed to infused IL-1β, where there is down-regulation of β_2-receptors, uncoupling and a reduction in bronchodilator responses to β-agonists. This is related to increased expression of G_i [103]. Transforming growth factor-β_1 (TGF-β_1) is produced by several cells in the airways, including macrophages and epithelial cells. TGF-β_1 reduces the density of β_2-receptors in cultured human airway smooth muscle cells through a mechanism that involves protein synthesis (possibly a transcription factor) [104].

5.4. Asthmatic Airways

There is evidence that β-receptors may be dysfunctional in asthmatic airways, because the bronchodilator response to β-agonists *in vitro* is impaired in airways taken from asthmatic patients who have died during an acute exacerbation [105]. In an autoradiographic study of a single patient with asthma who died from an asthmatic attack, no change in β-receptor density in airway smooth muscle was seen, despite a reduced relaxant response to isoprenaline [106]. Similarly, a normal airway distribution of β-receptors was reported in four patients with fatal asthma [107]. Surprisingly, an increase in both β-receptor density and affinity was observed in airway smooth muscle in seven cases of fatal asthma [108], and there is an inverse relationship between the impairment in relaxation response to isoprenaline and the increase in β-receptor density. These studies suggest that there is uncoupling of airway smooth muscle β-receptors in fatal asthma. The increase in β-receptor density may be the result of increased β_2-receptor gene transcription in response to some loss of negative feedback control of transcription. In the lungs of patients with mild asthma (transplantation donors) there was no difference either in β_1- or β_2-receptor density or in β-receptor mRNA compared with lungs of non-asthmatic lung donors [109]. Similarly in postmortem lung tissue there is no clear evidence for any difference in the amount of β_2-receptor mRNA in asthmatic patients compared with non-asthmatic controls [23]. Thus, although uncoupling of β-receptors may occur in fatal asthma (and may be a terminal event), it is unlikely that this is important in well-controlled asthmatic patients, because they respond so well to low doses of inhaled β-agonists. Recently, β_2-receptors have been assessed in biopsies from patients with asthma before and after segmental allergen challenge, which resulted in a small but insignificant reduction in β-agonist-induced cAMP production [80].

6. β_2-Receptor Polymorphisms

Several genetic polymorphisms of the human β_2-receptor gene have been reported and these may have clinical significance [110]. In a group of 51 asthmatic and 56 normal individuals, nine different point mutations in nucleic acid sequence were detected. Four of these polymorphisms resulted in a change in amino acid sequence, the most frequent of which were arginine 16 to glycine (Arg 16 → Gly) and glutamine 27 to glutamic acid (Gln 27 → Glu) [111]. The polymorphisms at codons 16 and 27 are relatively frequent and appear to be linked. In cells transfected with these mutant receptors, the Gln 27 → Glu mutation is resistant to β-agonist-induced down-regulation, whereas the Arg 16 → Gly mutation shows increased down-regulation compared with wild-type β_2-receptors [112]. As there is no difference in transcription rate between these receptors, the increased propensity to down-regulation of the Arg 16 → Gly mutation may reflect decreased receptor stability or increased degradation of mRNA. The incidence of β_2-receptor polymorphisms was no greater in asthmatic patients than in controls, although within the asthma group the polymorphism Arg 16 → Gly is associated with more severe asthma with increased nocturnal symptoms [113], whereas the Gln 27 → Glu polymorphism is associated with reduced airway hyperresponsiveness [114]. The Arg 16 → Gly polymorphism is also associated with an increased tendency to develop tolerance to inhaled β_2-agonists [115]. It is not yet certain whether there are also polymorphisms in the promoter region of the β_2-receptor gene in asthmatic patients that may predict altered regulation of the receptor.

References

1 Nijkamp FP, Engels F, Henricks PAJ, van Oosterhout AJM (1992) Mechanisms of β-adrenergic receptor regulation in lung and its implication for physiological responses. *Phys Rev* 72: 323–367
2 Barnes PJ (1995) Beta-adrenergic receptors and their regulation. *Am J Respir Crit Care Med* 152: 838–860
3 Frielle T, Collins S, Daniel KW, Capron MG, Lefkowitz RJ, Kobilka BK (1987) Cloning of the cDNA for the β₁-adrenergic receptor. *Proc Natl Acad Sci USA* 84: 7920–7924

4 Dixon RAP, Kobilka BK, Strader D, Benovic JL (1986) Cloning of the gene and cDNA for mammalian β-adrenergic receptor and homology with rhodopsin. *Nature* 321: 75–79

5 Chung F, Lentes K, Gocayne J et al. (1987) Cloning and sequence analysis of the human brain β-adrenergic receptor. *FEBS Lett* 211: 200–206

6 Emoring LJ, Marullo S, Briend-Sutren M, Patey G, Tate K, Delavier-Klutchko C, Strosberg AD (1989) Molecular characterization of the human β_3-adrenergic receptor. *Science* 245: 1118–1121

7 Ostrowski J, Kjelsberg MA, Caron MG, Lefkowitz RJ (1992) Mutagenesis of the β_2-adrenergic receptor: how structure elucidates function. *Annu Rev Pharmacol Toxicol* 32: 167–183

8 Kriff S, Lonnqvist F, Raimbault S et al. (1993) Tissue distribution of β_3-adrenergic receptor mRNA in man. *J Clin Invest* 91: 344–349

9 Thomas RF, Liggett SB (1993) Lack of beta$_3$-adrenergic receptor mRNA expression in adipose and other metabolic tissue in the adult human. *Mol Pharmacol* 43: 343–348

10 Strader CD, Sigal IS, Dixon RAF (1989) Structural basis of β-adrenergic receptor function. *FASEB J* 3: 1825–1832

11 Fraser CM, Chung F, Wang C, Venter JC (1988) Site-directed mutagenesis of human β-adrenergic receptors: substitution of aspartic acid-130 by asparagine produces a receptor with high-affinity agonist binding that is uncoupled for adenylate cyclase. *Proc Natl Acad Sci USA* 85: 5478–5482

12 Dixon RAF, Sigal IS, Rands E, Register RB, Candelore MR, Blake AD, Strader CD (1987) Ligand binding to the β-adrenergic receptor involves its rhodopsin-like core. *Nature* 326: 73–77

13 Fraser CM (1989) Site-directed mutagenesis of β-adrenergic receptors. *J Biol Chem* 264: 9266–9270

14 Chung F, Wang C, Potter PC, Venter JC, Fraser CM (1988) Site-directed mutagenesis and continuous expression of human β-adrenergic receptors. *J Biol Chem* 263: 4052–4055

15 Tota MR, Strader CD (1990) Characterization of the binding domain of the β-adrenergic receptor with the fluorescent antagonist carazolol. *J Biol Chem* 265: 16891–16897

16 Kobilka BK, Kobilka TS, Daniel K, Regan JW, Caron MG, Lefkowitz RJ (1988) Chimeric α_2 and β_2-adrenergic receptors: delineation of domains involved in effector coupling and ligand specificity. *Science* 240: 1310–1316

17 Nials AT, Sumner MJ, Johnson M, Coleman RA (1993) Investigations into factors determining duration of action of the β-adrenoceptor agonist salmeterol. *Br J Pharmacol* 108: 507–515

18 Green SA, Spasoff AP, Coleman RA, Johnson M, Liggett SB (1996) Sustained activation of a G protein-coupled receptor via "anchored" agonist binding. Molecular localization of the salmeterol exosite within the β_2-adrenergic receptor. *J Biol Chem* 271: 24029–24035

19 Anderson GP, Linden A, Rabe KF (1994) Why are long acting beta-adrenoceptor agonists long acting? *Eur Respir J* 7: 569–578

20 O'Dowd BF, Hnatowich M, Regan JW, Leader WM, Caron MG, Lefkowitz RJ (1988) Site-directed mutagenesis of the cytoplasmic domains of the human β_2-adrenergic receptor. *J Biol Chem* 263: 15985–15992

21 Samma P, Cotecchia S, Costa T, Lefkowitz RJ (1993) A mutation induced activated state of the β-adrenergic receptor. Extending the ternary complex model. *J Biol Chem* 268: 4625–4636

22 Hamid QA, Mak JC, Sheppard MN, Corrin B, Venter JC, Barnes PJ (1991) Localization of β_2-adrenoceptor messenger RNA in human and rat lung using *in situ* hybridization: correlation with receptor autoradiography. *Eur J Pharmacol* 206: 133–138

23 Bai TR, Zhou D, Aubert J, Lizee G, Hayashi S, Bondy GP (1993) Expression of β_2-adrenergic receptor mRNA in peripheral lung in asthma and chronic obstructive pulmonary disease. *Am J Respir Cell Mol Biol* 8: 325–333

24 Mak JCW, Nishikawa M, Haddad E-B, Kwon OJ, Hirst SJ, Twort CHC, Barnes PJ (1996) Localization and expression of β-adrenergic receptor subtype mRNAs in human lung. *Eur J Pharmacol (Mol Section)* 302: 215–221

25 Carstairs JR, Nimmo AJ, Barnes PJ (1985) Autoradiographic visualization of β-adrenoceptor subtypes in human lung. *Am Rev Respir Dis* 132: 541–547

26 Mak JCW, Nishikawa M, Barnes PJ (1994) Localization of β-adrenoceptor subtype mRNAs in human lung. *Am J Resp Crit Care Med* 149: 1027

27 Thomas RF, Liggett SB (1993) Lack of β_3 adrenergic receptor mRNA expression in adipose and other metabolic tissues in the adult human. *Mol Pharmacol* 43: 343–348

28 Torphy TJ (1994) β-Adrenoceptors, cAMP and airway smooth muscle relaxation: challenges to the dogma. *Trends Pharmacol Sci* 15: 370–374

29 Giembycz MA, Raeburn D (1991) Putative substrates for cyclic nucleotide-dependent protein kinases and the control of airway smooth muscle tone. *J Auton Pharmacol* 166: 365–398

30 Kume H, Hall IP, Washabau RJ, Takagi K, Kotlikoff MI (1994) Adrenergic agonists regulate K_{Ca} channels in airway smooth muscle by cAMP-dependent and -independent mechanisms. *J Clin Invest* 93: 371–379

31 Jones TR, Charette L, Garcia ML, Kaczorowski GJ (1993) Interaction of iberiotoxin with β-adrenoceptor agonists and sodium nitroprusside on guinea pig trachea. *J Appl Physiol* 74: 1879–1884

32 Miura M, Belvisi MG, Stretton CD, Yacoub MH, Barnes PJ (1992) Role of potassium channels in bronchodilator receptors in human airways. *Am Rev Respir Dis* 146: 132–136

33 Lalli E, Sassone-Corsi P (1994) Signal transduction and gene regulation: the nuclear response to cAMP. *J Biol Chem* 269: 17359–17362

34 Chrivia JC, Kwok RPS, Lamb N, Hagiwara M, Montminy MR, Goodman RH (1993) Phosphorylated CREB specifically binds to the nuclear factor CBP. *Nature* 365: 855–859

35 Foulkes NS, Sassone-Cursi P (1992) More is better: activators and repressors from the same gene. *Cell* 68: 411–414

36 Peters MJ, Adcock IM, Brown CR, Barnes PJ (1993) β-Agonist inhibition of steroid-receptor DNA binding activity in human lung. *Am Rev Respir Dis* 147: A772

37 Peters MJ, Adcock IM, Brown CR, Barnes PJ (1995) β-Adrenoceptor agonists interfere with glucocorticoid receptor DNA binding in rat lung. *Eur J Pharmacol (Mol Pharmacol Section)* 289: 275–281

38 Nishikawa M, Mak JCW, Shirasaki H, Barnes PJ (1993) Differential down-regulation of pulmonary β_1- and β_2-adrenoceptor messenger RNA with prolonged *in vivo* infusion of isoprenaline. *Eur J Pharmacol (Mol Section)* 247: 131–138

39 Collins S, Altschmied J, Herbsman O, Caron MG, Mellon PL, Lefkowitz RJ (1990) A cAMP element in the β_2-adrenergic receptor gene confers autoregulation by cAMP. *J Biol Chem* 265: 19930–19935

40 Collins S, Ostrowski J, Lefkowitz RJ (1993) Cloning and sequence analysis of the human β_1-adrenergic receptor 5′-flanking promoter region. *Biochim Biophys Acta* 1172: 171–174

41 Thomas RF, Holt BD, Schwinn DA, Liggett SB (1992) Long-term agonist exposure induces upregulation of β_3-adrenergic receptor expression via multiple cAMP response elements. *Proc Natl Acad Sci USA* 89: 4490–4494

42 Fernandes LB, Fryer AD, Hirshman CA (1992) M_2 muscarinic receptors inhibit isoproterenol-induced relaxation of canine airway smooth muscle. *J Pharmacol Exp Ther* 262: 119–126

43 Roffel AF, Meurs M, Elzinga CRS, Zaagsma J (1993) Muscarinic M_2 receptors do not participate in the functional antagonism between methacholine and isoprenaline in guinea pig tracheal smooth muscle. *Eur J Pharmacol* 249: 235–238

44 Rousell J, Haddad E-B, Webb BLJ, Giembycz MA, Mak JCW, Barnes PJ (1996) β-adrenoceptor-mediated down-regulation of M_2-muscarinic receptors: role of cAMP-dependent protein kinases and protein kinase C. *Mol Pharmacol* 49: 629–635

45 Kume H, Graziano MP, Kotlikoff MI (1992) Stimulatory and inhibitory regulation of calcium-activated potassium channels by guanine nucleotide binding proteins. *Proc Natl Acad Sci USA* 89: 11051–11055

46 Hall IP, Hill SJ (1988) $Beta_2$ adrenoceptor stimulation inhibits histamine-stimulated inositol phospholipid hydrolysis in bovine tracheal smooth muscle. *Br J Pharmacol* 95: 1204–1212

47 Pyne NJ, Freissmuth M, Palmer S (1992) Phosphorylation of the spliced variant forms of the recombinant stimulatory guanine-nucleotide-binding regulatory protein (G_{sa}) by protein kinase C. *Biochem J* 285: 333–338

48 Grandordy BM, Mak JCW, Barnes PJ (1994) Modulation of airway smooth muscle β-receptor function by a muscarinic agonist. *Life Sci* 54: 185–191

49 Masquilier D, Sassone-Corsi P (1992) Transcriptional cross talk: nuclear factors CREM and CREB bind to AP-1 sites and inhibit activation by Jun. *J Biol Chem* 267: 22460–22466

50 Imai F, Minger JN, Mitchell JA, Yamamoto KR, Granner DK (1993) Glucocorticoid receptor-cAMP response element-binding protein interaction and the response of the phosphoenolpyruvate carboxykinase gene to glucocorticoids. *J Biol Chem* 268: 5353–5356

51 Adcock IM, Stevens DA, Barnes PJ (1996) Interactions between steroids and β_2-agonists. *Eur Respir J* 9: 160–168

52 Bouvier M, Collins S, O'Dowd BF et al. (1989) Two distinct pathways of cAMP-mediated down-regulation of the β_2-adrenergic receptor. *J Biol Chem* 264: 16786–16792

53 Bouvier MW, Hausdorff A, DeBlasi A, O'Dowd BF, Kobilka BK, Caron MG, Lefkowitz RJ (1988) Removal of phosphorylation sites from the β-adrenergic receptor delays the onset of agonist-promoted desensitization. *Nature* 333: 370–373

54 Benovic JL, Strasser RH, Daniel K, Lefkowitz RJ (1986) Beta-adrenergic receptor kinase: identification of a novel protein kinase that phosphorylates the agonist-occupied form of the receptor. *Proc Natl Acad Sci USA* 83: 2797–2801

55 Inglese J, Freedman NJ, Koch WJ, Lefkowitz RJ (1993) Structure and mechanism of the G protein-coupled receptor kinases. *J Biol Chem* 268: 23735–23738

56 Koch WJ, Inglese J, Stone WC, Lefkowitz RJ (1993) The binding site for the beta gamma subunits of heterotrimeric G proteins on the β-adrenergic receptor kinase. *J Biol Chem* 268: 8256–8260

57 Loshe MJ, Benovic JL, Codina J, Caron MG, Lefkowitz RJ (1990) Beta arrestin: a protein that regulates beta-adrenergic receptor function. *Science* 248: 1547–1550

58 Pippig S, Andexinger S, Daniel K, Puzicha M, Caron MG, Lefkowitz RJ, Lohse MJ (1993) Overexpression of beta-arrestin and beta-adrenergic receptor kinase augment desensitization of beta 2-adrenergic receptors. *J Biol Chem* 268: 3201–3208

59 Pitcher J, Lohse MJ, Codina J, Caron MG, Lefkowitz RJ (1992) Densitization of the isolated β-adrenergic receptor β-adrenergic receptor kinase, cAMP-dependent protein kinase and protein kinase C occurs in distinct molecular mechanisms. *Biochemistry* 31: 3193–3197

60 Kelsen SG, Higgins NC, Zhou S, Mardini IA, Benovic JL (1995) Expression and function of the beta-adrenergic receptor coupled-adenylate cyclase system on human airway epithelial cells. *Am J Respir Crit Care Med* 152: 1774–1783

61 Hadcock JR, Port JD, Gelman MS, Malbon CC (1992) Cross-talk between tyrosine kinase and G protein-linked receptors. *J Biol Chem* 267: 26017–26022

62 Barak LS, Tiberi M, Freedman NJ, Kwatra MM, Lefkowitz RJ, Caron MG (1994) A highly conserved tyrosine residue in G-protein coupled receptors is required for agonist-mediated β_2-adrenergic receptor sequestration. *J Biol Chem* 269: 2790–2795

63 Hadcock JR, Wang HY, Malbon CC (1989) Agonist-induced destabilization of β-adrenergic receptor mRNA: attenuation of glucocorticoid-induced up-regulation of β-adrenergic receptors. *J Biol Chem* 264: 19928–19933

64 Nishikawa M, Mak JCW, Barnes PJ (1996) Effect of short- and long-acting β_2-agonists on pulmonary β_2-adrenoceptor expression in human lung. *Eur J Pharmacol* 318: 123–130

65 Kelsen SG, Anakwe OO, Aksoy MA, Reddy PJ, Dhanesekaran N, Penn R, Benovic JL (1997) Chronic effects of catecholamines on the beta 2-adrenoreceptor system in cultured human airway epithelial cells. *Am J Physiol* 272: L916–924

66 Port JD, Huang L, Malbon CC (1992) β-Adrenergic agonists that down-regulate receptor mRNA up-regulate a MR 35,000 protein(s) that selectively binds to β-adrenergic receptor mRNAs. *J Biol Chem* 267: 24103–24108

67 Huang LY, Tholanikunnel BG, Vakalopoulou E, Malbon CC (1993) The M(r) 35,000 beta-adrenergic receptor mRNA binding protein induced by agonists requires both an AUUUA pentamer and U-rich domains for RNA recognition. *J Biol Chem* 268: 25769–25775

68 Collins S, Caron MG, Lefkowitz RJ (1992) From ligand binding to gene expression: new insights into the regulation of G-protein-coupled receptors. *Trends Pharmacol Sci* 17: 37–39

69 Nishikawa M, Mak JCW, Shirasaki H, Harding SE, Barnes PJ (1994) Long term exposure to norepinephrine results in down-regulation and reduced mRNA expression of pulmonary β-adrenergic receptors in guinea pigs. *Am J Respir Cell Mol Biol* 10: 91–99

70 Suzuki T, Nguyen CT, Nantel F, Bovin H, Valiquette M, Frielle T, Bouvier M (1992) Distinct regulation of β_1- and β_2-adrenergic receptors in Chinese hamster fibroblasts. *Mol Pharmacol* 41: 542–551

71 Grove A, Lipworth BJ (1995) Tolerance with β_2-adrenoceptor agonists: time for reappraisal. *Br J Clin Pharmacol* 39: 109–118

72 Boulet L (1994) Long versus short-acting β_2-agonists. *Drugs* 47: 207–222

73 Newnham DM, McDevitt DG, Lipworth BJ (1994) Bronchodilator subsensitivity after chronic dosing with eformoterol in patients with asthma. *Am J Med* 97: 29–37

74 Yates DH, Sussman H, Shaw MJ, Barnes PJ, Chung KF (1995) Regular formoterol treatment in mild asthma: effect on bronchial responsiveness during and after treatment. *Am J Respir Crit Care Med* 152: 1170–1174

75 McGraw DW, Liggett SB (1997) Heterogeneity in beta-adrenergic receptor kinase expression in the lung accounts for cell-specific desensitization of the beta$_2$-adrenergic receptor. *J Biol Chem* 272: 7338–7344

76 Hayes MJ, Qing F, Rhodes CG et al. (1996) *In vivo* quantification of human pulmonary beta-adrenoceptors: effect of beta-agonist therapy. *Am J Respir Crit Care Med* 154: 1277–1283

77 O'Connor BJ, Fuller RW, Barnes PJ (1994) Non-bronchodilator effects of inhaled β_2-agonists. *Am J Respir Crit Care Med* 150: 381–387

78 O'Connor BJ, Aikman SL, Barnes PJ (1992) Tolerance to the non-bronchodilator effects of inhaled β_2-agonists. *N Engl J Med* 327: 1204–1208

79 Turki J, Green SA, Newman KB, Meyers MA, Liggett SB (1995) Human lung cell β_2-adrenergic receptors desnsitize in response to *in vivo* administered β-agonist. *Am J Physiol* 269: L709–L714

80 Penn RB, Shaver JR, Zangrilli JG, Pollice M, Fish JE, Peters SP, Benovic JL (1996) Effects of inflammation and acute β-agonist inhalation on β_2-AR signaling in human airways. *Am J Physiol* 271: L601–L608

81 Kobilka BK, Frielle T, Dohlman HG et al. (1987) Dilineation of the intronless nature of the genes for the human and hamster β_2-adrenergic receptor and their promoter regions. *J Biol Chem* 262: 7321–7327

82 Emorine LJ, Marullo S, Delavier-Klutchko C, Kaveri SV, Durieu-Trautmann O, Strusberg AD (1987) Structure of the gene for human β_2-adrenergic receptor: expression and promoter characterization. *Proc Natl Acad Sci USA* 84: 6995–6999

83 Malbon CC, Hadcock JR (1988) Evidence that glucocorticoid response elements in the 5' non-coding region of the hamster β_2-adrenergic receptor gene are obligative for glucocorticoid regulation of hamster mRNA levels. *Biochem Biophys Res Commun* 154: 676–681

84 Hui KKP, Conolly ME, Tashkin DP (1982) Reversal of human lymphocyte β-adrenoceptor desensitization by glucocorticoids. *Clin Pharmacol Ther* 32: 566–571

85 Brodie O, Brinkmann M, Schemuth R, O'Hara N, Daul A (1985) Terbutaline-induced desensitization of human lymphocyte β_2-adrenoceptors. Accelerated restoration of β-adrenoceptor responsivenes by prednisolone and ketotifen. *J Clin Invest* 1096: 1101

86 Davis AO, Lefkowitz RJ (1984) Regulation of beta-adrenergic receptors by steroid hormones. *Annu Rev Physiol* 46: 119–130

87 Collins S, Caron MG, Lefkowitz RJ (1988) β-Adrenergic receptors in hamster smooth muscle cells are transcriptionally regulated by glucocorticoids. *J Biol Chem* 263: 9067–9070

88 Hadcock JR, Williams DL, Malbon CC (1989) Physiological regulation at the level of mRNA: analysis of steady state levels of specific mRNAs by DNA-excess solution hybridization. *Am J Physiol* 256: C457–C465

89 Mak JCW, Nishikawa M, Barnes PJ (1995) Glucocorticosteroids increase β_2-adrenergic receptor transcription in human lung. *Am J Physiol* 12: L41–L46

90 Mak JCW, Nishikawa M, Shirasaki H, Miyayasu K, Barnes PJ (1995) Protective effects of a glucocorticoid on down-regulation of pulmonary β_2-adrenergic receptors *in vivo*. *J Clin Invest* 96: 99–106

91 Baraniuk JN, Ali M, Brody D et al. (1997) Glucocorticoids induce β_2-adrenergic receptor function in human nasal mucosa. *Am J Respir Crit Care Med* 155: 704–710

92 Yates DH, Kharitonov SA, Barnes PJ (1996) An inhaled glucocorticoid does not prevent tolerance to salmeterol in mild asthma. *Am J Respir Crit Care Med* 154: 1603–1607

93 Kalra S, Swystun VA, Bhagat R, Cockcroft DW (1996) Inhaled corticosteroids do not prevent the development of subsensitivity to salbutamol after twice daily salmeterol. *Chest* 109: 953–956

94 Tan KS, Grove A, McLean A, Gnosspelius Y, Hall IP, Lipworth BJ (1997) Systemic corticosteroid rapidly reverses bronchodilator subsensitivity induced by formoterol in asthmatic patients. *Am J Respir Crit Care Med* 156: 28–35

95 Bouvier M, Leeb-Lundberg LM, Benovic JL, Caron MG, Lefkowitz RJ (1987) Regulation of adrenergic receptor function by phosphorylatioin. II. Effects of agonist occupancy on phosporylation of α_1- and β-adrenergic receptors by protein kinase C and cyclic AMP-dependent protein kinase. *J Biol Chem* 262: 3106–3113

96 Mardini IA, Higgins NC, Zhou S, Benovic BL, Kelsen SG (1994) Functional behavior of the β-adrenergic receptor-adenyl cyclase system in rabbit airway epithelium. *Am J Respir Cell Mol Biol* 11: 287–295

97 Nakane T, Szentendrei L, Stern L, Virmani M, Seely J, Kunos G (1990) Effects of IL-1 and cortisol on beta-adrenergic receptors, cell proliferation and differentiation in cultured human A 549 lung tumor cells. *J Immunol* 145: 260–266

98 Szentendrei T, Lazar-Wesley C, Nakane T, Virmani M, Kunos G (1992) Selective regulation of β-adrenergic receptor gene expression by interleukin-1 in cultured human lung tumor cells. *J Cell Physiol* 152: 478–485

99 van Oosterhout AJM, Stam WB, Vanderscheueren RGJRA (1992) The effects of cytokines on β-adrenoceptor function of human peripheral blood mononuclear cells and guinea pig trachea. *J Allergy Clin Immunol* 90: 304–308

100 Wills-Karp M, Uchida Y, Lee JY, Jinot J, Hirata A, Hirata F (1993) Organ culture with pro-inflammatory cytokines reproduces impairment of the β-adrenoceptor-mediated relaxation in tracheas of a guinea pig antigen model. *Am J Respir Cell Mol Biol* 8: 153–159

101 Kelsen SG, Anakwe O, Zhou S, Benovic J, Aksoy M (1994) Interleukins impair beta adrenergic receptor-adenyl cyclase system function in human airway epithelial cells. *Am J Respir Crit Care Med* 149: A479

102 Hakanarson H, Herrick DJ, Serrano PG, Grunstein MM (1996) Mechanism of cytokine-induced modulaton of β-adrenoceptor responsiveness in airway smooth muscle. *J Clin Invest* 97: 2593–2600

103 Koto H, Mak JCW, Haddad E-B, Xu WB, Salmon M, Barnes PJ, Chung KF (1996) Mechanisms of impaired β-adrenergic receptor relaxation by interleukin-1β *in vivo* in rat. *J Clin Invest* 98: 1780–1787

104 Nogami M, Romberger DJ, Rennard SI, Toews ML (1994) TGF-β1 modules β-adrenergic receptor number and function in cultured human tracheal smooth muscle cells. *Am J Physiol* 266: L187–191

105 Bai TR (1991) Abnormalities in airway smooth muscle in fatal asthma: a comparison between trachea and bronchus. *Am Rev Respir Dis* 143: 441–443

106 Spina D, Rigby PJ, Paterson JW, Goldie RG (1989) Autoradiographic localization of beta-adrenoceptors in asthmatic human lung. *Am Rev Respir Dis* 140: 1410–1415

107 Sharma RK, Jeffery PK (1990) Airway β-adrenoceptor number in cystic fibrosis and asthma. *Clin Sci* 78: 409–417

108 Bai TR, Mak JCW, Barnes PJ (1992) A comparison of beta-adrenergic receptors and *in vitro* relaxant responses to isoproterenol in asthmatic airway smooth muscle. *Am J Respir Cell Mol Biol* 6: 647–651

109 Haddad E-B, Mak JCW, Barnes PJ (1996) Expression of β-adrenergic and muscarinic receptors in human lung. *Am J Physiol* 270: L947–L953

110 Hall IP (1996) β_2-Adrenoceptor polymorphisms: are they clinically important? *Thorax* 51: 351–353

111 Reihsaus E, Innis M, Macintyre N, Liggett SB (1993) Mutations in the gene encoding for the β_2-adrenergic receptor in normal and asthmatic subjects. *Am J Respir Cell Mol Biol* 8: 334–339

112 Green SA, Turi J, Innis M, Liggett SB (1994) Amino-terminal polymorphisms of the human β_2-adrenergic receptor impart distinct agonist-promoted regulatory properties. *Biochemistry* 33: 9414–9419

113 Turki J, Pak J, Green S, Martin R, Liggett SB (1995) Genetic polymorphism of the β_2-adrenergic receptor in nocturnal and non-nocturnal asthma: evidence that Gly 16 correlates with the nocturnal phenotype. *J Clin Invest* 95: 1635–1641

114 Hall IP, Wheatley A, Wilding P, Liggett SB (1995) Association of Glu 27 β_2-adrenoceptor polymorphism with lower airway reactivity in asthmatic subjects. *Lancet* 345: 1213–1214

115 Tan S, Hall IP, Dewar J, Dow E, Lipworth BJ (1997) Association between β_2-adrenoceptor polymorphism and susceptibility to bronchodilator desenitisation in moderately severe stable asthmatics. *Lancet* 350: 995–999

Molecular Biology of the Lung
Vol. 2: Asthma and Cancer
ed. by R.A. Stockley
© 1999 Birkhäuser Verlag Basel/Switzerland

CHAPTER 7
Regulation of Eosinophil Migration

Peter J. Jose, Anne Burke-Gaffney and Timothy J. Williams

Leukocyte Biology, Biomedical Sciences Division, Imperial College School of Medicine, London, UK

1   Introduction
2   Eosinophil Chemoattractants and Chemokines
2.1 CC Chemokines
3   Adhesion Pathways Involved in Eosinophil Migration
3.1 Rolling and Tethering
3.2 Firm Adhesion
3.3 Transmigration
4   Conclusions
     Acknowledgements
     References

1. Introduction

Eosinophils were first recognized about 100 years ago as cells with granules that display an affinity for eosin and other acidic dyes [1]. It was soon realized that the presence of eosinophils in tissue was associated with helminthic parasite infection, allergy, asthma and certain cancers. It is now generally believed that eosinophils are important effector cells in the beneficial host defence inflammatory response against helminthic parasites, and yet they can also play a major role in the excessive and inappropriate inflammatory responses seen in allergy and asthma.

Eosinophils can synthesize and secrete reactive oxygen species, platelet-activating factor (PAF), prostaglandins, leukotrienes (LTs), cytokines and enzymes which contribute to their inflammatory activity [2, 3]. The most prominent of the eosinophil granules contains basic proteins which are toxic to helminths and airway epithelium alike [4, 5]. These proteins are major basic protein, eosinophil cationic protein (ECP), eosinophil-derived neurotoxin and eosinophil peroxidase, which oxidizes halides to form reactive hypohalous acids. Release of basic proteins is generally taken as a sign of eosinophil activation and can be detected by morphological changes or by staining with monoclonal antibodies such as EG2, which recognizes the secreted form of ECP [6]. Eosinophil granule proteins have been detected in bronchoalveolar lavage (BAL) fluid of patients with symptomatic asthma [7].

Eosinophils are predominantly tissue-dwelling cells, which are formed in the bone marrow, and migrate into the blood and then into tissues, parti-

stages of eosinophil recruitment

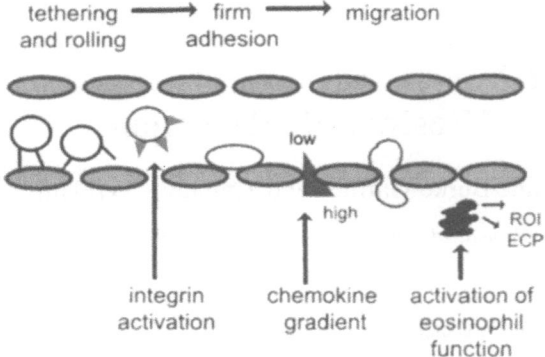

stages of chemokine action

Figure 1. Eosinophil recruitment showing tethering/rolling, firm adhesion, migration and the stages of chemokine action.

cularly those with a mucosal surface in contact with the environment: airways, gastrointestinal tract and genitourinary tract. As with other leukocytes, eosinophil movement from the bloodstream into tissue is mediated by chemoattractant molecules and follows sequential stages of interaction with the microvascular endothelium (Figure 1). Some cytokines, e.g. the interleukin IL-5, are known to increase eosinophil survival once they enter the tissue. Eosinophil accumulation in the absence of a concomitant accumulation of neutrophils is frequently described as "selective" or "preferential". Selective eosinophil accumulation in asthma suggests the involvement of specific pathways. These eosinophil-specific mechanisms may be: (1) the generation of eosinophil-selective chemoattractants or (2) the expression of eosinophil-selective adhesion molecules. These two mechanisms are the subject of this chapter.

2. Eosinophil Chemoattractants and Chemokines

Many of the classic chemoattractants influence both neutrophils and eosinophils. Thus, the generation of complement C5a, PAF and LTB$_4$ in the lung would not explain the selective eosinophilia seen in asthma, and there have been many attempt to find eosinophil-selective chemoattractants. As long ago as 1971, Kay et al. described an eosinophil chemotactic factor (ECF-A) released during anaphylaxis in the guinea-pig [8]. This was first identified as a tetrapeptide, although later it was suggested to be a lipoxygenase product of arachidonic acid [9], but it is now doubtful if it is as eosinophil selective as was first thought.

In the last 12 years, we have seen the discovery of the chemokines [10] starting with IL-8, primarily a neutrophil chemoattractant, although now known to be active on some other leukocytes including eosinophils, provided that they are first primed by the eosinophil-selective cytokine, IL-5. Chemokines are small, structurally-related and frequently heparin-binding chemotactic cytokines. Chemokines are synthesized with a hydrophobic signal sequence of about 20–25 amino acids which is cleaved to permit secretion of the relatively hydrophilic, basic mature protein; this is frequently about 70–80 amino acids (8–10-kDa). Occasionally chemokines may be larger and the molecular size may also be increased by glycosylation, which usually has little effect on biological activity *in vitro* but may serve to alter the stability or reactivity of these proteins *in vivo*.

It has been estimated that there may be up to 100 chemokines that can act on up to 30 chemokine receptors. Many chemokines are at present only identified as "expressed sequence tags" and thus the biological activity remains to be determined [10, 11]. Similarly, many of the receptors are "orphans" where the ligand still requires identification. It is expected that many of these gaps in our knowledge will soon be answered. Thus, selective chemokine production in the tissues and selective expression of receptors on the target cells offer the possibility of delicate control of inflammatory cell accumulation.

A common feature of chemokines is a motif of four cysteines which forms two intramolecular disulphide bonds [10]. The arrangement of the two cysteines near the amino terminus provides a structural basis for the classification of chemokines into four groups (Figure 2):

1. The CC chemokines have a pair of adjacent cysteines and are encoded on human chromosome 17. Monocyte chemoattractant protein-1 (MCP-1)

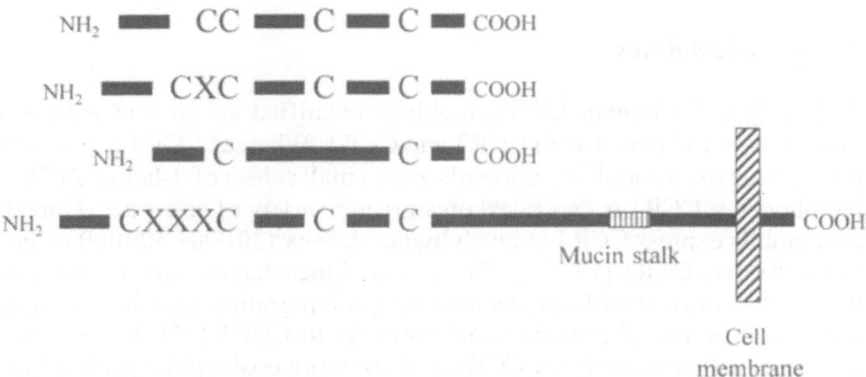

Figure 2. The four groups of chemokines showing differences in the arrangement of cysteines at the amino (NH$_2$) terminus. A large mucin stalk connects the CX$_3$C chemokine to a transmembrane segment and an intracellular domain.

was the first identified member of this class and has been shown to stimulate monocytes, lymphocytes and basophils. However, MCP-1 has little or no activity on eosinophils which lack its receptors. There are nine CC chemokine receptors (CCR1−9) so far identified. With the exception of IL-8, which has some effect on primed eosinophils, all known eosinophil-stimulating chemokines are of the CC class and signal through CCR3, CCR1 or both, which are the only CC chemokine receptors identified on eosinophils so far [12−14].

2. In the CXC chemokines, encoded on chromosome 4, there is an intervening amino acid (X) between the pair of amino-terminal cysteines. This apparently small structural difference makes the CXC chemokines sufficiently distinct from the CC chemokines that their actions are mediated via a different set of receptors (CXCR1−4). IL-8 is the most well described CXC chemokine.

3. In the C chemokines, the first and third cysteines have been lost such that there is only a single intramolecular disulphide bond. Lymphotactin [15] which acts on lymphocytes is the only published example of this class of chemokines. It is encoded on chromosome 1 and its receptor(s) has not yet been identified.

4. The most recently described class of chemokines, CX_3C, has three intervening amino acids between the amino-terminal pair of cysteines. Fractalkine [16], encoded on chromosome 16, is so far the only published member of this class and a receptor (CX_3CR1) has recently been identified. Fractalkine is an unusual molecule in that its complementary DNA (cDNA) predicts that the chemokine protein is attached to a mucin-like stalk which traverses the cell membrane. The cell-bound protein promotes strong adhesion of mononuclear leukocytes and a soluble form of fractalkine is a potent chemoattractant for these target cells.

2.1. CC Chemokines

Table 1 lists the human CC chemokines identified so far and indicates those known to interact with CCR3 and CCR1. Whereas CCR3 expression is restricted to eosinophils, basophils and a small subset of T-helper 2 (Th2) lymphocytes, CCR1 is expressed on a greater variety of cell types. Human eosinophils express CCR3 at much higher density (30 000−300 000 receptors/cell) than CCR1 [12−14]. Thus, chemokines that act on CCR3 are of the greatest interest with respect to eosinophil migration, and this has been confirmed by use of a monoclonal antibody to CCR3 [17]. Eotaxin and eotaxin-2 act exclusively on CCR3 and are more eosinophil specific than the other eosinophil-stimulating chemokines, which also interact with other receptors expressed on other cell types. RANTES and MCP-3 act on both CCR3 and CCR1, whereas in humans MIP-1α acts on CCR1 but not

Table 1. Interaction of human CC chemokines with receptors expressed on eosinophils

Receptor	CCR3	CCR1
Expression	High	Low
CC chemokine		
Eotaxin	++	
Eotaxin-2	++	
MIP-1α		+
MIP-1β		
MIP-3		
MIP-4		
MIP-5	+	+
RANTES	+	+
MCP-1		
MCP-2	+	+
MCP-3	+	+
MCP-4	++	
HCC-1		
I-309		
STCP-1		
TARC		
LARC		
ELC		

Original references and databank accession numbers for most of these human CC chemokines are given in Coulin et al. [11] and Baggiolini et al. [10]. For eotaxin-2, see Forssmann et al. [32].

CCR3 (although there is a species difference because in mouse MIP-1α signalling via CCR3 is more important than via CCR1).

Some of the major breakthroughs in chemokine biology have come from identification, characterization, purification and then sequencing of novel activities. Such an approach led to the discovery of IL-8 [18] and MCP-1 [19], the first described CXC and CC chemokines, respectively. Meanwhile other chemokines were discovered by molecular biological techniques. RANTES was first identified by use of subtractive hybridization and later found to stimulate memory T lymphocytes of the CD45RO+ phenotype [20]. However, Kameyoshi et al. made the important discovery that RANTES is also a chemoattractant for human eosinophils [21]. These authors were looking for eosinophil chemoattractants released from T lymphocytes and discovered that the major activity was, in fact, RANTES released from contaminating platelets. They also demonstrated probable glycosylation of the platelet-derived RANTES.

In contrast to the above work using cell culture supernatants, eotaxin was discovered by analysis of an *in vivo* animal model of allergic airway inflammation [22, 23]. Guinea-pigs were sensitized to ovalbumin and then exposed to an aerosolized ovalbumin challenge. Bronchoalveolar lavage (BAL) fluid collected 3–6 h after exposure to the allergen contained eosinophil chemoattractant activity when tested *in vivo* in naive guinea-pigs [23]. This assay involved injecting ^{111}In-labelled eosinophils intravenously, followed by intradermal injection of the BAL fluid. The accumulation of radioactivity in the injected skin sites provided a sensitive detection of eosinophil migration. Purification of the eosinophil chemoattractant, monitored throughout by the *in vivo* bioassay, was followed by amino acid sequencing which revealed a novel CC chemokine. As a result of its eosinophil selectivity and its chemotactic activity *in vitro*, we termed the protein "eotaxin". Eotaxin mRNA [24, 25] and protein [26] are expressed constitutively in guinea-pig lung and upregulated within 3–6 h of allergen challenge. The time course of eotaxin protein generation correlates well with the onset of eosinophil infiltration into the lung tissue, although there is a delay before large numbers of eosinophils are found in the airway lumen [26].

Degenerate primers based on the guinea-pig protein sequence permitted the cloning of guinea-pig eotaxin [24, 25]. The nucleotide sequence information was then used to clone mouse [27, 28], human [14, 29, 30] and rat [31] eotaxin. This work has now provided reagents to study eotaxin generation and action in greater depth. Eotaxin up-regulation after allergen challenge has been demonstrated in mouse and humans and it has been confirmed that eotaxin is more selective than other CC chemokines for eosinophils. Human eotaxin-2 has also been identified and shown to act only through CCR3 with a similar potency to eotaxin [32].

All of the eosinophil chemoattractant activity in BAL fluid of allergen-challenged guinea-pigs is neutralized by anti-eotaxin antibodies, suggesting that eotaxin is the major eosinophil chemoattractant generated. However, the situation is more complex for allergic airway inflammation in the mouse, where antibodies to eotaxin [33], MIP-1α [34], RANTES [34], MCP-3 [35] and MCP-5 [36] have all been shown, at least partially, to inhibit eosinophil accumulation. Some of this diversity of chemokines may be the result of differences in the strain of mouse or the protocols used for sensitization and challenge. It is also possible that some of the effects of these antibodies is primarily an inhibition of the influx or activation of leukocytes other than eosinophils. For example, MCP-5, which has been identified only in the mouse, is a good chemoattractant for lymphocytes and monocytes [36, 37], yet its reported ability as an eosinophil chemoattractant [36] has been disputed [37, 38]. As MCP-5 is up-regulated earlier than eotaxin [36], it may contribute to eosinophil accumulation by inducing an influx of mononuclear cells which then secrete eotaxin. Nevertheless, it is clear that a number of chemokines can contribute to eosinophil accumulation in the mouse which may explain why eosinophil accumulation is not completely abolished in eotaxin knock-out mice [39]. Clearly, CCR3 knock-outs are required to see if chemoattractants acting on other receptors will mediate allergic eosinophil accumulation. Given the plethora of CC chemokines acting on eosinophils, it is notable that eosinophil accumulation 18 h after allergen challenge was reduced by 70% in the eotaxin knock-outs [39] which suggests that, in mouse as well as in guinea-pig, eotaxin is a major eosinophil chemoattractant.

Lymphocytes play a role in controlling eosinophil accumulation in asthma via the generation of Th2 cytokines such as IL-4 and IL-5 [40]. IL-4 induces CC chemokines in some cells [41, 42] and we have found that anti-eotaxin antibodies partially inhibit IL-4-induced eosinophil accumulation [42]. IL-4 also induces expression of vascular cell adhesion molecule 1 (VCAM-1) on endothelial cells (see below) and so acts on two arms of the cell accumulation process. IL-5 has potent effects on eosinophils and we have found that IL-5 and eotaxin can act synergistically to induce eosinophil accumulation [43]. Elimination of T lymphocyte accumulation in murine models of allergic airway inflammation results in a reduction in eosinophil recruitment associated with eotaxin down-regulation [33, 44]. However, whereas MacLean et al. [44] proposed that the T cells were required for control of eotaxin synthesis, Gonzalo et al. [33] reported that T cell depletion reduced adhesion molecule expression rather than eotaxin generation.

In humans, as in mice, there are several CC chemokines that induce eosinophil migration, mostly through interaction with CCR3 (Table 1). Eotaxin, eotaxin-2 and MCP-4 are approximately equipotent and ten times more potent than RANTES and MCP-3, whereas MIP-1α is active on the less abundant CCR1. Alam et al. [45] found small increases in the levels of RANTES and MIP-1α in ten times concentrated BAL fluid from asthma patients compared with non-asthmatic controls. Eosinophil chemotactic activity was strongly inhibited by a polyclonal anti-RANTES antibody. However, the antibody was as active against MCP-3 (and perhaps other CC chemokines) as against RANTES, which makes it difficult to make firm conclusions as to the identity of the eosinophil chemoattractant(s). Venge et al. [46] found that the very weak chemotactic activity for eosinophils in BAL fluid taken from asthmatic patients during the season of high birch pollen allergen levels was partially blocked by antibodies to RANTES.

Segmental allergen challenge of people with asthma has proved to be a valuable model to investigate inflammatory mechanisms and a prominent influx of leukocytes, including eosinophils, was detected in biopsies taken 5–6 h after challenge [47]. Given that the generation of chemoattractants precedes eosinophil infiltration, Teran et al. [48] examined BAL fluid 4 h after segmental challenge. They purified an eosinophil chemoattractant and identified it as RANTES. Measurement of RANTES in ten times concentrated BAL fluid showed an increase from 4 pmol/l after instillation of saline to approximately 20 pmol/l after allergen. These authors looked for, but could not detect, eosinophil chemoattractant activity other than RANTES.

Eotaxin expression in the bronchial mucosa of people with asthma is higher than in non-asthmatic controls, and the cell sources of this increased expression include epithelial cells, endothelial cells, macrophages, T cells and eosinophils [49–51]. Lamkhioued et al. [51] reported levels of approximately 60 pmol/l eotaxin in ten times concentrated BAL fluid from asthmatic patients compared with 15 pmol/l in non-asthmatic controls. These are much higher levels of eotaxin than we have found (PJ Jose et al., unpublished data) and, given the greater potency of eotaxin than RANTES in the chemotactic assay, it is difficult to see how Teran et al. [48] could have missed such high levels of eotaxin. Nevertheless, Lamkhioued et al. [51] also found that eosinophil chemotactic activity in asthmatic BAL fluid was partially blocked by antibodies to eotaxin, RANTES and MCP-4. A combination of all three antibodies blocked the chemotactic response by approximately 50% [51], which suggests that all three CC chemokines, as well as other unidentified mediators, contribute to eosinophil accumulation in asthma. Clearly, more work remains to be done.

3. Adhesion Pathways Involved in Eosinophil Migration

For more than 150 years, it has been known that leukocyte recruitment into areas of inflammation starts with the binding of leukocytes to the endothelial lining of blood vessels, followed by their transmigration into tissues. In contrast, an understanding of the molecular mechanisms responsible for leukocyte recruitment has only become possible in the last 15 years, with the identification of leukocyte and endothelial adhesion molecules and leukocyte chemoattractant/activator molecules. Three families of cell adhesion molecules play a key role in leukocyte recruitment: the selectins, the integrins and the immunoglobulin superfamily [52]. It is now recognized that these different types of adhesion molecules, together with chemoattractants, must interact in a programmed, sequential manner for leukocyte recruitment to occur [52, 53]. The purpose of this section of the chapter is to summarize the adhesion pathways involved in leukocyte recruitment to areas of inflammation, with particular emphasis on eosinophil-selective pathways and recruitment into the airways.

Leukocyte recruitment occurs in the postcapillary venules of most tissues including the bronchial circulation of the airways. There are three distinct phases described as: (1) rolling and tethering, (2) firm adhesion, and (3) transmigration, as shown in Figure 1 [52, 53]. The first phase involves a slowing of the circulating leukocytes within the venule, with the leukocytes becoming loosely attached, or tethered, to the endothelium. The making and breaking of contacts between the leukocytes and the endothelial cells then give the impression of leukocytes rolling along the vessel wall. After a variable period of rolling, many leukocytes firmly adhere to the endothelial cell surface and change shape from a spherical to a flattened form. Leukocytes may also attach to each other, in addition to the endothelium, and form aggregates or "strings" of leukocytes. Adherent cells then move through the junction between the endothelial cells and migrate into the surrounding tissue. Each step of leukocyte recruitment is associated with specific adhesion molecules (Figure 3).

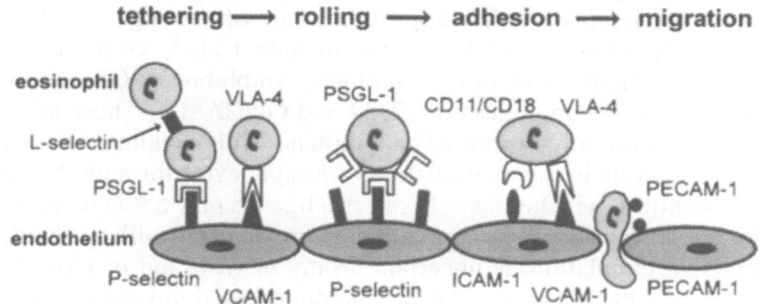

Figure 3. Adhesion molecules and their interactions involved in eosinophil recruitment (see text for details).

3.1. Rolling and Tethering

The selectin family of adhesion molecules plays a key role in the early phase of leukocyte rolling (Figure 3). The selectins are a family of three closely related cell surface molecules: E-selectin, expressed exclusively on endothelial cells; P-selectin, expressed on endothelial cells and platelets; and L-selectin which is constitutively expressed on most leukocytes but not on endothelial cells [54].

The molecular structure of selectins makes them the most ideally suited of the adhesion molecule families to mediate leukocyte-endothelial interactions under conditions of flow. The selectins have a unique and characteristic extracellular region made up of an amino-terminal calcium-dependent lectin domain, an epidermal growth factor (EGF)-like domain and a varying number of short consensus repeats (SCR) similar to those found in complement regulatory proteins [54]. Although these domains are found in numerous other proteins, the selectins are the only known example in which the three types of domain are found in immediate juxtaposition. This suggests that the spatial arrangement is important for receptor function [54]. The lectin domain plays an essential role in selectin-mediated adhesion because it binds to specific carbohydrate sugar residues, such as sialic acid and fucose, known to be essential components of selectin ligands [54]. The EGF-like domain is thought to contribute structural information required for the correct presentation of the lectin domain [54]. The SCR domain extends the ligand-binding domain away from the cell surface and thus may facilitate contact with selectin ligands presented on moving leukocytes [54].

As suggested above, the selectin ligands are, at least in part, carbohydrate. The prototype ligand for selectins is sialyl Lewis X, a tetrasaccharide of which two residues are fucose and sialic acid [54]. Selectin adhesion is uniformly dependent on sialic acid and there is strong evidence that all three selectins require fucose. It is now also apparent that L- and P-selectins, but not E-selectin, require a sulphate group on one of the sugar residues for adhesion [54]. Ligands for L-selectin include CD34, GlyCAM-1 and MAdCAM-1, originally identified in mouse lymph nodes. Of these, there are known human homologues of CD34 and GlyCAM-1. These adhesion molecules are normally expressed on lymph node high endothelial venules and play a key role in the recirculation of lymphocytes through the lymph nodes. In contrast, whether these L-selectin ligands play a role in leukocyte recruitment during airway inflammation, from the postcapillary venules of the bronchial circulation, is uncertain. Many *in vitro* and *in vivo* studies have suggested the existence of a carbohydrate-based inducible ligand for L-selectin on activated vascular endothelium, although its identity has still to be defined. Several glycoprotein ligands for E-selectin have been identified on leukocytes, including E-selectin ligand-1 (ESL-1). P-selectin glycoprotein-1 (PSGL-1), expressed on all leukocytes, is a counter-receptor for P-selectin and also for E-selectin which it binds with a lower affinity [54].

Small changes in blood flow and/or release of inflammatory mediators induce the endothelial expression of P- and E-selectin. P-selectin is thought to mediate the earliest leukocyte rolling because this stage is absent in P-selectin knock-out mice [54]. This early rolling is probably triggered after the release of histamine from tissue mast cells because histamine is known rapidly to mobilize P-selectin from the Weibel–Palade bodies to the cell surface [52]. Thrombin, complement fragments, free radicals and cytokines can also cause a rapid (peaks at 10 min), but transient (returns to basal levels by 20–30 min), increase in P-selectin [52]. In addition to the rapid expression of P-selectin at the cell surface, cytokines elevated during airway inflammation (e.g. tumour necrosis factor-α or TNF-α) and lipopolysaccharide (LPS) can up-regulate P-selectin at the transcriptional level [52]. P-selectin-deficient mice show reduced lung eosinophilia compared with wild-type controls at 3 h after allergen challenge, which suggests an important role for P-selectin in eosinophil recruitment into the lungs during inflammation [55]. However, the degree of inhibition declines at 24 h post-challenge, suggesting that other adhesion molecules may play a more prominent role than P-selectin at later times [55].

E-selectin also supports leukocyte rolling at sites of inflammation; however, because of the requirement for gene transcription for E-selectin expression, it does not contribute to rolling at the earliest phase of leukocyte recruitment. E-selectin is detected after stimulation with inflammatory cytokines, such as IL-1 and TNF-α, or bacterial products including LPS. E-selectin expression peaks at 4–6 h on cultured endothelial cells, for example, human lung microvascular endothelial cells (HLMVECs), and returns to basal levels within about 24 h [56]. E-selectin expression is also increased in bronchial biopsy tissue from patients with rhinitis compared with control patients [57], which may indicate a role for E-selectin in this upper airway inflammatory process. Also, monoclonal antibodies (mAbs)

against E-selectin blocked neutrophil influx and late-phase bronchoconstriction, after a single inhalation challenge, in a primate model of asthma
[57]. In contrast, however, E-selectin mAb did not reduce either acute
allergen-induced, or chronic allergen exposure-induced, eosinophilia in
this primate model [57]. Thus, E-selectin appears to be primarily involved
in neutrophil, rather than eosinophil, airway recruitment.

The apparent difference between the involvement of E-selectin in neutrophil and eosinophil rolling can also be seen *in vitro*. Eosinophils, compared
with neutrophils, show markedly less binding to E-selectin-coated plates in a
flow chamber, but significantly stronger avidity for P-selectin [58]. Stronger
avidity of eosinophils for P-selectin may result from the higher levels of
expression of PSGL-1, the P-selectin ligand, on eosinophils than neutrophils
[59]. In contrast, sialyl Lewis X, to which E-selectin may bind, is expressed at
lower levels on eosinophils than neutrophils and to our knowledge ESL-1, the
E-selectin ligand originally identified on murine neutrophils, has not been
detected on eosinophils. Similar studies carried out using TNF-α-stimulated
human umbilical vein endothelial cells (HUVECs) suggest that eosinophil
tethering to the endothelium is strongly dependent on P-selectin, but not E-
selectin, under physiological conditions of shear [58]. Also, the finding that
eosinophils have a higher avidity for P-selectin than neutrophils suggests that
the selective induction of P-selectin compared with E-selectin, for example, by
histamine and thrombin, may favour preferential eosinophil accumulation.

In contrast to the differential use of E- and P-selectin in the early phase
of neutrophil and eosinophil recruitment, L-selectin is involved equally in
both [58]. This suggests that eosinophils express L-selectin ligands equally to neutrophils. Leukocyte tethering through L-selectin is usually divided
into two different categories: direct tethering of leukocytes on the underlying
substrate (primary tethering) and interactions between flowing leukocytes
and leukocytes already attached to the endothelium (secondary tethering).
In this way strings of leukocytes accumulate on the endothelium. Anti-L-
selectin mAb appears to block interactions between leukocytes and prevents the formation of eosinophil or neutrophil strings *in vitro* [58]. This
suggests that one important function of L-selectin in eosinophil recruitment into the airways may be to mediate leukocyte–leukocyte, rather than
leukocyte–endothelial, interactions.

As suggested above, the lack of inhibition of eosinophil rolling at 24 h
after allergen challenge in P-selectin-deficient mice [58] suggests that
other adhesion molecules may play a more prominent role than P-selectin
at later time points. At 24 h after allergen challenge the lung endothelium
is likely to express intracellular adhesion molecule-1 (ICAM-1) and
VCAM-1, members of the immunoglobulin superfamily of adhesion molecules. These are the endothelial ligands for leukocyte β_2-integrins and the
β_1-integrin, VLA-4 ($\alpha_4\beta_1$), respectively [52]. Eosinophils and mononuclear
cells, but not neutrophils, express VLA-4 [52]. Under non-flow conditions
the major role of VLA-4 is to mediate firm adhesion of eosinophils to the

endothelium (as will be discussed later). VLA-4 has, however, been shown to contribute to eosinophil tethering interactions *in vivo* [60].

The nature of VLA-4's contribution to tethering can be seen *in vitro*. Eosinophils tether on VCAM-1-coated plates under conditions of flow, although at a lower shear stress than on selectins [58]. Also, in contrast to selectins, when eosinophils tether on VCAM-1 they appear not to roll along the endothelium but to arrest or stop immediately after the initial tethering. Tethered eosinophils may then detach within seconds unless stimulated with a chemokine, such as eotaxin, to increase the avidity of VLA-4 for its ligands [58]. After eotaxin stimulation, all tethered eosinophils arrest. When, however, TNF-α-stimulated HUVECs were used instead of VCAM-1-coated plates in similar experiments, an anti-VLA-4 mAb did not significantly reduce tethering to HUVECs [58]. This suggests that, when P-selectin and VCAM-1 are present together, such as on TNF-α-activated HUVECs, VLA-4 may have only a minor role to play in initial tethering [58]. In the absence of P-selectin, however, for example, in P-selectin-deficient mice, VLA-4 may play a more dominant role and account for the lack of inhibition of leukocyte recruitment 24 h after allergen challenge seen in these knock-out mice [55].

3.2. Firm Adhesion

When selectin-mediated rolling has slowed the leukocytes down sufficiently, firm adhesion can occur. Firm adhesion of eosinophils requires the interaction of endothelial immunoglobulin (Ig)-like adhesion molecules, ICAM-1, ICAM-2 and VCAM-1, with their respective leukocyte integrin counterligands (Figure 3) [52, 61]. Integrins are transmembrane cell surface proteins which consist of a heterodimer of non-covalently linked α and β chains; these together determine ligand-binding specificity [52]. The α chain also binds divalent cations and this has an important role to play in increasing the avidity of integrins for their ligands [52]. There are at least eight known α subunits and 15 known β subunits which combine to give about 21 different integrins; these are expressed on many different cell types. Those known to be expressed on eosinophils include several members of the β_1-integrin family: $\alpha_4\beta_1$ (VLA-4), $\alpha_6\beta_1$ (VLA-6; laminin receptor) and possibly $\alpha_5\beta_1$ (VLA-5; fibronectin receptor) [62]. Members of the β_2-integrin family, $\alpha_L\beta_2$ (CD11a/CD18), $\alpha_M\beta_2$ (CD11b/CD18) and $\alpha_x\beta_2$ (CD11c/CD18) are also expressed on eosinophils [52]. Of these, the integrins that play a key role in the firm adhesion of eosinophils to endothelial cells are considered to be VLA-4, CD11a/CD18 and CD11b/CD18 [52].

CD11a/CD18 binds to ICAM-1 and ICAM-2 [52]. In contrast, CD11b/CD18 only binds to ICAM-1 [52]. ICAM-1, unlike E-selectin, is expressed under non-inflammatory basal conditions on leukocytes, epithelial cells and smooth muscle cells, in addition to endothelial cells [63]. TNF-α,

IL-1, LPS, thrombin and exposure to oxygen radicals up-regulate ICAM-1 expression [52, 63]. In general, expression is detectable at 2–4 h, maximal at 24 h and may be sustained up to 72 h; this has been shown for HLM-VECs [56]. In contrast to ICAM-1, inflammatory stimuli do not up-regulate expression of ICAM-2. Compelling evidence showing that ICAM-1 is up-regulated 5–6 h after allergen challenge in human asthma [57], and that ICAM-1 mAbs inhibit airway eosinophilia and hyperresponsiveness in a primate model of asthma [64] suggests an involvement of ICAM-1 in eosinophil recruitment in the airways.

VLA-4 binds to VCAM-1 expressed on endothelial cells, as discussed above for eosinophil tethering, and also to fibronectin associated with the extracellular matrix [52]. VCAM-1 is the third member of the Ig family, expressed on endothelial cells and involved in firm adhesion of eosinophils [52]. There are two known forms of VCAM-1: one, with six Ig domains, is an alternatively spliced variant of the predominant seven-domain form [52, 61]. VCAM-1, like ICAM-1, is expressed on other cell types in addition to endothelial cells but, like E-selectin, VCAM-1 is not normally constitutively expressed. The stimuli that induce VCAM-1 include those that also induce ICAM-1 and E-selectin expression, for example, IL-1, TNF-α and LPS [56]. Increased expression can usually be detected within 2 h of stimulation and often reaches maximal expression at 16–24 h; up-regulation may last for 72 h, although this is dependent on the induction stimulus [56].

IL-4, a 20-kDa glycoprotein secreted by activated T lymphocytes [40] and mast cells [65], also induces VCAM-1 expression on endothelial cells derived from several vascular sites including HLMVECs [56]. Unlike IL-1, TNF-α or LPS, IL-4 does not increase ICAM-1 or E-selectin expression [56], although it may decrease expression of these adhesion molecules induced by other cytokines [66]. In contrast, IL-4 enhances LPS, IL-1 or TNF-α-induced VCAM-1 expression [56, 66]. The presence of IL-4 may thus result in selective VCAM-1 expression. Raised levels of IL-4, detected in asthma, may therefore contribute to the preferential recruitment of eosinophils to the airways in this disease. IL-13 has similar activities to IL-4 on endothelial cells because both cytokines bind to the IL-4 receptor α chain expressed on endothelial cells [67]. Thus, IL-13 also preferentially increases VCAM-1 expression [68]. Evidence for the involvement of VCAM-1 in airway inflammation comes from studies showing that VCAM-1 expression is increased in nasal biopsies from patients with rhinitis [58]. Also increased VCAM-1 expression and subsequent eosinophil and T lymphocyte accumulation are found after bronchial allergen challenge in asthmatic patients [57].

In addition to selective expression of endothelial adhesion molecules, up-regulation of expression and/or ligand affinity of β_1- and β_2-integrins by eosinophil-selective chemokines may also contribute to preferential eosinophil recruitment. An important characteristic of leukocyte integrins, in particular β_2-integrins, is that under non-inflammatory conditions they exist in a relatively inactive conformation, rendering the leukocytes non-adhesive. One of the key events of leukocyte recruitment is the activation and up-regulation, followed by deactivation, of these integrins at the proper time and place. The CC chemokines eotaxin, RANTES, MCP-3 and MCP-4 increase CD11b expression [69–72]. Eotaxin has also been shown to increase eosinophil adhesion to HLMVECs [73] and RANTES has been shown to increase adhesion to plates coated with soluble ICAM-1 [74]. Furthermore, RANTES and MCP-3 have been shown rapidly to increase the adhesiveness of eosinophil VLA-4 for VCAM-1 [71]. Monoclonal antibodies against VLA-4 and CD18 inhibit eotaxin-stimulated eosinophil adhesion to cytokine-activated HLMVECs [73] and eosinophil recruitment *in vivo* [42], consistent with the hypothesis that CC chemokines increase avidity of VLA-4 for VCAM-1 in addition to increasing CD11b expression.

One important way in which leukocyte integrins are activated is as the result of leukocyte interaction with chemoattractants bound to the surface of the endothelium. This manner of activation has been described for the CXC chemokine, IL-8. Presentation of IL-8 in this way may facilitate CD11b/CD18 up-regulation on leukocytes, because blood flow is less likely to remove or dilute it [53]. The kinetics of IL-8 production are similar to E-selectin expression and it is thought that simultaneous expression of an adhesion molecule involved in leukocyte rolling, and a chemokine that activates leukocyte integrins, is instrumental in converting rolling to firm adhesion [53]. The extent to which endothelial-bound CC chemokines may contribute to eosinophil integrin activation is unknown. It is possible, however, that endothelial presentation of these chemokines, with simultaneous expression of endothelial adhesion molecules, such as P-selectin or VCAM-1, may play a similar role in eosinophil recruitment.

Fractalkine is a recently identified chemokine that is known to be expressed on the endothelial surface. To date, this is the only known CX_3C chemokine and it is unique in that the chemokine domain sits on a mucin-like stalk [16]. Fractalkine is induced on cultured endothelial cells and is known to promote adhesion of monocytes and activated T cells *in vitro*. It is not clear whether, in addition to activating adhesion molecules on the leukocyte, the unique structure of fractalkine means that its binding to leukocyte receptors can contribute to the adhesive interactions in the absence of transduction signals. It will be interesting to see whether similar transmembrane chemokines with activity on eosinophils are identified.

3.3. Transmigration

Finally, after firm adhesion of leukocytes to the endothelium, leukocytes undergo dramatic shape change which allows them to pass through the interendothelial junction of the vessel wall and migrate into the surrounding tissue. For transmigration to occur a chemotactic gradient is thought to be necessary. In addition to facilitating firm adhesion, ICAM-1 and VCAM-1 are also thought to aid transmigration. Another member of the Ig family is platelet endothelial cell adhesion molecule-1 (PECAM-1; CD31) which is not involved in firm adhesion but plays a key role in transmigration (see Figure 3) [52, 75]. PECAM-1 has six Ig-like domains and is expressed in large amounts on resting endothelium where it is specifically located at the endothelial junctions. This localization is thought to facilitate its role in migration and it may act to guide leukocytes through the interendothelial junction [75]. Migration is mediated via homotypic binding to PECAM-1 expressed on leukocytes [52] and heterotypic binding to the leukocyte integrin $\alpha_v\beta_3$.

4. Conclusions

This chapter has described some of the mechanisms underlying eosinophil recruitment in the lung. Compelling, but still circumstantial, evidence in humans suggests that blocking eosinophil recruitment or activation would have an important therapeutic effect in diseases such as asthma, by preventing the pathogenesis associated with the release of toxic eosinophil products within the lung tissue.

Three clear therapeutic targets emerge from the analysis of basis mechanisms. First, animal models strongly suggest that eotaxin and related CC chemokines are of central importance for eosinophil recruitment. Therefore, blockade of the eotaxin, receptor, CCR3, with a small molecule antagonist is an attractive target. Second, IL-5 is a pivotal cytokine with respect to eosinophil biology, both in its actions alone on eosinophilopoiesis and eosinophil survival, but also acting in synergy with other mediators such as eotaxin. Humanized antibodies to IL-5 are now in clinical trials. Third, VLA-4 is important for the attachment of eosinophils to both microvascular endothelial cells during eosinophil recruitment and extravascular cells relating to leukocyte activation and subsequent airway hyperresponsiveness. Small molecule VLA-4 antagonists are currently being tested.

Therapeutic strategies based on these targets will provide the acid test in humans of the precise inter-relationship of eosinophil recruitment, airway damage and lung dysfunction.

Acknowledgements

We are grateful to the National Asthma Campaign and the Wellcome Trust for support.

References

1 Ehrlich P, Lazarus A, Meyers W (eds) (1900) *Normal and pathological.* Cambridge University Press, Cambridge, 148

2 Wardlaw AJ, Moqbel R, Kay AB, Kay AB (eds) (1997) *Allergy and allergic diseases,* Blackwell Science vol 10, *Eosinophils and the allergic inflammatory response.* Oxford, 171–197

3 Weller PF (1997) Human eosinophils. *J Allergy Clin Immunol* 100: 283–287

4 Butterworth AE (1984) Cell-mediated damage to helminths. *Adv Parasitol* 23: 143–235

5 Frigas E, Loegering DA, Gleich GJ (1980) Cytotoxic effects of the guinea pig eosinophil. Major basic protein on tracheal epithelium. *Lab Invest* 42: 35–43

6 Tai PC, Spry CJ, Peterson C, Venge P, Olsson I (1984) Monoclonal antibodies distinguished between storage and secreted forms of eosinophil cationic protein. *Nature* 309: 182–184

7 Wardlaw AJ, Dunnette S, Gleich GJ, Collins JV, Kay AB (1988) Eosinophils and mast cells in bronchoalveolar lavage in subjects with mild asthma. Relationship to bronchial hyperreactivity. *Am Rev Respir Dis* 137: 62–69

8 Kay AB, Stechschulte DJ, Austen KF (1971) An eosinophil leukocyte chemotactic factor of anaphylaxis. *J Exp Med* 133: 602–619

9 Sehmi R, Cromwell O, Taylor GW, Kay AB (1991) Identification of guinea pig eosinophil chemotactic factor of anaphylaxis as leukotriene B$_4$ and 8(S)-dihydroxy-5,9,11,13 (Z,E, Z,E)-eicosatetraenoic acid. *J Immunol* 147: 2276–2283

10 Baggiolini M, Dewald B, Moser B (1997) Human cytokines: An update. *Annu Rev Immunol* 15: 675–705

11 Coulin F, Power CA, Alouani S, Peitsch MC, Schroeder J, Moshizuki M, Clark-Lewis I, Wells TNC (1997) Characterisation of macrophage inflammatory protein-5/human CC cytokine-2, a member of the macrophage-inflammatory-protein family of chemokines. *Eur J Biochem* 248: 507–515

12 Daugherty BL, Siciliano SJ, DeMartino J, Malkowitz L, Sirontino A, Springer MS (1996) Cloning, expression and characterization of the human eosinophil eotaxin receptor. *J Exp Med* 183: 2349–2354

13 Ponath PD, Qin S, Post TW, Wang J, Wu L, Gerard NP, Newman W, Gerard C, Mackay CR (1996) Molecular cloning and characterization of a human eotaxin receptor expressed selectively on eosinophils. *J Exp Med* 183: 2437–2448

14 Kitaura M, Nakajima T, Imai T, Harada S, Combadiere C, Tiffany HL, Murphy PM, Yoshie O (1996) Molecular cloning of human eotaxin, an eosinophil-selective CC chemokine, and identification of a specific eosinophil eotaxin receptor, CC chemokine receptor 3. *J Biol Chem* 271: 7725–7730

15 Kelner GS, Kennedy J, Bacon KB, Kleyensteuber S, Largaespada DA, Jenkins NA, Copeland NA, Bazan JF, Moore KW, Schall TJ et al. (1994) Lymphotactin: A cytokine that represents a new class of chemokine. *Science* 266: 1395–1399

16 Bazan JF, Bacon KB, Hardiman G, Wang W, Greaves DR, Zlotnik A, Schall TJ (1997) A new class of membrane-bound chemokine with a CX$_3$C motif. *Nature* 385: 640–644

17 Heath H, Qin S, Wu L, LaRosa G, Kassam N, Ponath PD, Mackay CR (1997) Chemokine receptor usage by human eosinophils. The importance of CCR3 demonstrated using an antagonistic monoclonal antibody. *J Clin Invest* 99: 178–184

18 Yoshimura T, Matsushima K, Tanaka S, Robinson EA, Appella E, Oppenheim JJ, Leonard EJ (1987) Purification of a human monocyte-derived neutrophil chemotactic factor that has peptide sequence similarity to other host defense cytokines. *Proc Nat Acad Sci USA* 84: 9233–9237

19 Matsushima K, Larsen CG, Dubois GC, Oppenheim JJ (1989) Purification and characterization of a novel monocyte chemotactic and activating factor produced by a human myelomonocytic cell line. *J Exp Med* 169: 1485–1490

20 Schall TJ, Bacon K, Toy KI, Goeddel DV (1990) Selective attraction of monocytes and T lymphocytes of the memory phenotype by cytokine RANTES. *Nature* 347: 669–671

21 Kameyoshi Y, Dorschner A, Mallet AI, Christophers E, Schröder J (1992) Cytokine RANTES released by thrombin-stimulated platetets is a potent attractant for human eosinophils. *J Exp Med* 176: 587–592

22 Griffiths-Johnson DA, Collins PD, Rossi AG, Jose PJ, Williams TJ (1993) The chemokine, Eotaxin, activates guinea-pig eosinophils *in vitro,* and causes their accumulation into the lung *in vivo. Biochem Biophys Res Commun* 197: 1167–1172

23 Jose PJ, Griffiths-Johnson DA, Collins PD, Walsh DT, Moqbel R, Totty NF, Truong O, Hsuan JJ, Williams TJ (1994) Eotaxin: A potent eosinophil chemoattractant cytokine detected in a guinea-pig model of allergic airways inflammation. *J Exp Med* 179: 881–887

24 Jose PJ, Adcock IM, Griffiths-Johnson DA, Berkman N, Wells TNC, Williams TJ, Power CA (1994) Eotaxin: Cloning of an eosinophil chemoattractant cytokine and increased mRNA expression in allergen-challenged guinea-pig lungs. *Biochem Biophys Res Commun* 205: 788–794

25 Rothenberg ME, Luster AD, Lilly CM, Drazen JM, Leder P (1995) Constitutive and allergen-induced expression of eotaxin mRNA in the guinea pig lung. *J Exp Med* 181: 1211–1216

26 Humbles AA, Conroy DM, Marleau S, Rankin SM, Palframan RT, Proudfoot AEI, Wells TNC, Dechun L, Jeffery PK, Griffiths-Johnson DA et al. (1997) Kinetics of eotaxin generation and its relationship to eosinophil accumulation in allergic airways disease: analysis in a guinea pig model *in vivo*. *J Exp Med* 186: 601–612

27 Rothenberg ME, Luster AD, Leder P (1995) Murine eotaxin: An eosinophil chemoattractant inducible in endothelial cells and in interleukin 4-induced tumor suppression. *Proc Natl Acad Sci USA* 92: 8960–8964

28 Gonzalo J, Jia G, Aguirre V, Friend D, Coyle AJ, Jenkins NA, Lin G, Katz H, Lichtman A, Copeland N et al. (1996) Mouse eotaxin expression parallels eosinophil accumulation during lung allergic inflammation but it is not restricted to a Th2-type response. *Immunity* 4: 1–14

29 Ponath PD, Qin S, Ringler DJ, Clark-Lewis I, Wang J, Kassam N, Smith H, Shi X, Gonzalo J, Newman W et al. (1996) Cloning of the human eosinophil chemoattractant, eotaxin. Expression, receptor binding and functional properties suggest a mechanism for the selective recruitment of eosinophils. *J Clin Invest* 97: 604–612

30 Garcia-Zepeda EA, Rothenberg ME, Ownbey RT, Celestin J, Leder P, Luster AD (1996) Human eotaxin is a specific chemoattractant for eosinophil cells and provides a new mechanism to explain tissue eosinophilia. *Nature Med* 2: 449–456

31 Williams CMM, Newton DJ, Wilson SA, Williams TJ, Coleman JW, Flanagan BF (1998) Conserved structure and tissue expression of rat eotaxin. *Immunogenetics* 47: 178–180

32 Forssmann U, Uguccioni M, Loetscher P, Dahinden CA, Langen H, Thelen M, Baggiolini M (1997) Eotaxin-2, a novel CC chemokine that is selective for the chemokine receptor CCR3, and acts like eotaxin on human eosinophil and basophil leukocytes. *J Exp Med* 185: 2171–2176

33 Gonzalo J, Lloyd CM, Kremer L, Finger E, Martinez-A C, Siegelman MH, Cybulsky MI, Gutierrez-Ramos J (1996) Eosinophil recruitment to the lung in a murine model of allergic inflammation. The role of T cells, chemokines and adhesion receptors. *J Clin Invest* 98: 2332–2345

34 Lukacs NW, Strieter RM, Warmington K, Lincoln P, Chensue SW, Kunkel SL (1997) Differential recruitment of leukocyte populations and alteration of airway hyperreactivity by C-C family chemokines in allergic airway inflammation. *J Immunol* 158: 4398–4404

35 Stafford S, Li H, Forsythe PA, Ryan M, Bravo R, Alam R (1997) Monocyte chemotactic protein-3 (MCP-3)/fibroblast-induced cytokine (FIC) in eosinophilic inflammation of the airways and the inhibitory effects of an anti-MCP-3/FIC antibody. *J Immunol* 158: 4953–4960

36 Jia G, Gonzalo J, Lloyd C, Kremer L, Lu L, Martinez-A C, Wershil BK, Gutierrez-Ramos J (1996) Distinct expression and function of the novel mouse chemokine monocyte chemotactic protein-5 in lung allergic inflammation. *J Exp Med* 184: 1939–1951

37 Sarafi MN, Garcia-Zepeda EA, MacLean JA, Charo IF, Luster AD (1997) Murine monocyte chemoattractant protein (MCP)-5: a novel CC chemokine that is a structural and functional homologue of human MCP-1. *J Exp Med* 185: 99–109

38 Teixeira MM, Wells TNC, Lukacs NW, Proudfoot AEI, Kunkel SL, Williams TJ, Hellewell PG (1997) Chemokine-induced eosinophil recruitment. Evidence of a role for endogenous eotaxin in an *in vivo* allergy model in mouse skin. *J Clin Invest* 100: 1657–1666

39 Rothenberg ME, MacLean JA, Pearlman E, Luster AD, Leder P (1997) Targeted disruption of the chemokine eotaxin partially reduces antigen-induced tissue eosinophilia. *J Exp Med* 4: 785–790

40 Corrigan CJ, Kay AB (1992) T cells and eosinophils in the pathogenesis of asthma. *Immunol Today* 13: 501–507

41 Kishimoto TK, Jutila MA, Butcher EC (1990) Identification of a human peripheral lymph node homing receptor: a rapidly down-regulated adhesion molecule. *Proc Natl Acad Sci USA* 87: 2244–2248

42 Sanz M, Ponath PD, Mackay CR et al. (1998) Human eotaxin induces α_4 and β_2 integrin-dependent eosinophil accumulation in rat skin *in vivo*: delayed generation of eotaxin in response to IL-4. *J Immunol* 160: 3566–3576

43 Collins PD, Marleau S, Griffiths-Johnson DA, Jose PJ, Williams TJ (1995) Co-operation between interleukin-5 and the chemokine eotaxin to induce eosinophil accumulation *in vivo*. *J Exp Med* 182: 1169–1174

44 MacLean JA, Ownbey R, Luster AD (1996) T cell-dependent regulation of eotaxin in antigen-induced pulmonary eosinophilia. *J Exp Med* 184: 1461–1469

45 Alam R, York J, Boyars M, Stafford S, Grant JA, Lee J, Forsythe P, Sim T, Ida N (1996) Increased MCP-1, RANTES, and MIP-1a in bronchoalveolar lavage fluid of allergic asthmatic patients. *Am J Respir Crit Care Med* 153: 1398–1404

46 Venge J, Lampinen M, Håkansson L, Rak S, Venge P (1996) Identification of IL-5 and RANTES as the major eosinophil chemoattractants in the asthmatic lung. *J Allergy Clin Immunol* 97: 1110–1115

47 Montefort S, Gratziou C, Goulding D, Polosa R, Haskard DO, Howarth PH, Holgate ST, Carroll MP (1994) Bronchial biopsy evidence for leukocyte infiltration and upregulation of leukocyte–endothelial cell adhesion molecules 6 hours after local allergen challenge of sensitized asthmatic airways. *J Clin Invest* 93: 1411–1421

48 Teran LM, Noso N, Carroll M, Davies DE, Holgate S, Schroder J (1996) Eosinophil recruitment following allergen challenge is associated with the release of the chemokine RANTES into asthmatic airways. *J Immunol* 157: 1806–1812

49 Ying S, Robinson DS, Meng Q, Rottman J, Kennedy R, Ringler DJ, Mackay CR, Daugherty BL, Springer MS, Durham SR et al. (1997) Enhanced expression of eotaxin and CCR3 mRNA and protein in atopic asthma. Association with airway hyperresponsiveness and predominant co-localization of eotaxin mRNA to bronchial epithelial and endothelial cells. *Eur J Immunol* 27: 3507–3516

50 Mattoli S, Stacey MA, Sun G, Bellini A, Marini M (1997) Eotaxin expression and eosinophilic inflammation in asthma. *Biochem Biophys Res Commun* 236: 299–301

51 Lamkhioued B, Renzi PM, Younes A, Garcia-Zepeda EA, Allakhverdi Z, Ghaffar O, Rothenberg MD, Luster AD, Hamid QA (1997) Increased expression of eotaxin in bronchoalveolar lavage and airways of asthmatics contributes to the chemotaxis of eosinophils to the site of inflammation. *J Clin Immunol* 159: 4593–4601

52 Carlos TM, Harlan JM (1994) Leukocyte-endothelial adhesion molecules. *Blood* 84: 2068–2101

53 Albelda SM, Smith CW, Ward PA (1994) Adhesion molecules in inflammatory injury. *FASEB J* 8: 504–512

54 Kansas GS (1996) Selectins and their ligands: current concepts and controversies. *Blood* 88: 3259–3287

55 Broide DH, Sullivan S, Gifford T, Sriramarao P (1998) Inhibition of pulmonary eosinophilia in P-selectin-and ICAM-1-deficient mice. *Am J Respir Cell Mol Biol* 18: 218–225

56 Blease K, Seybold J, Adcock IM, Hellewell PG, Burke-Gaffney A (1998) Interleukin-4 and lipopolysaccharide synergise to induce vascular cell adhesion molecule-1 expression in human lung microvascular endothelial cells. *Am J Respir Cell Mol Biol* 18: 620–630

57 Montefort S, Holgate ST, Howarth PH (1993) Leukocyte-endothelial adhesion molecules and their role in bronchial asthma and allergic rhinitis. *Eur Respir J* 6: 1044–1054

58 Kitayama J, Fuhlbrigge RC, Puri KD, Springer TA (1997) P-selectin, L-selectin, and α_4 integrin have distinct roles in eosinophil tethering and arrest on vascular endothelial cells under physiological flow conditions. *J Immunol* 159: 3929–3939

59 Symon FA, Lawrence MB, Williamson ML, Walsh GM, Watson SR, Wardlaw AJ (1996) Functional and structural characterization of the eosinophil P-selectin ligand. *J Immunol* 157: 1711–1719

60 Sriramarao P, von Andrian UH, Butcher EC, Bourdon MA, Broide DH (1994) L-selectin and very late antigen-4 integrin promote eosinophil rolling at physiological shear rates *in vivo*. *J Immunol* 153: 4238–4246

61 Malik AB, Lo SK (1996) Vascular endothelial adhesion molecules and tissue inflammation. *Pharmacol Rev* 48: 213–229

62 Kuijpers TW, Mul FPJ, Blom M, Kovach NL, Gaeta FCA, Toliefson V, Elices MJ, Harlan JM (1993) Freezing adhesion molecules in a state of high-avidity binding blocks eosinophil migration. *J Exp Med* 178: 279–284

63 van de Stolpe A, van der Saag PT (1996) Intercellular adhesion molecule-1. *J Mol Med* 74: 13–33

64 Wegner CD, Gundel RH, Reilly P, Haynes N, Letts LG, Rothlein R (1990) Intercellular adhesion molecule-1 (ICAM-1) in the pathogenesis of asthma. *Science* 247: 456–459

65 Bradding P, Feather IH, Howarth PH, Mueller R, Roberts JA, Britten K, Bews JPA, Hunt TC, Okayama Y, Heusser CH et al. (1992) Interleukin 4 is localised to and released by human mast cells. *J Exp Med* 176: 1381–6

66 Thornhill MH, Haskard DO (1990) IL-4 regulates endothelial cell activation by IL-1, tumor necrosis factor, or IFN-gamma. *J Immunol* 145: 865–872

67 Synder B, Lugli S, Feng N, Etter R, Lutz A, Ryffel B, Sugamura K, Wunderli-Allenspach H, Moser R (1996) Interleukin-4 (IL-4) and IL-13 bind to a shared heterodimeric complex on endothelial cells mediating vascular cell adhesion molecule-1 induction in the absence of the common gamma chain. *Blood* 87: 4286–4295

68 Bochner BS, Klunk DA, Sterbinsky SA, Coffman RL, Schleimer RP (1995) IL-13 selectively induces vascular cell adhesion molecule-1 expression in human endothelial cells. *J Immunol* 154: 799–803

69 Elsner J, Hochstetter R, Kimmig D, Kapp A (1996) Human eotaxin represents a potent activator of the respiratory burst of human eosinophils. *Eur J Immunol* 26: 1919–1925

70 Tenscher K, Metzner B, Schöpf E, Norgauer J, Czech W (1996) Recombinant human eotaxin induces oxygen radical production, Ca^{2+}-mobilization, actin reorganization, and CD11b upregulation in human eosinophils via a Pertussis toxin-sensitive heterotrimeric guanine nucleotide-binding protein. *Blood* 88: 3195–3199

71 Weber C, Kitayama J, Springer TA (1996) Differential regulation of β1 and β2 integrin avidity by chemoattractants in eosinophils. *Proc Natl Acad Sci USA* 93: 10939–10944

72 Tenscher K, Metzner B, Hofmann C, Schopf E, Norgauer J (1997) The monocyte chemotactic protein-4 induces oxygen radical production, actin reorganization, and CD11b upregulation via a pertussin toxin-sensitive G-protein in human eosinophils. *Biochem Biophys Res Commun* 240:32–35

73 Burke-Gaffney A, Hellewell PG (1996) Eotaxin stimulates eosinophil adhesion to human lung microvascular endothelial cells. *Biochem Biophys Res Commun* 227: 35–40

74 Alam R, Stafford S, Forsythe P, Harrison R, Faubion D, Lett-Brown MA, Grant JA (1993) RANTES is a chemotactic and activating factor for human eosinophils. *J Immunol* 150: 3442–3447

75 Wakelin MW, Sanz M-T, Dewar A, Albelda SM, Larkin SW, Boughton-Smith NK, Williams TJ, Nourshargh S (1996) An anti-PECAM-1 antibody inhibits leukocyte extravasation from mesenteric microvessels *in vivo* by blocking the passage through the basement membrane. *J Exp Med* 184: 229–239

Molecular Biology of the Lung
Vol. 2: Asthma and Cancer
ed. by R. A. Stockley
© 1999 Birkhäuser Verlag Basel/Switzerland

CHAPTER 8
Proteinase Allergens of House Dust Mites: Molecular Biology, Biochemistry and Possible Functional Significance of Their Enzyme Activity

Clive Robinson, Hong Wan, Helen L. Winton, David R. Garrod[1], Geoffrey A. Stewart[2] and Philip J. Thompson[3]

Department of Pharmacoloy & Clinical Pharmacology, St George's Hospital Medical School, London, UK
[1] *School of Biological Sciences, University of Manchester, Manchester, UK*
[2] *Department of Microbiology, University of Western Australia, Nedlands, Western Australia*
[3] *Department of Medicine, Universiy of Western Australia, Nedlands, Western Australia*

1   Introduction
2   Proteinase Allergens
3   House Dust Mite Allergens
3.1 HDM Allergens in Groups 3, 6, and 9
4   Other Sources of Allergens with Enzymatic Activity
5   Interactions of Proteinase Allergens and the Airway Epithelium
6   Concluding Comments
     Acknowledgements
     References

1. Introduction

Asthma is a debilitating and life-threatening disease which is now the most common chronic disease of childhood. Sensitization of the lung to airbone allergens such as faecal pellet proteins of the house dust mite (HDM) is a primary risk factor for the development of asthma [1–5]. Allergic sensitization involves detection of an allergen by antigen-presenting cells [6–8] of the pulmonary immune system and subsequent activation of the immunoglobulin IgE production by B lymphocytes. In the lung, dendritic antigen-presenting cells are shielded from direct contact with the external environment by the protective lining created by the lung epithelium [6, 8]. How the immune system is exposed to allergens is therefore central to the development of asthma, but the mechanism is unclear.

The HDM represents a particularly important risk factor for asthma [2–4]. As human lifestyles become increasingly affluent and create domestic conditions favourable to HDMs, their spread may, in part, explain the increasing prevalence of the disease [5]. HDM faecal pellets present in the environment are inspired during breathing. The diameter of these pellets typically ranges from 10 to 40 μm [1]; consequently, when inhaled the large majority are likely to impact upon the surface lining of the first three generations of the airway tree [9]. Upon impaction on the airway surface, the pellets will be hydrated by epithelial lining fluid, causing leakage of their contents onto the airway lining. A high concentration of allergen is probably achieved initially at the site of impaction because HDM faecal pellets rapidly discharge their contents when they become hydrated [1]. It seems reasonable to propose that what follows in the process of allergic sensitization is heavily dependent upon the interactions that occur between allergens and the airway epithelium. However, this subject has been the topic of remarkably little study and is only now really gaining attention following the growing awareness that allergens may behave in a wider sense as pharmacologically activ proteins [6].

One of the defining characteristics of epithelia is that they are sophisticated barriers which separate compositionally distinct environments [10–13]. The epithelial lining of the airways is no exception in this regard; it acts as an interface between the pulmonary immune system and external environment [13]. The presence of a diverse variety of potentially threatening agents (viruses, bacteria, fungal spores, toxic chemicals and allergens) in inspired air results in the airway epithelium being under particularly heavy assault from substances likely to trigger either innate or adaptive responses in the host immune system. The airways have evolved specialized defences to cope with many types of external threat, but there is still a surprisingly poor understanding of how events at the airway mucosal interface lead to pathophysiological responses and disease [13]. In this chapter we consider the implications that recent advances in allergen biology have for understanding the key events in sensitization. In particular, we will concentrat upon recent studies that have highlighted the possible significance of the proteolytic activity of major HDM allergens which are prominent risk factors for allergic asthma.

2. Proteinase Allergens

Several airborne allergens associated with asthma are now known to have putative proteolytic activity (reviewed in Robinson et al. [6]). Most work in this area has concentrated on allergens from HDM, particularly the mite *Dermatophagoides pteronyssinus*, but allergens from non-mite sources have also been identified whose amino acid sequences have some similarity with proteolytic enzymes. This review will give most consideration to the possible significance of proteinase activity in HDM allergens because these have been the subject of recent study, but brief reference will also be made to some airborne allergens of non-mite origin which may also have enzymatic activity.

3. House Dust Mite Allergens

At least nine groups of HDM allergen have been characterized to date [6, 14–36]. Four groups of allergens from mites of the genus *Dermatophagoides* are known to have proteinase activity (reviewed in Robinson et al. [6]). Of the remaining dermatophagoides HDM allergens that are classified, some may be associated with other types of enzymatic activity (reviewed in [6]).

Allergens belonging to group 1 are currently the best characterized of the HDM allergens [6]. Der p 1 is the most extensively studied and its nucleic acid sequence predicts a 320 amino acid protein with molecular mass of about 36 kDa [15, 18]. However, the first 98 residues consist of signal and propeptide sequences which must be cleaved to generate the mature form of the protein. Similar propeptide cleavage occurs with the other group 1 allergens. The mature forms of the group 1 HDM allergens constitute a related family of 25-kDa acidic-neutral proteins, consisting of 222–223 amino acids which show some evidence of minor sequence polymorphisms within a given mite species [6, 14, 18]. Whole or partial amino acid sequences have been obtained for group 1 allergens from *D. pteronyssinus*, *D. farinae* and *Europglyphus maynei* (Der p 1, Der f 1 and Eur m 1, respectively) and these show approximately 80% conservation of identity between them [6, 14–17]. The group 1 allergens also show conserved sequence identity with C1 family cysteine proteinases [6, 37] whose archetypes are the plant proteinases papain and actinidin. Overall, the conservation of sequence identity between the HDM group 1 allergens and the plant enzymes is only 25–30%, but the existence of a familial relationship is more convincing when residues bounding the charge relay system of the cysteine proteinases are considered in isolation (Table 1).

Table 1. Conservation of catalytic site residues in the archetypal C1 family cysteine proteinases papain and actinidin and the HDM allergen Der p 1

Enzyme	19[a]	22				26	64					69	133
Papain	Q	C	G	S	C	W	N	G	G	Y	P	W	V
Actinidin	Q	C	G	S	C	W	D	G	G	Y	I	T	A
Der p 1	Q[c]	C	G	S	C[c]	W	H[d]	G[d]	D[b]	T[b]	I[b]	P[b]	I

Enzyme	157			160		175		177	205		207
Papain	V	X[e]	D	H	A	N	S	W·	S	S	F
Actinidin	V	X[e]	D	H	A	N	S	W	M	P	S
Der p 1	P[b]	N	Y	H[c]	A[b]	N[c]	S	W[d]	Y[b]	P	Y[b]

[a] Residue numbering based on papain sequence.
[b] Non-polar side-chain binding pocket.
[c] Catalytic site residues.
[d] Walls of acive site cleft.
[e] Deleted residue site X.

Although crystallographic coordinates are not yet available for these allergens and rigorous assignment of structure cannot be made, the existence of the amino acid sequence with enzymes for which detailed information exists has allowed the application of knowledge-based homology modelling to the examination of the Der p 1 molecule [38]. On the basis of this comparative modelling, Der p 1 is proposed to consist of a single polypeptide chain (Figure 1) which is folded to create two domains that delimit a central cleft (Figure 2). A cysteine residue (C34, using the single letter amino acid notation) on one wall of the cleft acts to initiate nucleophilic attack on the substrate, with a histidine residue (H170) on the opposite wall of the cleft acting as the second component of the charge relay system. The imidazole side chain of H170 is maintained in correct orientation by hydrogen bonding to asparagine N190 which is the final critical residue of the cysteine proteinase catalytic triad. Der p 1 exhibits some similarities and differences in structure to the C1 proteinase family archetype, papain. The wall of the active site of Der p 1 contains a prominent tryptophan residue (W192) which is conserved in papain (W177 in the papain sequence) where it is in close contact with P_1 subsite non-polar residues in the binary complex with the substrate. However, an aspartic acid residue (D158) which is important for catalysis in papain is not present in Der p 1. Differences such as these remain to be explored further. However, they raise the possibility that selective inhibition of the catalytic activity of Der p 1 may be possible, and some early indications confirm the feasibility of this [39].

There is no doubt that, by amino acid sequence, Der p 1 is a putative cysteine proteinase [6, 15, 38] and it behaves accordingly when biochemical criteria are examined *in vitro* [38, 40]. However, a claim has recently been advanced that Der p 1 may be a polyfunctional enzyme [41, 42], having some serine proteinase activity that can be inhibited by the serine proteinase inhibitor 4-[amidinophenyl]methanesulphonyl fluoride (APMSF). However, this observation has not been replicated by others [43] and it might

---→

Figure 1. Alignment of the sequences of cysteine proteinases of known tertiary structure and Der p 1. The structural environment at every residue position is represented using the program JoY [72]. Structural environments at the residues of Der p 1 correspond to the modelled structure [72]. Der p 1 numbering is shown. Conserved secondary structural elements are indicated. The isoforms of Der p 1 are indicated in the last row. The ! corresponds to the active site residues. Key to proteins: 9pap (papain); 2act (actinidin); 1ppo (papaya proteinase Ω); 1dpi (Der p 1). Key to JoY alignments:

solvent inaccessible:	UPPER CASE	X;
solvent accessible:	lower case	x;
positive ∅:	italic	*x*;
cis-peptide:	breve	x̆;
hydrogen bond to other side chain:	tilde	x̃;
hydrogen bond to main chain amide:	**bold**	x;
hydrogen bond to main chain carbonyl:	*underline*	*x*;
disulphide bond:	cedilla	x̧;

```
9pap    i p e y V d̲ w̲ f̄ q̣ k g A V T̄ p V k̲ n q̣ g s C̣ g S̃ C̃ W̲A̲F̲ S̲A V v T̲I E̊ G I i k i ẕ
2act    l p s ȳ v d̲ w̲ f̄ s a g A V v d I k̲ s Q̣ g e C̣ g G C̃ W̲A̲F̲ S̲A I a T̲V E̊ G i N̲k i t̲
1ppo    l p e n V d̲ w̲ f̄ k k g A V T̄ p V f̄ h q̣ g s C̣ g S̃ ẽ W̲A̲F̲ S̲A a T̲V E̊ G I n k i f̲

                10              20              30              40              50
1dpi    t ñ a ç s̃ i ñ g n̲ a p e i D̲L f̄ q m r̲ t V ī p I f̄ m q̣ g g C̣ g S̲ e W̲A f S̲ G V A A T̲E̲S̲ a y l a h̲
        β β              ϕ                   ϕ          α α α α α α α α α α α α α α α α α
                        • •       •                   • • • • • •     • • • •
        G                                        !                                       Y


9pap    t̲ g n l ñ q̣ Ÿ S̲E̊ Q̊E̲L L D̲ç D̲f̄ f̄ - - s̃ - ȳ G ç n g Gȳ p w S̃ A L q̣ l V a q y - G I H̲ȳ f̄ n t̲ Ÿ p
2act    g g s l i s L S̲E̊ Q̊E̲L I D̲C g r t q ñ T̄ - I̲ G ç d g G y I t d̄ G F q̣ f l i ñ d̲ g G I Ñ f̄ s̄ e ñ Ÿ p
1ppo    t̲ g k l v e L S̲E̊ Q̊E̲L V D̲C E̲r f̄ - - s̃ - ñ G ç k g Gȳ p p y A L ē ȳ V a k n - G I L̲f̄ l f̄ s k Ȳ p

                60          A B C D   70              80          A       90
1dpi    r n q s L d̲ L A E̲Q̊E̲L V D̲C a - - - - S̲ g̲L̲G ç h g d̲ t I P f̄ G I S̲Ȳ I q h n - g V V Q̊e̲ s y Ȳ r̲
        α ϕ          α α α α α α α                   •       •       ϕ       α α α α α α α α    ϕ    • • •
        • • • • • • • • •                         •       •                               •
                S                       K


9pap    ȳ ē g v q̣ f̄ y ç f̄ S̃ r̲ e k g p ȳ a a k̲ T d g v r q v q̣ p y ñ q̣ g a L l y s̲ I A n̲q P V S̃ v v L Q A a
2act    ȳ f̄ a q̣ d g d ç d v a l q̣ d̲ q̣ k̲ ȳ V t I d t y e n V p y ñ E̲w a L q̣ t̲ a V f̄ y q P V S̲ V a L d̲ A a
1ppo    ȳ k a k q̣ g t ç r̲ A k q v g g p i v k T̲ s̲ g v g r v q p n ñ e g n̲ L l n a I A k̲ Q P V S̃ V v V E̲s̄ f̲

                100         110A B           120             130         A       140
1dpi    ȳ v a f̄ e q̣ s ç f̄ r p n̲ A q̣ r - - F g I s̲ m ȳ ç q̣ l ȳ p p n a n k I f̲ e̲ A L A - q̣ T̄ H̲S̲ A I A v I i
        ϕ                          β β β β         ϕ     α α α α α α α α α       β β β β
                        •                       •       • •     • • • •     • •
                V                                       T


9pap    g - k d F q l y̲ r g g - - - - i f v G p̃ ç g n k v d̲ - H̄ A V A A V G Y̲ G p - - - - n y I L I K Ñ s̄ w
2act    g - d a F k q y̲ a s g - - - - i f t G p̃ ç g t a v d̲ - H̄ A I V I V G Ȳ G f̄ ē g g v d̲ y W̄ I V K Ñ s̄ w
1ppo    g - r p F q l Ȳ k̲ g g - - - - i f ē G p̃ ç g t k v d̲ - H̄ A V T A V G Y̲ G k s g g f̄ g y I l I K Ñ s̄ w

                150             160             170             180             190
1dpi    g i k d̲ L d̲ a F r L̃ȳ d g f̄ t I I q r̲ d n g y q p n ȳ H̄ A v Ñ I V G Y̲ s̄ ñ a q g v d̲ y W̄ I V R̲̃ N S w̄
        α α α α          ϕ          β β  ϕ ω          β β β β β β ϕ β β β     ϕ    β β β β β β
                •                                   • • • • • • • • •            • • • • •


9pap    g t g w̲ G ē n G y I f̄ I k f̄ g t g n̲ s y G v C̣ G L Ȳ t̲ s S f y P v k n
2act    d t t w̲ G ē e̲ G y M f̄ I l R̲̃ñ v g - g a G t̲ C̣ G I A ĩ m P S y P v k̲ y
1ppo    g t a w̲ G ē k G y I f̄ I K̲f̄ a p g ñ s p G v C̣ G L Ȳ k s S y y P t̲ k ñ

                200             A B C D   210             220         A
1dpi    d̄ t ñ W̲G d̲ n G y G ȳ F A A n̲ - - - - i D l M̲M̲I̲ E̲ē ȳ P ȳ V V i l
        ϕ          ϕ      ϕ ϕ β β β β β          ϕ       ϕ 3 3 3      β β β β
                •     •      • • • • •          • • • • •
                                        Q
```

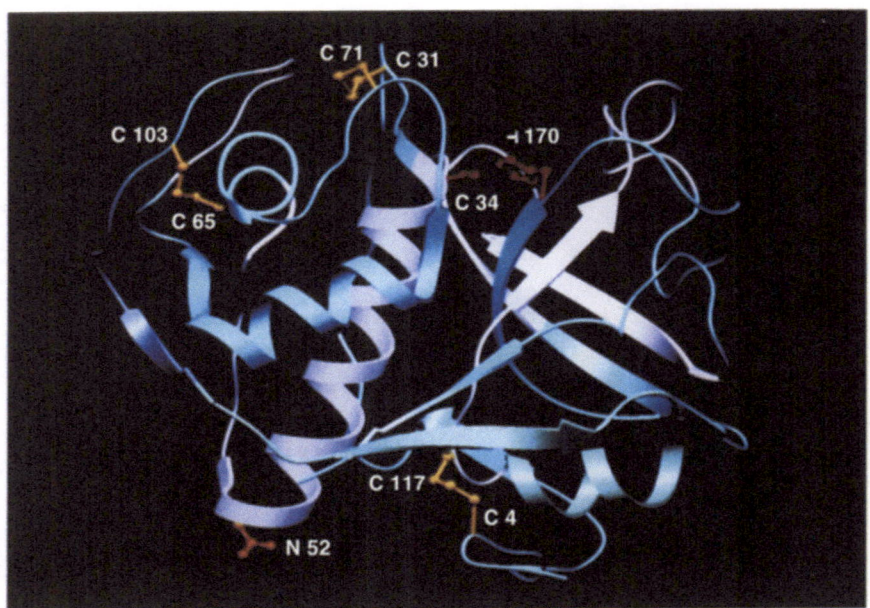

Figure 2. The structure of Der p 1 derived by homology modelling with the archetypal cysteine proteinases actinidin and papain. Der p 1 β-strands are indicated by arrows and α-helices as coils. Side chains of the three disulphides (yellow), the C34/H170 ion pair (red) and the glycosylation site (N52, orange) are shown explicitly. Human B cell epitopes (residues ranges 1–33, 60–94, 101–111, 155–187 and 209–222) are coloured light blue (and violet, residues 107–111). Overlapping T cell epitope sites (residue range 107–131) are coloured green and violet (spanning the B cell epitope site region). (The figure was constructed using the program SETOR and is reproduced from [38] by kind permission of Oxford University Press.)

simply reflect an effect of APMSF on serine residues that are not part of the active site itself, but that are located sufficiently adjacent to it so as to be able to influence catalysis after their reaction with APMSF [44]. Some experimental support for the non-specific inhibition of Der p 1 catalytic activity by APMSF has recently been presented. The sequencing and structural modelling of Der p 1 have also facilitated detailed epitope mapping of this allergen (Table 2) [45]. Major IgE-binding regions of Der p 1 comprise residues 15–33, 60–80, 81–94, 101–111 and 101–154 [46], with the last probably corresponding to the peptide segments that link the two domains of Der p 1.

The group 1 allergens of HDMs are derived from the digestive tracts of mites [47]. Their function in HDMs is probably to act as digestive enzymes responsible for degrading components of the desquamated flakes of mammalian skin on which the mites feed [48]. However, the "physiological" substrates of inhaled Der p 1 in humans are currently unknown, although some possibilities have been suggested. These include the 45-kDa CD23 low-affinity IgE receptor present on B lymphocytes [41, 49]. Der p 1 cleav-

Table 2. Peptide fragments corresponding to B cell and T cell epitopes of Der p 1

Peptide fragments (residue numbers)	T or B cell epitope	Net charge at pH 7.0	Isoelectric point pI
1–33	B	0.88	8.08
5–30	B	0.98	10.38
60–94	B	− 3.39	4.74
101–111	B	2.93	12.20
111–139	T	1.17	8.43
118–136	T	1.22	9.55
155–187*	B	1.21	9.50
209–222	B	− 3.02	3.47

* Terminal four residues removed from published sequence for epitope.

es CD23 *in vitro* to release a soluble 25-kDa fragment which is known from other studies to stimulate the growth and differentiation of plasma cells, T lymphocytes and basophils, as well as being an autocrine regulator of IgE synthesis [50]. It has been speculated that this effect may provide a basis for stimulation of IgE synthesis in susceptible individuals, but operation of this mechanism in lymphocytes would require high concentrations of Der p 1 to be achieved in blood or extracellular fluids. Given the small numbers of inhaled faecal pellets that are likely to enter the lung each day under normal breathing (about 200) and the barrier presented by lung epithelium, it is difficult to envisage how such high concentrations could be achieved under normal environmental exposures unless the target cell population is a pool of B lymphocytes in the airway which is capable of returning from the airway lumen. Although there may be bidirectional lymphocyte trafficking in the lung [51], these potentially interesting trafficking processes are poorly characterized and currently of unknown significance. Evidence has been presented that Der p 1 also degrades α_1-proteinase inhibitor [49], a major component of the anitproteolytic defences of the human respiratory tract. It is also noteworthy that Der p 1 is not inhibited by a range of other antiproteinases with the exception of α_2-macroglobulin [52], which is not normally present in epithelial lining fluid. The pathophysiological significance of this biochemical finding is not yet known, but it may be of potential relevance to the ability of this allergen to exert proteinase-dependent effects in the lung.

3.1. HDM Allergens in Groups 3, 6, and 9

Mite allergens belonging of these groups share their identity with serine proteinases (Table 3). HDM allergens belonging to group 3 are polymorphic proteins which in mature form have molecular masses of 25–30 kDa [6, 25]. Like those of group 1, group 3 allergens are preferentially found in the faecal components of mite cultures [19, 25, 29]. All of the known iso-

Table 3. N-Terminal sequences of *D. pteronyssinus* and *D. farinae* serine proteinase allergens deduced by protein and cDNA analyses

Proteinase allergen	Sequence

Mite trypsin

	1																			20
Der f 3	I	V	G	G	V	K	A	Q	A	G	D	X[a] P	Y	Q	I	S	L	Q	S
Der f 3	I	V	G	G	V	K	A	L	A	G	D	X[a] P	Y	E	I	S	L	E	V
Der f 3	I	V	G	G	V	K	A	K	A	G	D	X[a] P	Y	Q	I	S	L	Q	S
Der p 3	I	V	G	G	E	K	A	L	A	G	E	X[a] P	Y	Q	I	S	L[b]			
Der p 3	I	V	G	G	E	K	A	L	A	G	Q	X[a] P	Y	Q	I	S	L	Q	S
Der p 3 cDNA	I	V	G	G	E	K	A	L	A	G	E	C P	Y	Q	I	S	L	Q	S

Mite collagenolytic serine proteinase

Der p 9	I	V	G	G	S	N	A	S	P	G	D	A V	Y	Q	I	A	L[b]			

Mite chymotrypsin

Der f 6	(A)(V) G	G	Q	D	A	D	L	A	E	A	P	F	Q	I	S	L	L	K
Der p 6 cDNA	V I	G	G	Q	D	A	A	E	A	E	A	P	F	Q	I	S	L	M	K

[a] Idenity not established.
[b] End of sequence.
Brackets indicate assumed identity.

forms of these proteins appear to be strongly allergenic as judged by the radioallergosorbent test (RAST) [19, 25, 29]. Group 3 proteins express trypsin-like serine proteinase activity but lack the polyaspartyl-lysyl activation peptide of vertebrate trypsins [25]. The amino acid sequence identity is most conserved at the allergen amino acid residues corresponding to those that surround the charge relay system of trypsins [6, 25].

In contrast to allergens belonging to group 3, those of group 6 are 25-kDa proteins which share similar substrate properties and amino acid sequences with invertebrate chymotrypsins [29]. More recently, a third serine proteinase allergen has been isolated from *D. pteronyssinus* and designated Der p 9 [32]. Mature Der p 9 has a molecular mass of 24 kDa and shows approximately 60% identity with the group 3 and group 6 allergens [32]. However, its susceptibility to inhibitors and preferences for synthetic substrates show it to be functionally distinct from the group 3 and group 6 proteinase allergens. Der p 9 has a specificity profile similar to chymotrypsin and cathepsin G, and is capable of degrading type III collagen [32].

Much less is known about the biological effects of the serine proteinase HDM allergens than those of group 1. This partly reflects their more recent characterization and also the greater difficulty in purifying them from the complex mixtures of HDM allergens and other substances present in mite cultures. The complexity of the mixtures from which these sequenced proteins need to be purified is at present a considerable handicap in understanding the biology of these proteins. Greater progress in establishing the biological significance of both the cysteine and serine proteinase class allergens awaits the availability of fully characterized, catalytically competent, recombinant proteins. Attempts have been made to express HDM proteinase allergens, but the strategies and expression systems used to date have not been optimized to ensure production of correctly folded mature protein. This has resulted in the expressed proteins lacking full immunogenicity and proteolytic activity [53].

4. Other Sources of Allergens with Enzymatic Activity

Several other allergens have been putatively associated with proteolytic activity, either on the basis of functional studies or by comparison of their sequences with proteins of known function and/or structure. These include the cockroach allergen Bla g2 which shares some identity with aspartic proteinases [54]. The cockroach allergens Bla g1 and Per a1 exhibit proteolytic activity *in vitro* (unpublished observations). However, definitive demonstration of the proteolytic activity of cockroach allergens on mammalian cellular targets is still awaited.

A major difficulty in studying the biological effects of allergen proteins is obtaining homogeneous preparations of the allergen. This is further compounded by the need to do this on a relatively large scale. Investigations of the proteinase activity of HDM allergens has been greatly facilitated by amino acid sequencing which revealed that mite allergens of group 1 were putative cysteine proteinases [15, 37]. Thus the demonstration that Der p1 was catalytically competent was an interesting finding, but biochemically unexceptional given the sequence data. A more exciting question is the issue that follows logically from it, namely what is the pathophysiological significance of this activity.

Some other attempts to use sequence data to explore the biology of common domestic allergens associated with asthma have not enjoyed such simple predictive outcomes as has been the case with HDM. Allergy to domestic cats is found in 10–30% of patients with asthma [55, 56]. The major allergen from the saliva and sebaceous glands, Fel d 1 [57], has also been sequenced. Its structure is more complex than that of any of the known HDM allergens because it is a 38-kDa heterotetramer formed noncovalently from two disulphide-linked 18-kDa proteins which each consist of two chains [58]. Genomic cloning has established that chain 1 and chain 2 of the 18-kDa dimer are encoded by discrete genes [59]. Chain 1 is a nonglycosylated protein of 70 amino acid residues associated with two potential leader sequences. Chain 2 is a heavily glycosylated 90- or 92-residue peptide with a single leader sequence. The 90-residue form of chain 2 is predominantly expressed in cat skin, whereas the 92-residue form is expressed in salivary glands [59]. Examination of the amino acid sequence of Fel d 1 chain 1 reveals very weak similarity with uteroglobin [58] and the α subunit of a mouse salivary androgen-binding protein [60], whereas no evidence of similarity with known proteins has been established for chain 2. Database searches thus provide no *a priori* reason to anticipate, from the amino acid sequence, that Fel d 1 should exhibit proteinase activity. However, studies in this laboratory, using Fel d 1 subjected to extensive and rigorous purification and confirmation of identity by matrix-assisted laser desorption mass spectrometry and protein sequencing, have consistently found evidence of enzymatic activity in this allergen (Figure 3). The enzyme activity can be inhibited by agents that block the activity of serine proteinases. However, inhibition deviates from unimolecular stoichiometry, suggesting that the action of these compounds is not the result of inhibition of a classic serine proteinase and may instead result from non-specific binding of the inhibitors to serine residues near the active site. Furthermore, the absence of a histidine residue in the Fel d 1 heterotetramer precludes operation of the conventional histidine-aspartic acid-serine (HDS) catalytic triad of serine proteinases.

Pollens from grasses, weeds and trees are also major causes of allergic disorders and biochemical studies have been performed to identify the allergenic proteins involved (reviewed in [14]). Although many candidate allergens have now been seqenced there is, with few exceptions, little evidence of similarity with proteins of known function, regardless of whether they are enzymes or not. The allergens Amb a 1 and Amb a 2 of ragweed show some similarity with pectate lyases. Similarly, the birch pollen allergens Bet v 1 and Bet v 2 show similarity to plant pathogenesis-related protein and profilin, respectively, but the potential significance of all of these possible relationships has not been established (reviewed in [14]). However, pollens are rich sources of enzymes, such as lyases, esterases and polygalactouronases, and other potentially active proteins [61]. Allergenic proteins may thus be presented to humans in a complex milieu in which

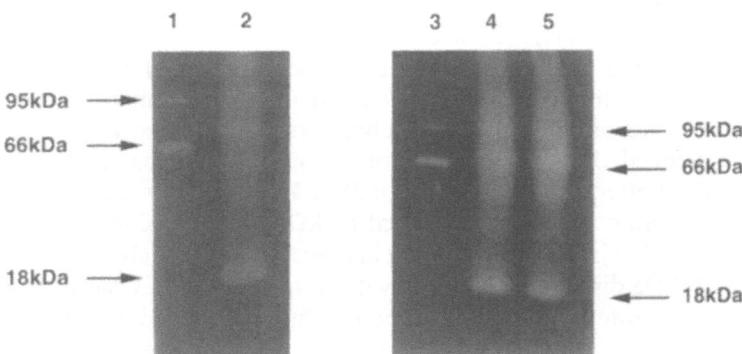

Figure 3. Proteolytic activity of the cat allergen Fel d 1. The figure illustrates two gelatin substrate zymograms electrophoresed at 4 °C and subsequently incubated at 37 °C to reveal enzymatic activity in the gel. Lanes 1 and 3 are controls showing markers of gelatinase A (apparent mass 66 kDa) and B (apparent mass 95 kDa); lanes 2, 4 and 5 are samples of highly purified Fel d 1. Note the band of gelatin-degrading activity front at an apparent mass of about 18 kDa, equivalent to Fel d 1 (chain 1 and chain 2), with a "comet tail" of activity behind.

these other factors may contribute significantly to the process of sensitization. This possibility is supported by a small but increasing body of studies which have examined this issue. Matheson et al. [62] have reported the identification of an 84-kDa arginine-specific enzyme from mesquite pollen which was capable of readily cleaving the vasoactive peptides angiotensin II and atrial natriuretic peptide. Interestingly, this enzyme was not inhibited by human plasma proteinase inhibitors, raising the possibility that any effects it might exert in humans may be partly dependent upon its ability to bypass host defences. Similarly, an 82-kDa serine endopeptidase has been reported in ragweed pollen [63] which inhibits α_1-proteinase inhibitor and which also degrades the neuropeptides vasoactive intestinal polypeptide and substance P [63]. These observations serve as important reminders that HDM proteinase allergens are likely to be presented to the airway embedded in a complex of other substances, which may themselves have biological effects that potentiate the action of the allergens.

5. Interactions of Proteinase Allergens and the Airway Epithelium

The difficulty in obtaining large amounts of highly purified, catalytically competent allergens has impeded progress in understanding the possible significance of their proteinase activity. This problem is further compounded by the fact that potential differences in substrate specificities make it unjustifiable to use proteinase class archetypes as surrogates to explore the biology of these allergens.

We have been particularly interested in examining the possible effects of Der p 1 on the airway epithelium because this is the site at which inhaled faecal pellets impact and the tissue surface at which the highest concentrations of proteinase are expected to the encountered. In the healthy airway, ingress of foreign proteins is prevented by the presence of mucosal defences comprising biochemical (e.g. antiproteinases) and physical (mucus, presence of intercellular tight junctions) components [13]. However, Der p 1 may be able to evade inhibition by or even degrade important antiproteinase defences of the respiratory tract [49, 52]. Furthermore, in the lung the protective covering of mucus is non-uniformly distributed and there are significant areas of epithelial lining devoid of mucus cover. It is thus easy to envisage that HDM faecal pellets landing upon mucus-laden areas of airway may exert little effect, whereas those impacting upon the watery lining of airway surface liquid will empty their contents directly on to structures that are potentially susceptible to proteolysis.

Our studies have shown that Der p 1 is able to initiate cleavage of epithelial cell adhesion [40, 64], raising the possibility that the proteinase is either directly or indirectly capable of increasing epithelial permeability. This was initially investigated using sheets of airway mucosa dissected from bronchial airways [40]. In these experiments, treatment of the mucosal sheets with either spent (i. e. faecally enriched) medium from HDM cultures (spent growth medium extract or SGME) or with purified Der p 1 produced an increase in the net apical to basal flux of albumin across the airway sheet [40, 64]. The action was not the result of gross cytotoxicity because the tisue released little lactate dehydrogenase activity under these conditions [40]. Treatment of epithelial cell monolayers cultured on substrata of biomatrix proteins with either SGME or Der p 1 resulted in detachment of cells, suggesting that the increase in albumin flux was probably the result of damage to the epithelial barrier caused by physical loss of cells [40]. The ability of SGME or Der p 1 to detach cells was caused entirely by the proteinase activity of Der p 1 because it was inhibited in a potent, concentration-dependent fashion by the cysteine proteinase inhibitor E-64 [40]. Intraluminal application of Der p 1 into intact airway segments *ex vivo* resulted in a clear disruption of epithelial architecture (Figure 4) [40]. Columnar cells were seen to become separated at their apical margins and evidence of a cleavage in basal cellular adhesion confirmed the findings of the studies in cultured cells. This cleavage of both basal and lateral adhesion created vacancies in the continuity of the airway epithelium where focally restricted loss of barrier functions would occur [40].

These studies show that the proteolytic activity of Der p 1 results in impaired adhesion in epithelial cells and that lateral cellular adhesion may initially be more susceptible to disruption than basal adhesion is [6, 40]. However, the treatment of epithelia with enzymes is actually a potentially complex experiment because there may be multiple targets for the enzymes on a single cell. Therefore, in the absence of an established mechanism to explain the apparent difference in susceptibility of the different sites of adhesion, it is impossible to know why such a difference could exist [6]. Epithelial architecture can be disrupted by enzymes other than the cysteine proteinase Der p 1, and these effects also appear to arise from mechanisms that are not dependent on cytotoxic effects [65–67]. Histologically, the disruption brought about by these other proteinases is grossly similar to that seen with Der p 1, but precise interpretation of the effects is difficult because there has been little investigation of the cellular mechanisms involved. However, the general pattern of changes suggests that disruption of intercellular junctions must be a crucial event in the process. This raises the question of how these changes occur. Tryptic cleavage of the extracellular domains of cell junctions results in characteristic ultrastructural changes in which electron-dense intercellular material is first degraded and junctional halves of adjacent cells separate [68]. The separated halves the become internalized in cytoplasmic vacuoles [68]. Whether or not similar changes occur with the proteinase allergen Der p 1 remains to be established, but early indicates suggest that breakdown of tight junctions may be an important effect of Der p 1 in epithelia [43, 69]. Tight junctions are the major regulators of paracellular permeability pathways in epithelia. Although low-molecular-weight solutes are able to permeate tight junctions and cross epithelial barriers [11–13], proteins such

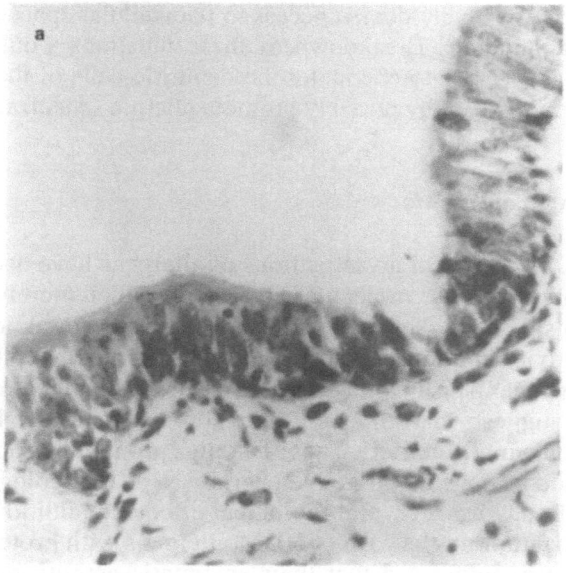

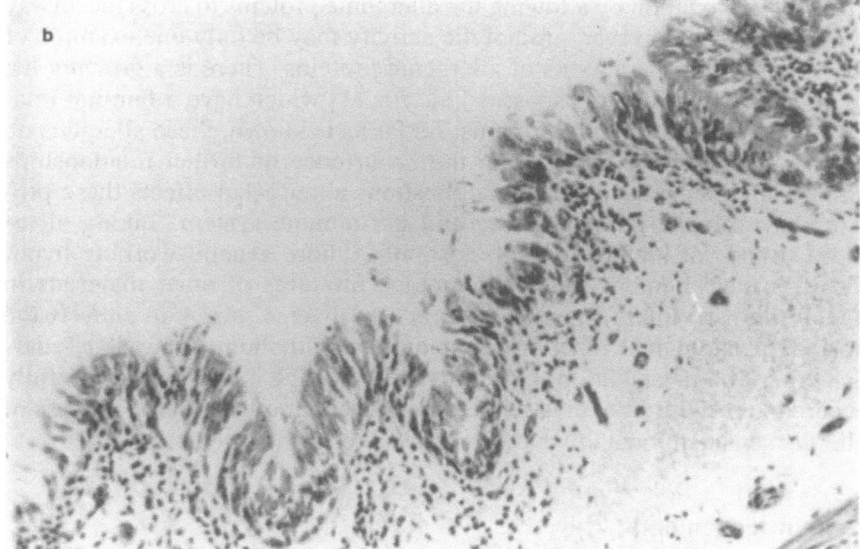

Figure 4. Sections of bovine bronchi after (a) sham treatment or (b) treatment with pure Der p 1. Note the evidence in (b) of the loss of intercellular adhesion and visual evidence indicating disruption of the epithelial barrier.

as allergens are effectively denied access to paracellular spaces by the presence of tight junctions. Breakdown of these junctions would enable an allergen such as Der p 1 to encounter the dendritic cells of the pulmonary immune system and thereby possibly promote allergic sensitization [6, 40].

6. Concluding Comments

Until recently, biochemical investigations of allergens have been restricted to a consideration of these molecules as proteins which merely evoke IgE-dependent sensitization, Several HDM allergens are now known to have proteolytic activity and to exert striking effects on airway epithelial cells, although the mechanisms involved are currently speculative. Accumulating evidence also suggests that some non-mite allergens may also have proteolytic or other enzymatic activity. These findings prompt the suggestion that allergens should be considered more generally as pharmacologically active proteins which may exert several biological effects in addition to evoking allergic sensitization. In the case of HDM allergens with proteolytic activity, it has been hypothesized that their enzymatic activity may facilitate allergic sensitization by allowing the allergenic proteins to cross the airway epithelium [6]. However, proteolytic activity may be only one example of the wider biological actions of allergenic proteins. There is a growing list of allergens from diverse sources [14, 70, 71] which have a familial relationship as ligand-binding proteins. As far as is known, these allergens do not have proteolytic activity, but the occurrence of further relationships among allergens raises intriguing questions about what effects these proteins have on the human airway and its immune system. Taking all of these strands of knowledge into account, a more general working hypothesis is that allergens (and the complex mixtures of other materials in which they are found) may actually act by diverse means to subvert the normal physiological function of the airway epithelium to facilitate allergen entry and presentation. Experimental evidence is now being carefully accured to test this hypothesis and to understand more about the process of allergic sensitization and what it is that makes an allergen an allergen.

Acknowledgements

We thank the National Asthma Campaign for supporting our research on proteinase allergens.

References

1 Tovery ER, Chapman MD, Platts-Mills TAE (1981) Mite faeces are a major source of house dust allergens. *Nature* 289: 592–593
2 Sporik K, Holgate ST, Platts-Mills TA, Cogswell JJ (1990) Exposure to house dust mite allergen (Der p 1) and the development of asthma in childhood. A prospective study. *N Engl J Med* 323: 502–507

3 Platts-Mills A, Thomas WR, Aalberse RC, Vervolet D, Chapman MD (1992) Dust mite allergens and asthma: report of a second international workshop. *J Allergy Clin Immunol* 89: 1046–1060

4 Peat JK, Tovey E, Toelle BG, Haby MM, Gray EJ, Mahmic A, Woolcock AJ (1996) House dust mite allergens. A major risk factor for childhood asthma in Australia. *Am J Respir Crit Care Med* 153: 141–146

5 Dowse GK, Turner KJ, Stewart GA, Alpers MP, Woolcock AJ (1985) The association between *Dermatophagoides* mites and the increasing prevalence of asthma in village communities within the Papua New Guinea highlands. *J Allergy Clin Immunol* 75: 75–83

6 Robinson C, Kalsheker NA, Srinivasan N, King CM, Garrod DR, Thompson PJ, Stewart GA (1997) On the potential significance of the enzymatic activity of mite allergens to immunogenicity. Clues to structure and function reveales by molecular characterization. *Clin Exp Allergy* 27: 10–21

7 Holt PG (1995) Macrophage and dendritic cell populations in the respiratory tract. In: ST Holgate (ed) Immunopharmacology of the respiratory system. Academic Press, London, 1–12

8 Holt PG (1997) Dendritic cell populations in the lung and airway wall. In: PJ Barnes, MM Grunstein, AR Leff, AJ Woolcock AJ (eds) *Asthma*. Lippincott-Raven, Philadelphia, 453–463

9 Weibel ER (1991) Design of airways and blood vessels considered as branching trees. In: RG Crystal et al. (eds) *The lung: scientific foundation*. Raven Press, New York, 711–720

10 Farquhar M, Palade GE (1963) Junctional complexes in various epithelia. *J Cell Biol* 17: 375–412

11 Anderson JM, Van Itallie CM (1995) Tight junctions and the molecular basis for regulation of paracellular permeability. *Am J Physiol* 269: G467–G475

12 Schneeberger EE, Lynch RD (1992) Structure, function and regulation of cellular tight junctions. *Am J Physiol* 262: L647–L661

13 Robinson C (1995) The airway epithelium: The origin and target of inflammatory airways disease and injury. In: ST Holgate (ed) *Immunopharmacology of the respiratory system*. Academic Press, London, 187–207

14 Stewart GA (1994) Molecular biology of allergens. In: WW Busse, ST Holgate (eds) *Asthma and Rhinitis*. Blackwell Scientific Publications, Oxford, 898–932

15 Chua KY, Stewart GA, Thomas WR, Simpson RJ, Dilworth RJ, Plozza TM, Turner KJ (1988) Sequence analysis of cDNA coding for a major house dust mite allergen, Der p I. Homology with cysteine proteases. *J Exp Med* 167: 175–182

16 Dilworth RJ, Chua KY, Thomas WR (1991) Sequence analysis of cDNA coding for a major house dust mite allergen, Der f I. *Clin Exp Med* 167: 25–32

17 Kent NA, Hill MR; Keen JN, Holland PWH, Hart BJ (1992) Molecular characterization of group I allergen Eur m I from house dust mite Euroglyphus maynei. *Int Arch Allergy Immunol* 99: 150–152

18 Chua KY, Kehal PK, Thomas WR (1993) Sequence polymorphisms of cDNA clones encoding the mite allergen Der p I. *Int Arch Allergy Immunol* 101: 364–368

19 Heymann PW, Chapman MD, Aalberse RC, Fox JW, Platts-Mills TAE (1989) Antigenic and structural analysis of group II allergens (Der f II and Der p II) from house dust mites (*Dermatophagoides* spp). *J Allergy Clin Immunol* 83: 1055–1067

20 Lind P (1985) Purification and partial characterization of two major allergens from the house dust mite *Dermatophagoides pteronyssinus*. *J Allergy Clin Immunol* 76: 753–761

21 Lombardero M, Heymann PW, Platts MT, Fox JW, Chapman MD (1990) Conformational stability of B cell epitopes on group I and group II *Dermatophagoides* spp. allergens. Effect of thermal and chemical denaturation on the binding of murine IgG and human IgE antibodies. *J Immunol* 144: 1353–1360

22 Yuuki T, Okumura Y, Ando T, Yamakawa H, Suko M, Haida M, Okudaira H (1990) Cloning and sequencing of cDNAs corresponding to major mite allergen Der f II. *Jpn J Allergol* 39: 557–561

23 Chua KY, Doyle CR, Simpson RJ, Turner KJ, Stewart GA, Thomas WR (1990) Isolation of cDNA coding for the major mite allergen Der p II by IgE plaque immunoassay. *Int Arch Allergy Appl Immunol* 91: 118–123

24 Trudinger M, Chua KY, Thomas WR (1991) cDNA encoding the major mite allergen Der f II. *Clin Exp Allergy* 21: 33–37

25 Stewart GA, Ward LD, Simpson RJ, Thompson PJ (1992) The group III allergen from the house dust mite *Dermatophagoides pteronyssinus* is a trypsin-like enzyme. *Immunology* 75: 29–35

26 Smith W-A, Chua K-Y, Kuo MC, Rogers BL, Thomas WR (1994) Cloning and sequencing of the *Dermatophagoides pteronyssinus* group III allergen, Der p III. *Clin Exp Allergy* 24: 220–228

27 Lake FR, Ward LD, Simpson RJ, Thompson PJ, Stewart GA (1991) House dust mite derived amylase: Allergenicity and physicochemical characterisation. *J Allergy Clin Immunol* 87: 1035–1042

28 Tovey ER, Johnson MC, Roche AL, Cobon GS, Baldo BA (1989) Cloning and sequencing of a cDNA expressing a recombinant house dust mite protein that binds human IgE and corresponds to an important low molecular weight allergen. *J Exp Med* 170: 1457–1462. (Published erratum appears in *J Exp Med* (1990) 171: 1387)

29 Yasueda H, Mita H, Akiyama K, Shida T, Ando T, Sugiyama S, Yamakawa H (1993) Allergens from Dermatophagoides mites with chymotyptic activity. *Clin Exp Allergy* 23: 384–390

30 Shen H-D, Chua K-Y, Lin K-L, Hsieh K-H, Thomas WR (1993) Molecular cloning of a house dust mite allergen with common antibody binding specificities with multiple components in mite extracts. *Clin Exp Allergy* 23: 934–940

31 O'Neill GM, Donovan GR, Baldo BA (1994) Cloning and characterization of a major allergen of the house dust mite, *Dermatophagoides pteronyssinus*, homologous with glutathione *S*-transferase. *Biochim Biophys Acta* 1219: 521–528

32 King CM, Simpson RJ, Thompson PJ, Stewart GA (1996) The isolation and characterization of a novel collagenolytic serine protease allergen (Der p 9) from the dust mite *Dermatophagoides pteronyssinus*. *J Allergy Clin Immunol* 98: 739–747

33 Aki T, Fujikawa A, Wada T, Jyo T, Shigeta S, Murooka T, Oka S, Ono K (1994) Cloning and expression of cDNA coding for a new allergen from the house dust mite. *Dermatophagoides farinae*: Homologoy with human heat shock cognate proteins in the heat shock protein 70 family. *J Biochem* 115: 435–440

34 Stewart GA, Simpson RJ, Moritz RL, Thomas WR, Turner KJ (1988) Physiochemical characterization of allergens Der p I (Dpt 12), Dpt 22 and Dpt 36 from the house dust mite. In: AL de Weck, A Todt (eds) *International Workshop Proceedings, Mite allergy, A world wide problem*, The UCB Institute for Allergy, Brussels, 35–38

35 Shen HD, Chua KY, Hsieh KH, Thomas WR (1996) Molecular cloning and immunological characterization of the group 7 allergens of house dust mites. *Adv Exp Med Biol* 409: 241–242

36 Bennett BJ, Thomas WR (1996) Cloning and sequencing of the group 6 allergen of *Dermatophagoides pteronyssinus*. *Clin Exp Allergy* 26: 1150–1154

37 Stewart GA, Thompson PJ, Simpson RJ (1989) Protease antigens from house dust mite. *Lancet* 2: 154–155. (Correction: *Lancet* 2: 462)

38 Topham CM, Srinivasan N, Thorpe CJ, Overington JP, Kalsheker NA (1994) Comparative modelling of major house dust mite allergen Der p I: Structure validation using an extended environmental amino acid propensity table. *Protein Engineering* 7: 689–894

39 Cysteine protease inhibitors for use in treatment of IgE mediated allergic diseases. *World Intellectual Property Organization* PCT application WO 97/04004 (1997)

40 Herbert CA, King CM, Ring PC, Holgate ST, Stewart GA, Thompson PJ, Robinson C (1995) Augmentation of permeability in the bronchial epithelium by the house dust mite allergen Der p 1. *Am J Respir Cell Mol Biol* 12: 369–378

41 Hewitt CRA, Brown AP, Hart BJ, Pritchard DI (1995) A major house dust mite allergen disrupts the immunoglobulin E network by selectively cleaving CD23: Innate protection by antiproteases. *J Exp Med* 182: 1537–1544

42 Hewitt CRA, Horton H, Jones RM, Pritchard DI (1997) Heterogeneous proteolytic specificity and activity of house dust mite proteinase allergen Der p 1. *Clin Exp Allergy* 27: 201–207

43 Winton HL, Wan H, Cannell MB, Thompson PJ, Garrod DR, Stewart GA, Robinson C (1998) Class specific inhibition of house dust mite proteinases which cleave cell adhesion, induce cell death and which increase the permeability of lung epithelium. Br J Pharmacol 124: 1048–1059

44 Chambers L, Suneal K, Sreedharan SD, Kalsheker N, Brocklehurst K (1997) Is the dust mite allergen Der p 1 a cysteine proteinase? *Biochem Soc Trans* 25: 85S

45 Higgins JA, Thorpe CJ, Hayball JD, O'Hehir RE, Lamb JR (1994) Overlapping T cell epitopes in the group I allergen of *Dermatophagoides* species restricted by HLA-DP and HLA-DR class II molecules. *J Allergy Clin Immunol* 93: 891–899

46 Green WK, Thomas WR (1992) IgE binding structures of the major house dust mite allergen Der p I. *Mol Immunol* 29: 257–262

47 Tovey ER, Baldo BA (1990) Localization of antigens and allergens in thin sections of the house dust mite, *Dermatophagoides pteronyssinus* (*Acari: Pyroglyphidae*): *J Med Entomol* 27: 368–376

48 Colloff MJ, Stewart GA (1997) House dust mites. In: PJ Barnes, MM Grunstein, AR Leff, AJ Woolcock (eds) *Asthma*. Lippincott-Raven, Philadelphia, 1089–1104

49 Schulz O, Laing P, Sewell H, Shakib F (1995) Der p I, a major allergen of the house dust mite, proteolytically cleaves the low-affinity receptor for human IgE (CD23). *Eur J Immunol* 25: 3191–3194

50 Yu P, Kosco-Vilbois M, Richards M, Kohler G, Lamers M (1994) Negative feedback regulation of IgE synthesis by urine CD23. *Nature* 369: 753–756

51 Pabst R, Binns RM (1995) Lymphocytes migrate from the bronchoalveolar space to regional bronchial lymph nodes. *Am J Respir Crit Care Med* 151: 495–499

52 Schulz O, Ramjee M, Sewell HF, Shakib F (1997) The cystene proteinase Der p 1, a major allergen of the house dust mite, is inhibited by human α2-macroglobulin and antipain but not by cystain. *ICACI XVI Proceedings* A539

53 Scobie G, Ravindran V, Deam SM, Thomas M, Sreeedharan SK, Brocklehurst K, Kalsheker N (1994) Expression cloning of a dust mite cysteine proteinase, Der p 1, a major allergen associated with asthma and hypersensitivity reactions. *Biochem Soc Trans* 22: 448S

54 Arruda LK, Vailes LD, Mann BJ, Shannon J, Fox JW, Vedick TS, Hayden ML, Chapman MD (1995) Molecular cloning of a major cockroach (*Blatella germanica*) allergen, Bla g 2. *J Biol Bhem* 270: 19563–19568

55 Bryant DH, Burns MW (1976) Skin test reactions to inhalant allergens in asthmatic patients. *Med J Aust* 1: 918–926

56 Sarsfield JK, Boyle AG, Rowell FC, Moriarty SC (1976) Pet sensitivities in asthmatic children. *Arch Dis Child* 51: 186–192

57 Ohman JL, Lowell FC, Bloch KJ (1974) Allergens of mammalian origin III. Properties of a major feline allergen. *J Allergy Clin Immunol* 113: 1668–1677

58 Morgenstern JP, Griffith IJ, Brauer AW, Rogers BL, Bond JF, Chapman MD, Kuo M-C (1991) Determination of the amino acid sequence of *Fel dI*, the major allergen of the domestic cat: protein sequence analysis and cDNA cloning. *Proc Natl Acad Sci USA* 88: 9690–9694

59 Griffith IJ, Craig S, Pollock J, Xu X-B, Morgenstern JP, Rogers BL (1992) Expression and genomic structure of the genes encoding FdI, the major allergen of the domestic cat. *Gene* 113: 263–268

60 Karn RC (1994) The mouse slaivary androgen-binding protein (ABP) alpha subunit closely resembles chain 1 of the cat allergen Fel dI. *Biochem Genet* 32: 271–277

61 Allen RL, Lonsdale DM (1971) Sequence analysis of three members of the maize polygalacturonase gene family expressed during pollen development. *Plant Mol Biol* 20: 343–345

62 Matheson N, Schmidt J, Travis J (1995) Isolation and properties of an angiotensin II-cleaving peptidase from Mesquite pollen. *Am J Respir Cell Mol Biol* 12: 441–448

63 Bagarozzi DA, Pike R, Potempa J, Travis J (1996) Purification and characterization of a novel endopeptidase in ragweed (*Ambrosia artemisiifolia*) pollen. *J Biol Chem* 271: 26227–26232

64 Herbert CA, Holgate ST, Robinson C, Thompson PJ, Stewart GA (1990) Effect of mite allergen on permeability of bronchial mucosa. *Lancet* 2: 1132

65 Herbert CA, Edwards D, Boot JR, Robinson C (1993) Stimulated eosinophils and proteinases augment the transepithelial flux of albumin in bovine bronchial mucosa. *Br J Pharmacol* 110: 840–846

66 Herbert CA, Arthur MJP, Robinson C (1996) Eosinophils augment gelatinase activity in the airway mucosa. Comparative effects as a putative mediator of epithelial injury. *Br J Pharmacol* 117: 667–674

67 Azghani AO, Gray LD, Johnson AR (1993) A bacterial protease perturbs the paracellular barrier function of transporting epithelial monolayers in culture. *Infect Immun* 61: 2681–2686

68 Overton J (1968) The fate of desmosomes in trypsinized tissue. *J Exp Zool* 168: 203–214

69 Winton HL, Wan H, Cannell MB, Gruenert DC, Thomson PJ, Garrod DR, Stewart GA, Robinson C (1998) Cell lines of pulmonary and non-pulmonary origin as tools to study the effects of house dust mite proteinases on the regulation of epithelial permeability. *Clin Exp Allergy*; in press

70 Arruda LK, Vailes LD, Hayden ML, Benjamin DC, Chapman MD (1995) Cloning of cockroach allergen, Bla g 4, identifies ligand binding proteins (or calycins) as a cause of IgE antibody responses. *J Biol Chem* 270: 31196–31201

71 Cavaggioni A, Sorbi RT, Keen JN, Pappin DJ, Findlay JB (1987) Homology between the pyrazine-binding protein from nasal mucosa and major urinary proteins. *FEBS Lett* 212: 225–228

72 Overington JP, Johnson MS, Sali A, Blundell TL (1990) Tertiary structural constraints on protein evolutionary diversity: templates, key residues and structure prediction. *Proc R Soc London* B241: 132–145

Cancer

Molecular Biology of the Lung
Vol. 2: Asthma and Cancer
ed. by R. A. Stockley
© 1999 Birkhäuser Verlag Basel/Switzerland

CHAPTER 9
Gene Expression in Lung Cancer

Tariq Sethi

Respiratory Medicine Unit, Department of Medicine (RIE), University of Edinburgh, Royal Infirmary, Edinburgh, UK

1   Introduction and Background
1.1   Classification of Lung Cancers
2   Genetic Susceptibility
2.1   Hereditary Predisposition
2.2   Chromosomal Abnormalities in Lung Cancer
3   Recessive Oncogenes
3.1   Retinoblastoma Gene
3.2   Gene p53
3.3   Chromosome 3p
3.4   Chromosome 9p Tumour-Suppressor Gene in NSCLC
3.5   Chromosome 5q Recessive Oncogene in Lung Cancer
3.6   Dominantly Acting Oncogenes
3.7   Genetic Changes in *myc* Oncogenes
3.8   The *ras* Oncogenes in Lung Cancer
3.9   The c-*Raf*-1 Proto-oncogene
3.10   The *bcl*-2 Oncogene
4   Conclusions
        References

1. Introduction and Background

Lung cancer is the most common fatal malignancy of both men and women in the developed world, killing over 40000 people in the UK per year [1]. The diagnosis of this disease is usually associated with a prognosis of a survival rate of less than 5%. The biggest risk factor for lung cancer is cigarette smoking. Besides smoking, other environmental and occupational exposures, such as to aromatic hydrocarbons, radon, asbestos, nickel, arsenic and chromium, are important determinants of lung cancer risk. Although lung cancer is largely preventable by elimination of these exposures, this disease will be a major public health problem for the foreseeable future because ex-smokers continue to have a significantly increased risk of developing lung cancer. In addition, the incidence of lung cancer deaths unrelated to smoking is expected to continue to rise over the next 20 years.

Lung carcinogenesis is a multi-stage process involving changes in 10–20 genes involved with DNA repair, cell growth, signal transduction and cell cycle control [2]. In combination with environmental exposures, inherited polymorphisms in a variety of genes, particularly the carcinogen metabolism genes, affect the susceptibility of an individual to develop lung cancer [3, 4]. A better understanding of the molecular mechanisms that cause lung cancer should lead to the development of new prospects for earlier diagnosis and more successful treatments.

1.1. Classification of Lung Cancers

Lung cancers arise from the respiratory epithelium and are classified on this basis of histological type. The two main types are small cell lung cancer (SCLC) and non-small cell lung cancer (NSCLC). A new hypothesis, which is becoming increasingly accepted, is that the main histological types of lung cancer are related through a common differentiation pathway in the bronchial epithelium, mediated by the consistent genetic abnormalities now being described for lung cancer (reviewed in Mabry et al. [5]). This model has been extended, linking differentiation of normal adult bronchial epithelial cells with interactive roles for the chromosome 3p, retinoblastoma (Rb) and *p53* genes, and interplay between the HER/2/neu, *myc*, *ras* and protein kinase C (PKC) gene products [5]. This is illustrated by experiments using a non-tumorigenic cell line, BEAS-2B, derived from normal bronchial epithelial cells transfected with simivian virus SV 40 to induce continuous growth [6–9]. Using this model it was shown that over-expression and point mutations of diffrent oncogenes produce different histological types of tumours. Thus, over-expression of *c-myc* and *raf* resulted in the development of SCLC cells, particularly the variant SCLC cell subtype. Transfection with H-*ras* and HER-2/neu led to the development of adenocarcinomas, whereas transfection of mutant p53 led to the development of squamous cell carcinomas. Furthermore, a cell culture model system for one of these transitions has been developed [10], in which over-expression of a mutated H-*ras* gene in a classic SCLC cell line in conjunction with high levels of *c-myc* expression causes transition to a large cell undifferentiated cancer phenotype. Hence, this *in vitro* model shows that the combination of two genetic abnormalities, which can occur in lung cancer, results in a transition of phenotype. These *in vitro* findings appear to be mirrored *in vivo*.

2. Genetic Susceptibility

2.1. Hereditary Predisposition

The genetic abilities to deactivate carcinogens may play an important role in preventing chromosomal damage. The long-term retention (up to 4 months) of a number of the more than 3000 compounds present in cigarette smoke points to the importance of an efficient deactivating systems as protection against potential carcinogens [11]. The spectrum of oncogene mutations seen in lung cancer is consistent with the carcinogens present in cigarette smoke. It is proposed that the formation of deoxyguanosine adducts by constituents of cigarette smoke including benzo(a)pyrene are responsible for the GC to TA transversion seen in a number of oncogenes in lung cancer. The mutated guanine residue usually resides on the non-transcribed strand of DNA, which is consistent with the model proposed for preferential repair of the transcribed strand in damage of DNA by carcinogens. Unlike other common cancers, the frequency of transition mutations of GC to AT at CpG sites is very low in lung cancers (9%). Such mutations are thought to arise in part from spontaneous deamination of 5-methylcytosine. The low frequency of this type of mutation in lung cancer has been used as evidene of exogenous agents as the source of DNA damage [12]. Enhanced formation of benzo(a)pyrene: DNA adducts has been detected in the monocytes of individuals predisposed to lung cancer, suggesting that enzyme systems responsible for DNA-adduct excision and repair might be defective in these individuals [13]. Cigarette smoke induces a number of enzyme systems associated with microsomes, including cytochrome P450-dependent aryl hydrocarbon hydroxylase and dimethylnitrosamine demethylase, epoxide hydrolase and UDP-glucuronyltransferase. The activation of these phase I enzymes is higher in lung cancer tissue from smokers than in that from non-smokers [11]. Cigarette smoke decreases the level of the phase II enzyme, glutathione-S-transferase [11]. Certain alleles of drug-metabolizing enzymes such as the cytochrome P450 enzymes [14] or other polymorphic markers, e.g. extensive metabolizers of debrisoquine, are associated with a significantly elevated risk of developing lung cancer [15].

The multistep model of carcinogenesis proposes that two or more genetic mutations are required to transform a cell and to enable its monoclonal expansion into a tumour. Inheritance of one or more of these mutations allows tumours to develop earlier than if several spontaneous mutations have to accumulate in a cell. Numerous studies have been conducted to assess the role of genetics in the development of lung cancer after exposure to long-term carcinogens, especially cigarette smoke [16]. That susceptibility has a genetic component is indicated by studies which show that: (1) that only 10% of individuals who smoke develop lung cancer; (2) some individuals who do not smoke develop lung cancer; and (3) there is a significantly increased risk of lung cancer as well as other tumours among blood relatives of lung cancer patients compared with controls. There are reports linking inherited mutations in the retinoblastoma gene on chromosome 13q14 [17], the *p53* gene at chromosome 17p13 [18], and a H-*ras* allele on chromosome 11p [16] to an increased risk of lung cancer. Inheritance of a major autosomal gene has been postulated to determine susceptibility to lung cancer at ages younger than 50 years [19]. A synergistic effect between hereditary predisposition and cigarette smoking has also been noted. This effect of heridity and environmental factors is strikingly demonstrated by the report of the deaths of 58-year-old identical male twins 2 months apart from smoking-related alveolar cell carcinoma. Lung cancer appeared in the individuals within months of each other, had similar histopathologies and metastasized to the brain [20].

2.2. Chromosomal Abnormalities in Lung Cancer

Progression of human cancer is characterized by an accumulation of genetic changes, resulting in activation of oncogenes and inactivation of tumour-suppressor genes and leading progressively to increased genetic instability. These molecular changes are not fully understood but a mutator phenotype leading to genomic instability may be an early step in the development of some cancers. A mutator or replication error (RER) phenotype appears to be important in hereditary non-polyposis colon cancer and characterized by a high frequency of microsatellite instability and defects in DNA mismatch repair genes. Studies on the occurrence of RER in lung cancer have demonstrated a high frequency of microsatellite instability in SCLC (20 of 43 tumours) [21, 22] but infrequent microsatellite instability in NSCLC (7 of 108 tumours) [23]. In both SCLC and NSCLC with associated microsatellite instability, the tumours were characterized by widespread allelic loss (loss of heterozygosity or LOH) as a result of loss of chromosomes or portions of chromosomes and poor prognosis. However, it still remains to be determined whether the high proportion of SCLC with microsatellite instability represents a true RER phenotype with a mismatch repair defect.

Sequential accumulation of LOH is a frequent event in lung cancer and occurs during progression from primary tumours to metastatic sites [24]. Dominant oncogenes require only one mutation for their tumorigenic potential to be activated, whereas the inactivation of recessive oncogenes usually requires genetic events in both alleles. These events are deletions or mutations in the tumour-suppressor gene. Deletions occur frequently in several chromosomal regions in lung cancer cells.

Although there is the high degree of aneuploid and chromosomal loss in late stages of all histological types of lung tumours, there are some noticeable differences between histological types. SCLC exhibits infrequent loss of 9p but more frequent losses of 3p, 5q, 13q and 17p than NSCLC [25–27]. Cytogenetic data obtained for 12 SCLC established cell lines and two fresh SCLC tumour specimens indicated that the region of chromosome 3p14–p23 was deleted in 100% of the cells analysed [28]. Further studies on 64 fresh lung tumours from 47 patients showed that a 100% LOH occurred on chromosomes 3p, 13q and 17p in SCLC [25]. These chromosomal losses occurred early in the development of the tumour before N-*myc* amplification, chromosome 11p deletion or clinical appearance of metastasis.

NSCLCs show consistent LOH at chromosomal regions 3p, 9p, 11p, 13q and 17p [24]. Within NSCLC, squamous cell carcinomas appear to have a larger number of genetic alterations than adenocarcinomas. LOH on 4q, 9q and 21q is common in squamous cell carcinoma [27], but infrequent in adenocarcinomas [28]. Putative oncogenes have been found at 13q (Rb gene) [29], 17p (*p53* gene) [30] and 11p (Wilms' tumour [31] and *ras* [32]). In contrast, a convincing candidate oncogene for the 3p, 5q and 9p regions has not yet been isolated. LOH on chromosome 2q, 18q and 22q is also a frequent but late event in lung cancer, but with increasing knowledge, timing and frequency of different molecular lesions, it will be possible to determine whether alterations are specific for different stages of lung cancer or a consequence of increased genetic instability.

3. Recessive Oncogenes

3.1. Retinoblastoma Gene

The existence of recessive oncogenes or tumour-suppressor genes, in 7cancers, was first proposed by Knudson to explain the early appearance and familial pattern of retinoblastomas in young children. This model proposed that two genetic lesions are required for tumour development. In the hereditary form of the disease, one lesion is transmitted through the germline, whereas the second lesion is acquired postnatally as a somatic mutation. In the sporadic forms of the disease, both lesions have to occur postnatally, thus explaining the relative rarity of this form of the disease. Later cytogenetic analyses on retinoblastoma cells demonstrated a deletion of chromosome 13 material at band q14, as well as loss of heterozygosity [29, 30]. The cloning and characterization of the retinoblastoma gene (*RB1*) showed that loss of the gene or its protein product by homologous deletion or mutation was the event that resulted in tumour development.

There is evidence that survivors of heriditary retinoblastoma are at a higher risk of developing lung cancers as adults and develop them at an earlier age than the general population [31]. Relatives of retinoblastoma patients, who are carriers of an *RB1* mutation, have a 15-fold increased risk of lung cancer than the general population [32]. Hence loss of the *RB1* gene appears also to play a role in the development of lung tumours. The retinoblastoma gene is mutated in more than 90% of SCLC cells but in only a fraction of NSCLC cells. Cytogenetic analyses of SCLC tumours and stablished cell lines indicate an increased number of deletions involving chromosome 13 in over 75% of cases, involving either loss of the entire chromosome 13 or loss of heterozygosity at 13q12–13q33 [25, 28, 33]. In fact, analysis of 50 established lung tumour cell lines and 8 primary SCLC lung tumour tissues revealed structural abnormalities at the DNA level and abnormalities in size and expression of the 4.7-kb RB1 mRNA in 65% of SCLC and 75% of carcinoid lines [34].

The Rb1 protein product, pRB, has a molecular mass of about 105 kDa and is located in the nucleus. The retinoblastoma gene-encoded nucleophosphoprotein is important in cell cycle regulation, binding to regulatory proteins including c-myc and their transcription factor E2f. This protein is expressed in all cell types and is phosphorylated at multiple sites just before DNA replication at the boundary between the G1 and S phases [35]. Both phosphorylated and non-phosphorylated forms of pRB complex with DNA viral proteins involved in cellular transformation, e.g. SV40 large T antigen, adenovirus E1a protein and the human papillomavirus E7 protein [36]. The picture that emerges is that each of these viral proteins specifically inactivates the RB1 gene product as a requisite to transforming the infected cell, a view consistent with the proposed role of pRB as a tumour suppressor. This is further supported by the demonstration that reintroduction of a cloned RB1 cDNA into retinoblastoma and osteosarcoma cells that lack active RB1 genes results in a decreased growth rate of these cells and loss of the ability to grow in soft agar [37].

3.2 Gene p53

The gene *p53* was originally cloned from chemically transformed mouse cells. The human *p53* recessive oncogene maps to chromosome 17p13 [30], a region that has been found to suffer loss of heterozygosity in colon, breast and brain tumours, and also in NSCLC and SCLC cell lines and primary tumours. Of the known tumour-suppressor genes, *p53* is the gene most frequently mutated in human malignancies. The highest number of *p53* mutations in lung cancer is in SCLC in which 70% of tumours have mutations, followed by 65% of squamous cell, 60% of large cell tumours, and 33% of adenocarcinomas [38]. Although *p53* alterations occur in the late stages of some cancers, they appear relatively early in lung cancer, suggesting that this gene may be damaged early in the pathogenesis of these tumours [39]. In one study, mutant *p53* was not detected in hyperplasia or squamous metaplasia but was detected in 13 of 17 carcinomas *in situ*, 20 of 30 invasive carcinomas and in distant metastases from the primary tumours [39]. Mutant *p53* protein accumulates in progressive stages of squamous dysplasia, providing further evidence that *p53* mutations occur before development of the fully invasive carcinoma [40]. Recent studies have described the detection of *p53* or *ras* mutations in sputum samples some of which were collected from patients before the development of clinically detectable tumours [41]. These results indicate the possibility of using molecular approaches for early detection of lung cancer.

Analysis of *p53* mutations in different cancers are furthering our understanding of the mechanisms of carcinogenesis. There are hot spots for mutations of *p53* within the conserved regions of the gene, codons 157, 248 and 273 in lung tumours, although mutations at many other codons have been indentified [38, 42–44]. Overall, the most prevalent type of mutation in lung cancers is a GC to TA transversion. This results in abnormal mRNAs encoding mutant p53 cells which have an increased half-life and bind to heat shock protein hsp70. A study of 30 lung cancer cell lines of all histological types detected mRNA abnormalities in 74% of cases, including changes in size, reduced or absent expression of message, as well as point or small mutations within the open reading frame. Gross abnormalities at the DNA level, rearrangements and two homozygous deletions were found in 75 of cases. Point mutations in *p53* mRNA and the resulting proteins of increased stability have been detected in primary lung tumour specimens [44, 45]. The range of p53 mutation in lung cancers reflects smoking habits. Tumours of smokers compared with those of non-smokers have a significantly higher frequency of GC to TA transversion in *p53*, with a bias towards the non-transcribed strand of DNA (29 vs 0%) and a lower frequency of all transitions, expecially GC to AT transitions (21 vs 69%) [38]. To understand mechanisms of carcinogen-induced lung cancers further, lung tumours from miners and other occupationally exposed populations have been examined for *p53* mutations [46, 47], including tumours from miners exposed to high doses of radon. The mutational hotspot (16 of 30 mutations) at codon 249 – AGG (Arg) to ATG (Met) – was identified in squamous and large cell carcinomas [46] but not in adenocarcinomas [47]. Three of these mutations occurred in tumours from miners who had never smoked, suggesting that this mutation is associated with a non-tobacco carcinogen. Epidemiological evidence implicates occupational exposure to radon in uranium miners as a cause of lung cancer, although miners are also exposed to a variety of other potential carcinogens [48]. The types of mutations found in lung cancers differ from those found in other tumours such as colon and liver cancers, and these differences are related to different carcinogen exposures. The p53 gene acquires oncogenic potential at the DNA level primarily as a result of a point mutations in the wild-type gene the normal function of which appears to be suppression of cellular transformation [49].

Acquired mutations in *p53* have been associated with both treatment resistance and relapse, through a defect in apoptosis; p53 is a nuclear phosphoprotein that is important in cell cycle control; it arrests cells in the check point for the G1/S cell cycle which controls genetic stability, growth arrest and cell death when there has been DNA damage. Loss of function of *p53*, or one of the genes in the *p53* pathway of cellular growth control, can lead to unchecked progression of the cell cycle before appropriate DNA repair can occur so that the DNA mutation is passed on to progeny. This may eventually lead to malignant transformation.

Increased genomic instability has been correlated with *p53* mutations, and such instability could generate multiple genetic alterations leading to cancer. Genetic instability (including gene amplification) increases the frequency in cells that lack a normal *p53* [50]. In one pathway of pro-grammed cell death (apoptosis) induced by DNA-damaging chemothera-peutic drugs or ionizing radiation, inactivation of *p53* could increase both the pool of proliferating cells and the probability of their neoplastic trans-formation by inhibition of programmed cell death [51]. There are several mechanisms to remove wild-type *p53*, which include homozygous dele-tions at the DNA level and point mutations in exons or introns that result in no or a mutated mRNA-encoding mutant or no p53 protein. Mutated p53 protein can sequester wild-type p53 in heteroduplexes, rendering the cells functionally homozygous for the mutant.

The importance of p53 inactivation to the development of lung cancers has been shown by the high incidence of lung adenocarcinomas that develop in transgenic mice carrying a mutant *p53* gene [52]. Furthermore, one study demonstrated germline p53 mutations in all five Li-Fraumeni syndrome families studied, lung cancer being one of the tumours that members of these families develop [18]. Transfection of wild-type p53 suppressed the growth of a human lung cancer cell line expressing p53 [53]. Transfection with wild-type *p53* cDNA caused a significant decrease in the cloning efficiency and reduced tumorigenic potential in nude mice compared with transfection with mutant p53 and controls [52]. The first clinical trial using a retroviral vector containing the wild-type *p53* gene to slow lung cancer growth and induce apoptosis has shown initial promise [54]. The induction of apoptosis by *p53* after genotoxic insult may act as a defence mechanism to protect the organism from propagation of cells that have sustained muta-tion. Abrogation of the *p53* pathway is the most common specific alteration in human cancer, and may be central to the progression of the disease and to its response to treatment by radiation and chemotherapeutic drugs [55].

3.3. Chromosome 3p

The consistent loss of three distinct regions of chromosome 3 – 3p25, 3p21.3 and 3p14-cen – in SCLC, has prompted speculation that these regions encode tumour-suppressor genes [56]. Loss of heterozygosity at chromo-some 3p in seen in SCLC [25], NSCLC [57], cervical cell cancer, sporadic renal cell carcinoma, hereditary renal cell carcinoma and breast cancer. This is one of the earliest lesions detected in lung cancer, appearing in about 75% of hyperplasias. A number of candidate tumour-suppressor genes have been proposed from these regions. The levels of the enzyme aminoacylase-1 (ACY-1), which maps to 3p21.1, are consistently decresed in SCLC [58]. The *c-erbAβ* proto-oncogene encodes a 55-kDa thyroid hormone receptor (THR-β) and is found on human chromosome 3p21−25. This region of chromosome 3 lies within the portion of the short arm found to be deleted in SCLC, and LOH for *c-erbAβ* was detected in six of six

SCLC cell lines examined [59]. The gene encoding the retinoic acid receptor-β is also within the chromosome 3p deleted region at 3p24 [60]. Some of the effects of retinoic acid on lung tumours might be related to alterations in this gene.

Deletion of the protein tyrosine phosphatase-γ gene on the short arm of chromosome 3 has also been described [61]. This gene may be important in regulating the level of protein phosphorylation on tyrosine residues. Tyrosine phosphorylation is a major pathway in signal transduction, which is activated by growth factors. Hence, deletions of the protein tyrosine phosphatase-γ gene localized to 3p21 could increase the level of protein phosphorylation on tyrosine residues within the cell, resulting in transformation. A new putative receptor protein tyrosine kinase of the *met* family, with strutural similarity to the product of the C-*MET* proto-oncogene, the receptor for hepatocyte growth factor and scatter factor, has been localized to 3p21 [62]. The von Hippel-Lindau tumour-suppressor gene maps to 3p25 but is mutated only rarely in lung cancer cell lines [63]. C-*raf* oncogene has been mapped to 3p25 and is frequently deleted in lung cancer [64]. The DNA mismatch repair gene hMLH1, associated with heriditary non-polyposis colon cancer, also maps to 3p [65]. In addition recent micro-cell fusion experiments have demonstrated that introduction of the normal chromosome 3 results in repression of telomerase expression in cancer cells but not in normal cells [66]. Despite identification of the above candidates, the specific lung tumour-suppressor genes on 3p have still to be identified, although fine mapping of the minimally deleted regions is being actively pursued.

3.4. Chromosome 9p Tumour-Suppressor Gene in NSCLC

The region most frequently deleted on chromosome 9p in lung cancers is 9p21 [67]. Candidate tumour-suppressor genes mapped to this region are p16 (MTS1/s1/p16-INK-4) and p15 (MTS2/p15-INK-4B) which code inhibitors of the cyclin-dependent kinase CDK4 which is involved in cell cycle control of the G1 checkpoint [68, 69]. The loss of this function could cause the cell cycle to become dysregulated, thereby leading to uncontrolled cell growth. The infrequent losses on chromosome 9p in SCLC suggest that p16 does not have a major role in SCLC [70]. Studies show that tumour-suppressor genes in this region in NSCLC are frequently inactivated (52% of cases) by homozygous deletions and not by point mutations [71, 72]. Homozygous deletion as a mechanism of loss of function is unusual among known tumour-suppressor genes, e.g. *p53* and *RB*, in which loss of function has previously been found to occur via a point mutation with subsequent loss of the remaining chromosome. As *p16* and *p15* were predicted to be tumour-suppressor genes, it was surprising that more intragenic mutations were not identified in the tumours exhibiting LOH. One possible explanation is the presence of another tumour-suppressor gene in the region which would also be deleted in those tumours exhibiting homozygous deletions of p16 and/or p15. it is also conceivable that mutations or hypermethylation exists in the promoter regions of the p16 or p15 genes. In support of this, it has recently been identified that the second allele of p16 can be inactivated by hypermethylation of the CpG island in the promoter region [73]. About 50% of murine lung adenocarcinomas, both spontaneous and chemically, induced, exhibit LOH on chromosome 4 in the region homologous with human 9p21 [74, 75]. LOH was detected in carcinomas but not adenomas, suggesting the late acquisition of this change in murine lung tumours in contrast to humans in which the LOH of 9p appears relatively early in carcinogenesis.

In SCLC 48 cell lines with absent or mutant *RB* all had detectable p16 protein. In contrast, about 10% of SCLC cell lines which had no *p16* expression had wild-type *RB*. Two-thirds of the NSCLC cell lines examined exhibited loss of *p16* and all but one of these had wild-type *RB*. The remaining cell lines with detectable p16 protein had absent or mutant *RB* [76, 77]. This inverse correlation between the presence and loss of these genes provides evidence for a common *p16/RB* pathway of growth suppression. Moreover these data suggest that *p16* rather than a gene with another function is the tumour-suppressor gene or chromosome 9p21.

3.5. Chromosome 5q Recessive Oncogene in Lung Cancer

Portions of 5p are also frequently deleted in lung cancer in an area that contains the *MCC* and *APC* genes, which are involved in the development of colon cancer. It is of interest, however, that lung and colonic cancers in general do not occur simultaneously. Neither of these genes, nor cytokine or cytokine receptor genes localized in their proximity, have any known function in the development of lung cancer. The loss of DNA from this chromosome has been observed with allelic loss in 87% of SCLC and 70% of NSCLC cases, suggesting that recessive oncogenes in lung carcinogenesis are located on chromosome 5q [78].

3.6. Dominantly Acting Oncogenes

Transforming genes are present and often expressed as proton-oncogenes in normal tissues and are highly conserved during evolution, suggesting that they are important cellular components. The identification of these proto-oncogenes as constituents of normal cells, and the elucidation of the mechanisms of genetic mutation, translocation, amplification and deletion by which they are activated to play dominant roles in oncogenesis, represent a major advance in understanding of the molecular basis of cancer. At least 11 of the known dominantly acting oncogenes have been shown to be activated in a variety of lung cancers. The precise stages at which these oncogenes become activated in the lung tumours, and the exact role they play in the development and progression of these lung tumours, has not been delineated.

3.7. Genetic Changes in myc Oncogenes

The *myc* family of proto-oncogenes c-, N- and L-*myc* (located on human chromosomes 8, 2 and 1p32, respectively), are overexpressed in the vast majority of SCLC cell lines in tumours [79]. The nuclear localization and *in vitro* DNA-binding properties of these proteins suggest that they play an important role in regulating cell growth. A c-*myc* antisense oligodeoxy-nucleotide inhibits entry into the S-phase but not progress from G0 to G1. The mRNA of c-*myc* is amplified after stimulation by growth factors or fetal calf serum [80]. This proto-oncogene is involved in the immorta-lization of primary cells in culture [32]. The c-, N-, L-*myc* proteins coope-rate with the Ha-*ras* and *raf* oncogenes in transforming primary rat fibro-blasts with L-*myc*, producing foci at 1–10% of the rate observed for c- and N-*myc* [32, 81]. Although the *myc* family members demonstrate a high degree of conservation at the nucleic acid and amino acid levels, sug-gesting common intracellular functions, the differential tissue expression of these genes during embryogenesis and adult life, and their different abilities to complement *ras* and *raf*, suggest that they each play important and unique roles.

Of the proto-oncogenes, c-*myc* was the first to be found to have altered expression in SCLC established lines and in lung tumours [79]; it is the only member of the *myc* family to correlate with clinical outcome. The DNA of this proto-oncogene was found to be amplified 20 to 76-fold in 8 of 18 SCLC cell lines examined [82]. In addition, c-*myc* mRNA was found to be over-expressed 15–35 times in these cells even in the absence of DNA amplification. This occurred via increased rates of transcription from the *myc* promoter because the cytoplasmic half-life of the c-*myc* mRNA was unchanged [83]. A block to normal c-*myc* transcription elongation is located in the first intron of the c-*myc* gene. This block is absent in some of those cell lines expressing elevated levels of c-*myc* mRNA without gene amplification [83]. The other members of the *myc* family also demonstrate the same uncoupling of DNA and mRNA amplification as was noted for c-*myc*. Over-expression can also be observed frequently in NSCLC. The *myc* family DNA amplication is found more frequently in tumour cell lines than in tumour specimens.

A number of studies have shown that amplification of c-*myc* is associa-ted with relative resistance to chemotherapy and radiotherapy. For example, one study showed that DNA amplification of one of the *myc* family genes occurred in 3 of 40 (8%) untreated patient specimens compared with 19 of 67 (28%) treated patient specimens [84]. It seems that DNA amplification of the c-*myc* family genes is unlikely to be a primary event in the pathogenesis of lung cancer. Amplification of these genes may render a growth advantage to an already transformed cell, which can subsequently become the dominant population in the tumour. Transfection of c-*myc* into a classic histological SCLC cell line caused a change in morphological features and growth patterns consistent with variant histology, but the cells retained some neuroendocrine markers [5]. Variant SCLC cell lines typically have a more rapid growth rate and a higher cloning efficiency in semi-solid agarose, and lack the markers of neuroendocrine differentiation when compared with the more classic SCLC cell lines. The DNA amplification of *myc* family genes, particularly c-*myc*, has been associated with shortened survival in patients with SCLC. These studies, however, use samples taken from patients after the initiation of therapy, so their applicability is currently uncertain. Prospective studies of gene expression may prove useful.

3.8. The ras Oncogenes in Lung Cancer

Members of the *ras* family of proto-oncogenes, consisting of K-, H- and N-*ras*, are inner plasma membrane-associated GTPases which bind GTP to cleave it to GDP. They play a critical role in the pathway of signal transduction from cell membrane to the nucleus, acting as a link between tyrosine kinases and serine/threonine kinases, and they appear to control cell growth [85]. Activated *ras* oncogenes have been found in a variety of human tumours. Activated H-*ras* can transform normal human bronchial epithelium after transcription *in vitro* [86] and induce lung adenomas in mice made transgenic for H-*ras* [87]. The involvement of *ras* proto-oncogenes in human lung tumours was first detected by transfection of tumour DNA into NIH3T3 mouse fibroblasts. K-*ras* restriction fragments were found in cells transformed by the DNA from SCLC, adenocarcinoma, squamous cell carcinoma and undifferentiated lung carcinoma cell lines; the K-*ras*-2 gene 12p12 was found to be mutated in some of the original tumour tissue [32]. Activating point mutations were localized predominantly in codons 12, 13 and 61. 14 of 77 NSCLC tumour samples were found to have K-*ras* mutations, all of which were single point mutations in codon 12 from adenocarcinomas [88]. H-*ras* mutated at codon 61 was detected in SQCC cell line. Loss of heterozygosity of the c-H-*ras* gene on chromosome 11p15 has been associated with more aggressive NSCLC tumours. N-*ras* was found in one undifferentiated lung cancer but most *ras* mutations in lung cancers are K-*ras* [89].

The activation of K-*ras* is thought to represent an early event in lung carcinogenesis. The K-*ras* proto-oncogene was one of the first genes found to be altered in lung cancers; it is activated by point mutation in about 30% of human lung adenocarcinomas and large cell carcinomas, but infrequently in squamous cell carcinomas and very rarely in SCLC [90]. The predominant K-*ras* mutation detected in human lung adenocarcinomas is a GC to TA transversion in the first base of codon 12 [91]. Lung tumours from mice treated with benzo(a)pyrene also have the same K-*ras* mutation, suggesting that this occurs in humans as a direct result of cigarette smoking. In these mouse models, K-*ras* mutations are detected in the earliest hyperplastic lesions, although in human lung adenocarcinomas *ras* activation seems to be a somewhat later event which appears in carcinomas *in situ* [93]. Furthermore, the involvement of *ras* proto-oncogenes in later stages of lung carcinogenesis is indicated by several studies, noting the association of activated *ras* proto-oncogenes, which have metastatic potential of transformed human bronchial epithelial cells [94] and differentiation of established SCLC lines, increased hormone production [10] or large cell lung cancer phenotype [95]. There is an association of *ras* activation in cancers with poor prognosis and survival of patients with adenocarcinoma [96]. In addition survival is even shorter when *ras* mutations occur in combination with other oncogenes, e. g. overexpression of erb B-2 [97].

3.9. The c-Raf-1 Proto-oncogene

The c-*Raf* protein, p74*Raf*, is a serine/threonine-specific kinase which is membrane localized and activated by *ras*. Phosphorylation at serine and threonine residues activates p74*Raf* kinase which transmits signals from the membrane of the cytoplasm [98]. The c-*Raf*-1 proto-oncogene maps to chromosome 3p25, a region of chromosome 3 frequently deleted in both SCLC and NSCLC lung tumours. Cytogenetic analyses of SCLC cell lines show that one c-*Raf*-1 allele is deleted in about 80% of the lines [99]. However, c-*Raf*-1 mRNA was expressed at high levels in 12 of 12 SCLC cell lines [100]. Transcriptional activation of c-*Raf*-1, along with other proto-oncogenes, is a common feature of NSCLC [101].

3.10. The bcl-2 Oncogene

The *bcl*-2 oncogene was the first oncogene to be identified that specifically prevented cells from dying. High levels of *Bcl*-2 protein prevent cells from undergoing apoptosis in response to a number of death-inducing stimuli, indicating that this protein blocks the final common pathway by which cells enter apoptosis. The oncogene *bcl*-2 can contribute to malignancy by blocking apoptosis and undergo synergy with other oncogenes. SCLC cells show a high level of *bcl*-2 expression in almost 100% of tumours. There is also a close correlation between *bcl*-2 and neuroendocrine marker expression in NSCLC. It is now realized that *bcl*-2 is only one of a family of related proteins; some of its members can protect cells whereas others may bind to *bcl*-2 and counteract its protective effect [102]. As a greater understanding of the *bcl*-2 families of proteins evolves, strategies will be developed to target these pathways.

4. Conclusions

Many oncogenic changes occur in growth factor receptors and signal transduction components which will give cells a growth advantage and explain how a tumour may survive the retention of wild-type p53. Alternatively the frequent loss of wild-type p53, overexpression of *bcl*-2 and *myc* or constitutive activation of *ras* may prevent a cell from dying and confer resistance to chemotherapy. The discovery of the cyclin-dependent kinase inhibitors *p16* and *p15*, and of *p53* and *Rb* as candidate tumour-suppressor genes in lung cancer, provides evidence for the importance of cell cycle check points in cancer. The study of gene function in different critical pathways, e.g. cell cycle and signal transduction, may have both therapeutic and prognostic importance and, with a greater understanding of the molecular events involved in the genesis and progresson of lung cancer, we may be able both to prevent and to treat this disease. As susceptibility factors for genetic alterations affecting lung cancer development are discovered, it might be practical to target anti-smoking and early detection efforts for those individuals with the highest risks.

Tests for the presence of certain oncogenes, e. g. *ras*, mutations in adenocarcinomas or loss of tumour-suppressor genes, e. g. LOH at certain low site mutations or functional analysis of genes such as *Rb* or *p16*, may suggest new treatment modalities and predictions of which therapies will be successful for a given patient. As the mechanism of action of these oncogenes is elucidated, it will be possible to develop novel therapies against this devastating disease.

References

1 Boring CC, Squires TS, Tong T (1995) Cancer statistics. *CA Cancer J Clin* 45: 8–30
2 Minna JD (1994) Summary of the role of dominant and recessive oncogenes in the pathogenesis of lung cancer and the application of this knowledge in translational research. In: H Pass et al. (eds) *Lung cancer: principles and practice*. JB Lippincott, Philadelphia
3 Caporaso N, Landi MT, Vineis P (1991) Relevance of metabolic polymorphisms to human carcinogenesis: evaluation of epidemiologic evidence. *Pharmacogenetics* 1: 4–19
4 Nakachi K, Imai K, Hayashi S et al. (1991) Genetic susceptibility to squamous cell carcinoma of the lung in relation to cigarette smoking dose. *Cancer Res* 51: 5177–5180
5 Mabry M, Nelkin DB, Falco JP, Barr LF, Baylin SB (1991) Transitions between lung cancer phenotypes – implications for tumor progression. *Cancer Cells* 3(2): 53–58
6 Sellers TA, Chen PL, Potter JD et al. (1994) Segregation analysis of smoking-associated malignancies: evidence for mendelian inheritance. *Am J Med Genet* 52: 308–314
7 Kawajiri K, Watanabe J, Eguchi H et al. (1995) Genetic polymorphisms of drug-metabolizing enzymes and lung cancer susceptibility. *Pharmacogenetics* 5: S70–S73

8 Gariboldi M, Manenti G, Canzian F et al. (1993) A major suscpetibility locus to murine lung carcinogenesis maps on chromosome 6. *Nature Genet* 3: 132–136

9 Devereux TR, Wiseman RW, Kaplan N et al. (1994) Assignment of a locus for mouse lung tumor susceptibility to proximal chromosome 19. *Mamm Genome* 5: 749–755

10 Mabry M, Nakagawa T, Nelkin BD, MyDowell E, Gesell M, Eggleston JC, Casero RA Jr, Baylin SB (1988) v-Ha-ras oncogene insertion: a model for tumor progression of human small cell lung cancer. *Proc Natl Acad Sci USA* 85: 6523–6527

11 Petruzzelli TS, Camus AM, Carrozzi L, Ghelarducci L et al. (1988) *Cancer Res* 48: 4695–4700

12 Rudiger W, Nowak D, Hartmann K, Cervitti P (1985) *Cancer Res* 45: 5890–5894

13 Bohr VA, Phillips DH, Hanawalt PC (1987) Heterogensous DNA damage and repair in the mammalian genome. *Cancer Res* 47: 6426–6436

14 Ayesh R, Idle JR, Ritchie JC, Crothers MJ, Hetzel MR (1984) Metabolic oxidation phenotypes as markers for susceptibility to lung cancer. *Nature* 312: 169–170

15 Nakachi K, Imai K, Hayashi S, Kawajiri K (1993) Polymorphisms of the CYP1A1 and glutathione *S*-transferase genes associated with susceptibility to lung cancer in relation to cigarette dose in a Japanese population. *Cancer Res* 53: 2994–2999

16 Heighway J, Thatcher N, Cerny T, Hasleton PS (1986) Genetic predisposition to human lung cancer. *Br J Cancer* 53: 453–457

17 Sanders BM, Jay M, Draper GJ, Roberts EM (1989) Non-ocular cancer in relatives of retinoblastoma patients. *Br J Cancer* 60: 358–365

18 Malkin D, Jolly KW, Barbier N, Look AT, Friend SH, Gebhard MC, Andersen TI, Borresen AL, Li FP, Garber J et al. (1992) Germline mutations of the p53 tumor-suppressor gene in children young adults with second malignant neoplasms. *N Engl J Med* 326: 1309–1315

19 Sellers TA, Chen PL, Potter JD, Bailey-Wilson JE, Rothschild H, Elston RC (1994) Segregation analysis of smoking-associated malignancies: evidence for Mendelian inheritance. *Am J Med Genet* 52: 308–314

20 Joishy SK, Cooper RA, Rowley PT (1977) Alveolar cell carcinoma in identical twins. Similarity in time of onset, histochemistry, and site of metastasis. *Ann Intern Med* 87: 447–450

21 Merlo A, Mabry M, Gabrielson E et al. (1994) Frequent microsatellite instability in primary small cell lung cancer. *Cancer Res* 54: 2098–2101

22 Mao L, Lee DJ, Tockman MS et al. (1994) Microsatellite alterations as clonal markers for the detection of human cancer. *Proc Natl Acad Sci USA* 91: 9871–9875

23 Fong KM, Zimmerman PV, Smith PJ (1995) Microsatellite instability and other molecular abnormalities in non-small cell lung cancer. *Cancer Res* 55: 28–30

24 Sheseki M, Kohno T, Nishikawa R et al. (1994) Frequent allelic losses on chromosomes 2q, 18q and 22q in advanced non-small cell lung carcinoma. *Cancer Res* 54: 5643–5648

25 Yokota J, Wada M, Shimosato Y et al. (1987) Loss of heterozygosity on chromosomes 3, 13, and 17 in small cell carcinoma and on chromosome 3 in adenocarcinoma of the lung. *Proc Natl Acad Sci USA* 84: 9252–9256

26 Hosoe S, Ueno K, Shigedo Y et al. (1994) A frequent deletion of chromosome 5q21 in advanced small cell and non-small cell carcinoma of the lung. *Cancer Res* 54: 1787–1790

27 Tsuchiya E, Nakamura Y, Weng S et al. (1992) Allelotype of non-small cell lung carcinoma – comparison between loss of heterozygosity in squamour cell carcinoma and adenocarcinoma. *Cancer Res* 52: 2478–2481

28 Whang-Peng J, Bunn PA Jr, Kao-Shan CS, Lee EC, Carney DN, Gazdar A, Minna JD (1982) A nonrandom chromosomal abnormality, del 3p(14–23), in human small cell lung cancer (SCLC). *Cancer Genet Cytogenet* 6: 119–134

29 Dryja TP, Mukai S, Petersen R, Rapaport JM, Walton D, Yandell DW (1989) Parental origin of mutations of the retinoblastoma gene. *Nature* 339: 556–558

30 Cavenee WK, Murphree AL, Shull MM, Benedict WF, Sparkes RS, Kock E, Nordenskjold M (1986) Prediction of familial predisposition to retinoblastoma. *N Engl J Med* 314: 1201–1207

31 Leonard RC, MacKay T, Brown A, Gregor A, Crompton GK, Smyth JF (1988) Small-cell lung cancer after retinoblastoma. *Lancet* 2: 1503

32 Birrer MJ, Alani R, Cuttitta F, Preis LH, Sabich AL, Sanders DA, Siegfried JM, Szabo E, Brown PH (1992) Early events in the neoplastic transformation of respiratory epithelium. *J Natl Cancer Inst Monogr* 13: 31–37

33 Johnson BE, Sakaguchi AY, Gazdar AF, Minna JD, Burch D, Marshall A, Naylor SL (1988) Restriction fragment length polymorphism studies show consistent loss of chromosome 3p alleles in small cell lung cancer patients' tumors. *J Clin Invest* 82: 502–507

34 Harbour JW, Lai SL, Whang-Peng J, Gazdar AF, Minna JD, Kaye FJ (1988) Abnormalities in structure and expression of the human retinoblastoma gene in SCLC. *Science* 241: 353–357

35 Hu QJ, Lees JA, Buchkovich KJ, Harlow E (1992) The retinoblastoma protein physically associates with the human cdc2 kinase. *Mol Cell Biol* 12: 971–980

36 Dyson N (1994) pRB, p107 and the regulation of the E2F transcription factor. *J Cell Sci* 18 (suppl) 81–87

37 Huang JH, Yee JK, Shew JY, Chen PL, Bookstein R, Friedmannn T, Lee EY, Lee WH (1988) Suppression of the neoplastic phenotype by replacement of the RB gene in human cancer cells. *Science* 242: 1563–1566

38 Greenblatt MS, Bennet WP, Hollstein M et al. (1994) Mutations in the p53 tumor suppressor gene: clues to cancer etiology and molecular pathogenesis. *Cancer Res* 54: 4855–4978

39 Fontanini G, Vignati S, Bigini D et al. (1994) Human non-small cell lung cancer: p53 protein accumulation is an early event and persists during metastatic progression. *J Pathol* 174: 23–31

40 Nuorva K, Soini Y, Kamel D et al. (1993) Concurrent p53 expression in vronchial dysplasias and squamous cell lung carcinomas. *Am J Pathol* 142: 725–732

41 Mao L, Hruban R, Boyle JO et al. (1994) Detectiion of oncogene mutations in sputum precedes diagnosis of lung cancer. *Cancer Res* 54: 1634–1637

42 Miller CW, Simon K, Aslo A et al. (1992) p53 mutations in human lung tumors. *Cancer Res* 52: 1695–1698

43 Kishimoto Y, Murakami Y, Shiraishi M et al. (1992) Aberrations of the p53 tumor suppressor gene in human non-small cell lung carcinomas of the lung. *Cancer Res* 52: 4799–4804

44 Takahashi T, Carbone D, Takahashi T, Nau MM, Hida I, Ueda R, Minna JD (1992) Wild-type but not mutant p53 suppresses the growth of human lung cancer cells bearing multiple genetic lesions. *Cancer Res* 52: 2340–2343

45 Takahashi T, Takahashi T, Suzuki H, Hida T, Sekido Y, Ariyoshi Y, Ueda R (1991) The p53 gene is very frequently mutated in small-cell lung cancer with a distinct nucleotide substitution pattern. *Oncogene* 6: 1775–1778

46 Taylor JA, Watson MA, Devereux TR et al. (1994) p53 mutation hotspot in radon-associated lung cancer [see comments]. *Lancet* 343: 86–87

47 McDonald JW, Taylor JA, Watson MA et al. p53 and K-*ras* in radon-associated lung adenocarcinoma. *Cancer Epidemiol Biomarkers Prev, in press*

48 Saccomanno G, Huth GC, Auerbach O et al. (1988) Relationship of radioactive radon daughters and cigarette smoking in the genesis of lung cancer in uranium miners. *Cancer* 62: 1402–1408

49 Hall PA, Lane DP (1997) Tumor suppressors: a developing role for p53? *Curr Biol* 7: R144–R147

50 Harris CC (1993) The p53 tumor suppressor gene: at the crossroads of molecular carcinogenesis, molecular epidemiology and cancer risk assessment. *Science* 262: 1980–1981

51 Vogelstein B, Kinzler KW (1992) p53 function and dysfunction. *Cell* 70: 523–526

52 Harvey M, Vogel H, Morris D, Bradley A, Bernstein A, Donehower LA (1995) A mutant p53 transgene accelerates tumour development in heterozygous but not nullizygous p53-deficient mice. *Nature Genet* 9: 305–311

53 Cajot JF, Anderson MJ, Lehman TA, Shapiro H, Briggs AA, Stanbridge EJ (1992) Growth suppression mediated by transfection of p53 in Hut292DM human lung cancer cells expressing endogenous wild-types p53 protein. *Cancer Res* 52: 6956–6960

54 Roth JA, Nguyen D, Lawrence DD, Kemp BL, Carrasco CH, Ferson DZ et al. (1996) Retrovirus-mediated wild-type p53 gene transfer to tumors of patients with lung cancer. *Nature Med* 2: 985–991

55 Cox LS, Lane DP (1995) Tumour suppressors, kinases and clamps: how p53 regulates the cell cycle in response to DNA damage. *Bioessays* 17: 501–508

56 Hibi K, Takahashi T, Yamakawa K et al. (1992) Three distinct regions involved in 3p deletion in human lung cancer. *Oncogene* 7: 445–449

57 Weston A, Willey JC, Modali R, Sugimura H, McDowell EM, Resau J, Light B, Haugen A, Mann DL, Trump BF et al. (1989) Differential DNA sequence deletions from chromosomes 3, 11, 13, and 17 in squamous-cell carcinoma, large-cell carcinoma, and adenocarcinoma of the human lung. *Proc Natl Acad Sci USA* 86: 5099–5103

58 Miller YE, Minna JD, Gazdar AF (1989) Lack of expression of aminoacylase-1 in small cell lung cancer. Evidence for inactivation of genes encoded by chromosome 3p. *J Clin Invest* 83: 2120–2124

59 Dobrovic A, Houle B, Belouchi A, Bradley WE (1988) erbA-related sequence coding for DNA-binding hormone receptor localized to chromosome 3p21–3p25 and deleted in small cell lung carcinoma. *Cancer Res* 48: 682–685

60 Gebert JF, Moghal N, Frangioni JV, Sugarbaker DJ, Neel BG (1991) High frequency of retinoic acid receptor beta abnormalities in human lung cancer. *Oncogene* 6: 1859–1868. (Published erratum appears in *Oncogene* 1992 7: 821)

61 LaForgia S, Morse B, Levy J, Barnea G, Cannizzaro LA, Li F, Nowell PC, Boghosian-Sell L, Glick J, Weston A et al. (1991) Receptor protein-tyrosine phosphatase gamma is a candidate tumor suppresor gene at human chromosome region 3p21. *Proc Natl Acad Sci USA* 88: 5036–5040

62 Ronsin C, Muscatelli F, Mattei MG, Breathnach R (1993) A novel putative receptor protein tyrosine kinase of the met family. *Oncogene* 8: 1195–1202

63 Sekido Y, Bader S, Latif F et al. (1994) Molecular analysis of the von Hippel-Lindau disease tumor suppressor gene in human lung cancer cell lines. *Oncogene* 9: 1599–1604

64 Graziano SL, Pfeifer AM, Testa JR (1991) Involvement of the RAF1 locus, at band 3p25, in the 3pdeletion of small cell lung cancer. *Genes Chromosome Cancer* 3: 283–293

65 Bronner CE, Baker SM, Morrison PT et al. (1994) Mutation in the DNA mismatch repair gene homologue hMLH1 is associated with hereditary nonpolyposis colon cancer linked to chromosome 3p. *Nature* 368: 258–261

66 Ohmura H, Tahara H, Suzuki M et al. Restoration of the cellular senescence program and repression of telomerase by human chromosome 3. *Cancer Res, in press*

67 Cairns P, Mao L, Merlo A et al. (1994) Rates of p16(MTS1) mutations in primary tumors with 9p loss. *Science* 265: 415–416

68 Kamb A, Gruis NA, Weaver-Feldhaus J et al. (1994) A cell cycle regulator potentially involved in genesis of many tumor types. *Science* 264: 436–440

69 Hannon GJ, Beach D (1994) p15^{INK4B} is a potential effector of TGF-β-induced cell cycle arrest. *Nature* 371: 257–260

70 Reid T, Peterson I, Holtgreve-Grez H et al. (1994) Mapping of multiple DNA gains and losses in primary small cell lung carcinomas by comparative genomic hybridization. *Cancer Res* 54: 1801–1806

71 Hayashi N, Sugimoto Y, Tsuchiya E et al. (1994) Somatic mutations of the MTS (multiple tumor suppressor) 1/CDK41 (cyclin-dependent kinase-4 inhibitor) gene in human primary non-small cell lung carcinomas. *Biochem Biophys Res Commun* 202: 1426–1430

72 Okamoto A, Hussain SP, Hagiwara K et al. (1995) Mutations in the p16-INK/MTSI/CDKN2, p15-INK4B/MTS2, and p18 genes in primary and metastatic lung cancer. *Cancer Res* 55: 1448–1451

73 Merlo A, Herman JG, Mao L et al. (1995) 5′ CpG island methylation is associated with transcriptional silencing of the tumour suppressor p16/CDKN2/MTS1 in human cancers. *Nature Med* 1: 686–692

74 Hegi ME, Devereux TR, Dietrich WF et al. (1994) Allelotype analysis of mouse lung carcinomas reveals frequent allelic losses on chromosome 4 and an association between allelic imbalances on chromosome 6 and K-*ras* activation. *Cancer Res* 54: 6257– 6264

75 Herzog CR, Wiseman RW, You M (1994) Deletion mapping of a putative tumor suppressor gene on chromosome 4 in mouse lung tumors. *Cancer Res* 54: 4007–4010

76 Ottarson GA, Kratzke RA, Coxon A et al. (1994) Absence of p16INK4 protein is restricted to the subset of lung cancer lines that retains wildtype Rb. *Oncogene* 9: 3375–3378

77 Shapiro GI, Edwards CD, Kobzik L et al. (1995) Reciprocal Rb inactivation and p16^{INK4} expression in primary lung cancers and cell lines. *Cancer Res* 55: 505–509

78 D'Amico D, Carbone DP, Johnson BE et al. (1992) Polymorphic sites within the MMC and APC loci reveal very frequent loss of heterozygosity in human small cell lung cancer. *Cancer Res* 52: 1996–1999

79 Johnson BE, Makuch RW, Simmons AD, Gazdar AF, Burch D, Cashell AW (1988) *Cancer Res* 48: 5163–5166

80 Heikkila R, Schwab G, Wickstrom E, Loke SL, Pluznik DH, Watt R, Neckers LM (1987) A c-myc antisense oligodeoxynucleotide inhibits entry into S phase but not progress from G0 to G1. *Nature* 328: 445–449

81 Schwab M, Varmus HE, Bishop JM (1985) Human N-myc gene contributes to neoplastic transformation of mammalian cells in culture. *Nature* 316: 160–162

82 Little CD, Nau MM, Carney DN, Gazdar AF, Minna JD (1983) Amplification and expression of the c-myc oncogene in human lung cancer cell lines. *Nature* 306: 194–196

83 Krystal G, Birrer M, Way J, Nau M, Sausville E, Thompson C, Minna J, Battey J (1988) Multiple mechanisms for transcriptional regulation of the myc gene family in small-cell lung cancer. *Mol Cell Biol* 8: 3373–3381

84 Johnson BE, Brennan JF, Ihde DC, Gazdar AF (1992) myc family DNA amplification in tumours and tumour cell lines from patients with small cell lung cancer. *J Natl Cancer Inst Monogr* 13: 39

85 Marshall CJ (1996) Ras effectors. *Curr Opin Cell Biol* 8: 197–204

86 Yoakum GH, Malan-Shibley L, Harris CC (1991) Malignant progression of harvey ras transformed normal human bronchial epithelial cells. *Basic Life Sci* 57: 341–351

87 Suda Y, Aizawa S, Hirai S, Inoue T, Furuta Y, Suzuki M, Hirohashi S, Ikawa Y (1987) Driven by the same Ig enhancer and SV40 T promoterras induced lung adenomatous tumors, myc induced pre-B cell lymphomas and SV40 large T gene a variety of tumors in transgenic mice. *EMBO J* 6: 4055–4065

88 Santos E, Martin-Zanca D, Reddy EP, Pierotti MA, Della Porta G, Barbacid M (1984) Malignant activation of a K-ras oncogene in lung carcinoma but not in normal tissue of the same patient. *Science* 223: 661–664

89 Suzuki Y, Orita M, Shiraishi M, Hayashi K, Sekiya T (1990) Detection of ras gene mutations in human lung cancers by single-strand conformation polymorphism analysis of polymerase chain reaction products. *Oncogene* 5: 1037–1043

90 Reynolds SH, Wiest JS, Devereux TR et al. (1992) Proto-oncogene activation in spontaneously occurring and chemically induced rodent and human lung tumors. In: A Klein-Szarto, M Anderson, JC Barrett et al. (eds). *Comparative molecular carcinogenesis*. John Wiley & Sons, New York, 303–320

91 You M, Candrian U, Maronpot RR et al. (1989) Activation of the K-*ras* proto-oncogene in spontaneously occurring and chemically induced lung tumors of the strain A mouse. *Proc Natl Acad Sci USA* 86: 3070–3074

92 Belinsky SA, Devereux TR, Foley JF et al. (1992) Role of the alveolar type II cell in the development and progression of pulmonary tumors induced by 4-(methylnitrosamino)-1-(3-pyridyl)-1-butanone in the A/J mouse. *Cancer Res* 52: 3164–3173

93 Sugio K, Kishimoto Y, Virmani AK et al. (1994) K-*ras* mutations are a relatively late event in the pathogenesis of lung carcinomas. *Cancer Res* 54: 5811–5815

94 Bonfil RD, Reddel RR, Ura H, Reich R, Fridman R, Harris CC, Klein-Szanto JP (1989) Invasive and metastatic potential of a v-Ha-ras-transformed human bronchial epithelial cell line. *J Natl Cancer Inst* 81: 587–594

95 Mabry M, Nakagawa T, Baylin S, Pettengill O, Sorenson G, Nelkin B (1989) Insertion of the v-Ha-ras oncogene induces differentiation of calcitonin-producing human small cell lung cancer. *J Clin Invest* 84: 194–199

96 Mitsudomi T, Steinberg SM, Oie HK et al. (1991) *ras* gene mutations in non-small cell lung cancers are associated with shortened survival irrespective of treatment intent. *Cancer Res* 51: 4999–5002

97 Kern JA, Filderman AE (1993) Oncogenes and growth factors in human lung cancer. *Clin Chest Med* 14: 31–41

98 Morrison DK, Cutler RE Jr (1997) Complexity of raf signalling. *Curr Opin Biol* 9: 174–179

99 Sithanandam G, Dean M, Brennscheidt U, Beck T, Gazdar A, Minna JD, Brauch H, Zbar B, Rap UR (1989) Loss of heterozygosity at the c-raf locus in small cell lung carcinoma. *Oncogene* 4: 451–455

100 Kiefer PE, Bepler G, Kubasch M, Havemann K (1987) Amplification and expression of protooncogenes in human small cell lung cancer cell lines. *Cancer Res* 47: 6236–6242

101 Kiefer PE, Wegmann B, Bacher M, Erbil C, Heidtmann H, Haveman K (1990) Different pattern of expression of cellular oncogenes in human non-small-cell lung cancer cell lines. *J Cancer Res Clin Oncol* 116: 29–37

102 Ben-Ezra JM, Kornstein MJ, Grimes MM, Krystal G (1994) Small cell carcinomas of the lung express the Bcl-2 protein. *Am J Pathol* 145: 1036–1040

Molecular Biology of the Lung
Vol. 2: Asthma and Cancer
ed. by R. A. Stockley
© 1999 Birkhäuser Verlag Basel/Switzerland

CHAPTER 10
Gene Therapy for Cancer: Prospects for the Treatment of Lung Tumours

Nicola K. Green, Moira G. Gilligan, David J. Kerr, Peter F. Searle
and Lawrence S. Young

CRC Institute for Cancer Studies, University of Birmingham, UK

1   Introduction
2   Methods of Gene Delivery
2.1   Viral Vectors
2.1.1 Retroviral vectors
2.1.2 Adenoviral vectors
2.1.3 Adeno-associated virus
2.1.4 Herpes simplex virus
2.2   Physical Methods
3   Gene Targeting
3.1   Selective Delivery of Therapeutic Genes to Tumour Cells
3.1.1 *Ex vivo* delivery
3.1.2 *In vivo* regional delivery
3.2   Selective Uptake Mechanisms
3.3   Tumour-Specific Promoters
3.4   Tumour-Specific Mechanisms
3.4.1 Tumour-Restricted Cytolytic Viruses
4   Gene Therapy Strategies for Lung Cancer
4.1   Restoration of Tumour-Suppressor Gene Expression
4.2   Pro-drug-Activating Enzymes
4.3   Immunological Approaches
4.4   Antisense Oligodeoxynucleotides
4.5   Ribozymes
5   Conclusion
       References

1. Introduction

Lung cancer is the most common fatal malignancy in the developed world, accounting for about 10% of all cancers, and increasing in incidence by about 0.5% per year in the UK [1]. Non-small cell lung cancer (NSCLC) comprises about 75% of all lung cancers and includes adenocarcinoma, squamous cell, large cell and bronchioalveolar carcinoma. Over the past 20 years, despite advances in medical and surgical intervention, there has been little change in the 5-year survival rates for lung cancer, with only 10% of patients surviving for 5 years after diagnosis.

Cancer is a genetic disease which results in abnormalities in the key processes of cellular proliferation, differentiation and apoptosis. The principal genetic aberrations include mutations in cellular proto-oncogenes and DNA repair genes, and the inactivation or loss of tumour-suppressor genes. Although there are inherited predispositions to cancer resulting from germ-line transmission of mutant tumour-suppressor genes, the harmful mutations are usually somatically acquired, accumulating in a clone of cells with progressive escape from normal regulatory constraints. It is currently believed that at least 10 such mutations are required to convert a normal lung cell into a malignant cell. As the reversal of a single genetic lesions can have a significant effect on tumour cell growth and tumorigenicity, this approach can be useful in tumour cells with multiple genetic lesions [2, 3].

The past two decades have witnessed a revolution in all branches of biology brought about by the development and application of recombinant DNA technology. The prospect of genetic intervention for the treatment of cancer is very appealing, because the development of sophisticated viral vectors as well as non-viral DNA delivery systems means that it is now possible to deliver genetic information to cells *in vivo*, although for many applications there are still substantial hurdles in terms of efficiency and selectivity. A variety of strategies has been suggested by which gene transfer to tumour cells may inhibit growth, promote cellular death (either directly or after prodrug administration) or enhance recognition of the tumour cells by the immune system. Other approaches envisage gene transfer to non-tumour cells to increase their resistance to cytotoxic drugs, or to augment immune responsiveness to tumours directly. The methods by which therapeutic genes are delivered to their target cells are independent of the mechanism of action of the encoded gene product. At present, and for the foreseeable future, the relatively low efficiency and selectivity of delivery systems impose strict constraints on what is achievable and therefore make greater demands on the effector mechanisms. Important parameters to consider for any gene therapy approach are: the mechanisms of cell killing; the efficiency of gene transfer that is required for the strategy to be effective; the degree of tumour selectivity achieved; and the duration of gene expression required. The best methods of gene delivery currently available are viral-mediated gene delivery using retroviral and adenoviral vectors. Of the 120 or so clinical trials under way using gene therapy for the treatment of cancer, about 70% are using retroviral vectors and 15% adenoviral vectors.

2. Methods of Gene Delivery

2.1. *Viral Vectors*

Recombinant viral vectors are produced by replacement of viral genes with therapeutic DNA sequences; such viruses are replication deficient because they lack some or all of the genes required for viral propagation. To produce the virus, the proteins are provided instead from chromosomally integrated genes in specially engineered packaging or produce cell lines.

2.1.1. Retroviral vectors: Recombinant retroviral vectors are produced by replacing the *gag, pol* and *env* viral genes with foreign DNA. Retroviruses provide the advantage of stable gene expression from an integrated proviral genome, but as integration is random there has been concern that vectors may integrate into an important cellular gene or the regulatory regions of such genes and be potentially oncogenic. As experience with these vectors accumulates, it is now considered that this represents a very unlikely event and the risk is considered to be quite small. The integration of retroviral genomes occurs only in actively dividing cells, which could therefore be used to limit delivery of the vector to rapidly dividing tumour cells as opposed to the more slowly replicating cells of normal tissues.

If retroviral vectors are to be used successfully in human gene therapy protocols, it is essential that secondary spread of the retrovirus from the target cells is prevented. During characterization of early versions of producer cell lines, generation of replication-competent virus (RCR) had been found to occur [4] and this became a key regulatory issue concerning the use of retroviral vectors. The development of new generation packaging cells, in which helper functions are present on separate constructs [5], means that it is now possible routinely to generate retroviral vectors without RCR. Other potential problems concerning the use of retroviruses include problems of low titre and rapid inactivation of viruses produced from murine packaging cells by human complement [6], but these problems are being addressed by the development of high-titre human packaging cell lines [7].

2.1.2. Adenoviral vectors: Replication-deficient adenoviral vectors are produced by replacement of up to 3.2 kilobases (kb) of the E1 region of the genome with foreign DNA. Another region of the viral genome that can be deleted if larger sequences of DNA need to be incorporated into the vector is the E3 region. Products of the E3 region have been shown to be involved in avoidance of host immunosurveillance and virus–cell interactions, protecting virus-infected cells from the effects of tumour necrosis factor (TNF) and reducing immunogenicity by inhibiting class I major histocompatibility complex (MHC) translocation to the cell membrane [8]. A new generation of adenoviral vectors has recently been developed which address the problems of limited insert capacity and the production of immunogenic viral proteins. These new vectors can package up to 30 kb of foreign DNA and contain no viral genes [9]. The vectors are propagated in 293 cells with the necessary viral functions provided by the cell line and a helper virus.

One advantge of adenoviral vectors compared with retroviral ones is the ability to produce higher titres: it is relatively easy to produce 10^{10} infectious units/ml compared with only 10^6-10^8/ml for retroviruses. Another advantage is that adenoviruses can infect cells regardless of their replication status, but the vectors remain episomal, so that gene expression is transient. This approach may be most suitable for therapeutic strategies where long-term gene expression is not required, for example, suicide gene therapy; if expression was required over an extended period, repeated administration of the adenoviral constructs would be required. Administration of adenovirus may lead to the development of an inflammatory response by the host, although this may be advantageous in cancer gene therapy by aiding the destruction of tumour cells. Other potential problems are concerns that repeated administration may lead to problems of virus neutralization by elevated antibody titres, and the possibility of complementation by wild-type virus if the patient has an infection at the time of treatment.

2.1.3. Adeno-associated virus: Adeno-associated virus (AAV) is a single-stranded DNA parvovirus that can only replicate when complemented by adenovirus or herpes virus. In the absence of these helper viruses it integrates into chromosomal DNA, preferentially at a defined region on chromosome 19. Integration is possible into non-replicating cells but is more efficient in the S phase of the cell cycle [10]. A recent report demonstrated that the transduction efficiency of immortalized cells with AAV was 50 times greater than transduction of primary cells [11], a feature that may give a degree of tumour specificity to a gene therapy protocol. AAVs are currently being used as vectors in two clinical trials in the USA, to introduce interleukin 2 (IL-2) cDNA into ovarian and prostate tumour cells [12].

2.1.4. Herpes simplex virus: Early reports using replication-compromised herpes simples virus (HSV) as a vector for gene therapy demonstrated significant toxic effects on infected cells [13, 14], preventing their use in human gene therapy trials. The recent identification of a mutant HSV (HSV-1716), which cannot produce the virulence factor ICP34.5, suggests that HSV may now be appropriate for use in gene therapy protocols [15]. Intraperitoneal injection of HSV-1716 into severe combined immunodeficient (SCID) mice bearing xenografts of human malignant mesothelioma cells reduced tumour burden and prolonged survival compared with control groups. No spread of virus outside the intraperitoneal cavity was observed, suggesting that HSV-1716 may be suitable for the treatment of localized human tumours [16].

2.2. Physical Methods

The efficiency of physical methods of gene transfer is significantly less than can currently be achieved by viral transfer. Nevertheless, research in this area is intense because there are many potential benefits of non-viral methods of gene delivery. The problems of immune responses against the viral vectors and unintentional replication and spread of viral vectors would be eliminated, and there are less stringent size restraints on the DNA inserted into the cell. Moreover, physical methods lend themselves readily to the stringent manufacturing criteria that would be required for large-scale production. Some cells can take up naked DNA after direct injection *in vivo* [17] or electroporation [18]. DNA can also be introduced into cells by bombardment with DNA-coated gold particles [19] or complexing the DNA with cationic lipid [20]. Liposome-mediated and receptor-mediated gene transfer are the physical methods most likely to be applicable to clinical use. A major disadvantage of liposome-mediated transfection is toxicity caused by the lipid components but this may be reduced to some extent by altering the composition of the lipid used [21].

3. Gene Targeting

A variety of strategies can be used to optimize the selectivity of gene delivery and expression in target tissues.

3.1. Selective Delivery of Therapeutic Genes to Tumour Cells

3.1.1. Ex vivo *delivery*: A limitation of both conventional and gene transfer cancer treatment approaches is the inability to deliver a sufficient concentration of therapeutic agent to the tumour cells without causing significant toxicity to normal cells. At present the optimal protocol for targeted gene delivery is the removal of tumour cells from the patient, retroviral transduction *in vitro* and administration of the genetically modified cells back into the patient (Figure 1). This method is, however, only really applicable for "cancer vaccine" type treatments and irradiated cells must be used.

3.1.2. In vivo *regional delivery*: For certain types of cancer that are localized to specific body cavities or are served by a dedicated blood supply, regional perfusion with therapeutic constructs/viruses would greatly enhance organ and tumour specificity. Selective arterial perfusion is possible for pancreatic cancer because the portal circulation can effectively be isolated at surgery during the time of arterial catheter insertion so that very high doses of virus could be given while minimizing the risk of systemic "spillover".

Regional delivery can also be achieved by direct intratumoral injection. Examples include administration of recombinant viruses directly into endobronchial lesions accessible by bronchoscopy [22, 23], stereotactic injection of HSV-TK-expressing producer cells into malignant brain

EX-VIVO TRANSDUCTION OF
TUMOUR CELLS

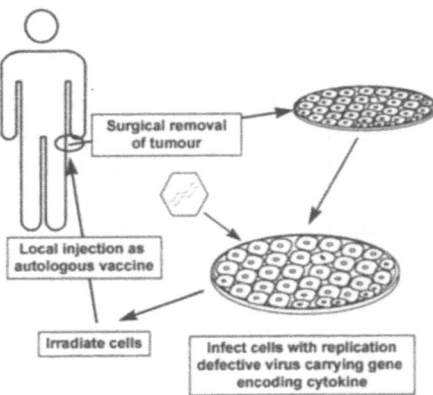

Figure 1. *Ex vivo* gene delivery: tumour cells are removed from the patient, retrovirally transduced and expanded *in vitro*, irradiated and administered back to the patient.

tumours followed by treatment with ganciclovir [24] and injection of HSV thymidine kinase (HSV-TK) expressing producer cells into metastatic malignant melanomas, followed by treatment with ganciclovir [25].

3.2. Selective Uptake Mechanisms

Another example of targeted gene delivery is the use of specific cell surface receptors; this approach requires that DNA be complexed to specific polypeptide ligands, which are recognized by cell surface receptors such as the use of asialoglycoprotein to transfer a human serum albumin gene into Nagrase rat repatocytes [26].

As the integration of retroviruses occurs only in actively dividing cells, this could be used to limit delivery of the vector to rapidly dividing tumour cells as opposed to the more slowly replicating cells of normal tissues. An example is the use of retroviruses to target HSV-TK expression to brain tumours in preference to normal brain tissue [27].

3.3. Tumour-Specific Promoters

Expression of therapeutic constructs can be limited to tumour cells using tumour-specific promoters. Carcinoembryonic antigen (CEA) is the most widely used tumour marker because elevated serum levels are found in a range of different tumours, including lung, pancreatic, colorectal and breast cancer. Overexpression of CEA occurs in up to 50% of lung cancers [28]. CEA functions *in vitro* as a cellular adhesion molecule [29], and belongs to a large and heterogeneous group of glycoproteins which are normally only expressed in fetal tissue [30]. The 5′-regulatory regions of the CEA gene have been characterized and several transcriptional regulatory consensus sequences identified [31]. The production of constructs containing a therapeutic gene under the control of the CEA promoter will allow tumour-specific expression in CEA-expressing tumours; however, other tumour-specific promoters would be required to target genes into non-CEA-expressing tumours.

Other tumour-selective promoters include those of the mucin (MUC) gene family [32, 33], the fibroblast growth factor/fibroblast growth factor receptor gene family [34], the c-*erb*B2 gene [35], the α-fetoprotein gene [36] and the prostate-specific antigen (PSA) gene [37]. To achieve expression of therapeutic enzymes in primary tumours and metastases the administration of several constructs, or the production of vectors containing two or more promoters, may be required. Once the promoters of tumour-specific antigens have been fully mapped and characterized, it may be possible to construct synthetic promoters which contain binding sites for several tumour-specific transcription factors, thus providing a vector that could be used in multiple tumour types. A synthetic promoter has been developed to drive HSV-TK gene expression in SCLCs which overexpress MYC proteins [38]. Four repeats of the MYC-MAX response element were linked to the HSV-TK promoter, and expression of HSV-TK was observed specifically in cells expressing high levels of MYC protein.

3.4. Tumour-Specific Mechanisms

3.4.1. Tumour-Restricted Cytolytic Viruses: The oncogene *p53* mediated cell cycle arrest and apoptosis in response to DNA damage. DNA tumour viruses encode proteins that inactivate *p53* and allow efficient viral replication [39]. The dl1520 (ONYX-015) virus is an adenovirus in which the gene for the 55-kDa protein that binds to and inactivates *p53* has been deleted from the E1B region [40]. Normal human cells are highly resistant to ONYX virus whereas tumour cells containing *p53* abnormalities show replication-dependent cytopathic effects when infected. Antitumoral effects of intratumoral injections of ONYX virus have been observed in nude mice with C33A (cervical carcinoma) and HLaC (laryngeal carcinoma) xenografts [41]. The efficacy of the ONYX virus plus chemotherapy using cisplatin or 5-fluorouracil has been shown to be significantly greater than either agent alone, and this regimen is currently being used in phase I clinical trials for the treatment of ovarian and head and neck tumours.

4. Gene Therapy Strategies for Lung Cancer

4.1. Restoration of Tumour-Suppressor Gene Expression

The conversion of an abnormal or malignant phenotype to a more normal non-tumorigenic phenotype can, in some instances, be achieved by the reintroduction of a normal allele into a defective cell. Such an approach for cancer therapy would involve the replacement of lost or mutated tumour-suppressor genes, cellular proto-oncogenes or DNA repair genes. Examples of such mutations which would be appropriate for gene therapy intervention include the tumour-suppressor gene *p53* [42, 43], which is a nuclear DNA-binding protein that is a transcription regulator. Cellular concentrations of *p53* increase after chromosomal damage; growth is arrested in the cell and the cell is prevented from entering mitosis (Figure 2). If the cellular damage cannot be repaired apoptosis is initiated [44]. Of the

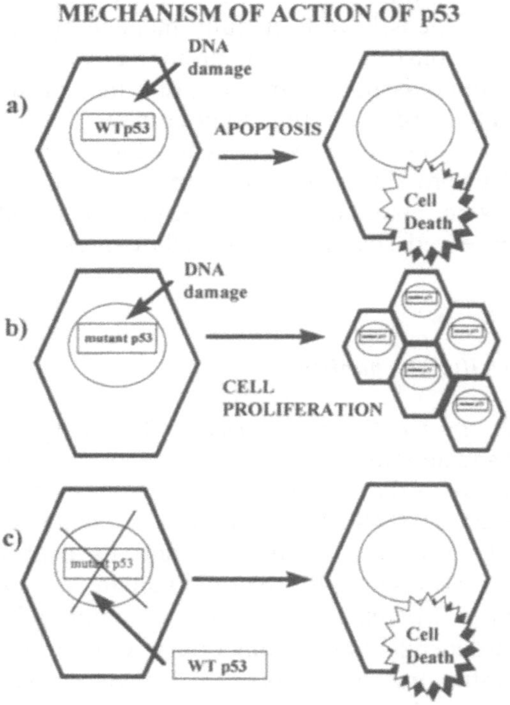

Figure 2. Mechanism of action of *p53*: (a) when a cell containing a wild-type *p53* gene is exposed to DNA damage cellular concentrations of *p53* increase, cell growth is arrested preventing it from entering mitosis. If the cellular damage cannot be repaired the cell is destroyed by apoptosis. (b) However, if the cell contains a mutant *p53* gene, mitosis continues generating a clonal population of cells containing chromosomal damage. (c) Blocking the action of the mutant *p53* gene (by antisense oligonucleotides or ribozymes) or the reintroduction of a wild-type *p53* gene can restore a normal phenotype.

1 million new cancer cases diagnosed annually in the USA, 50% are thought to carry a mutation in the *p53* gene and *p53* mutations have been identified in up-to 60% of NSCLCs and more than 95% of SCLCs.

Tumour growth is the result not of only abnormal cell proliferation but also of inhibition/suppression of the apoptotic pathways of cells. Resistance to chemotherapy also seems to relate to the suppression of apoptosis in tumour cells, resulting in an increased population of chemoresistant cells. High levels of the bcl-2 protein [45], which inhibits apoptosis, have been demonstrated in SCLCs that are particularly resistance to chemotherapy [46].

Retroviral vectors have been used to introduce wild-type *p53* genes into tumour cell lines *in vitro* and in animal models. Retroviral-mediated transfer of wild-type *p53* into an H226Br human NSCLC cell line containing a mutant *p53* gene inhibited cell growth, and a bystander effect was observed with unmodified cells being growth inhibited in a mixed population of parental and transduced cells [47]. This study was extended *in vivo* [48] using an orthotopic lung cancer model. H226Br cells were implanted into the right main stem bronchus of nude mice via a tracheotomy and 3 days later control retrovirus, wild-type p53 virus or mutant p53 virus was injected into the bronchus via the tracheotomy once daily for 3 days. At postmortem examination, 30 days after implantation of tumour cells, mice treated with wild-type *p53* had significantly fewer and smaller lung tumours than the mice in the control groups.

In the first clinical trial of gene therapy for SCLCs, patients were treated by intratumoral injection with a retroviral vector containing a wild-type *p53* gene [23]. Tumour regression was observed in three of nine patients, tumour growth was stabilized for up to 5 months in another three patients and, importantly, there were no toxic side effects from the vector. A significant increase in levels of apoptosis was observed in the post-treatment tumour biopsy specimens compared with pre-treatment.

Roth and colleagues are conducting another trial using a defective adenovirus vector to deliver wild-type *p53* (p53WT) locally into patients with unresectable local regional or isolated metastatic stage IV disease. This treatment is based on a combination therapy using cisplatin and the p53WT vector because previous studies had demonstrated synergy between the two treatments [49]. In this study, H1299 human NSCLC cell lines with a homozygous deletion of p53 were exposed to cisplatin for 24 hours then infected with Ad-p53WT 48 hours later. Cells exposed to cisplatin before adenoviral infection had a 31–60% greater inhibition of growth and higher levels of wild-type p53 protein and apoptosis compared with cells infected with adenovirus alone. The study was then extended in animal models. H1299 cells were grown as subcutaneous xenografts in nude mice, the mice were treated with cisplatin (5 µg/g body weight intraperitoneal injection) followed by injection of Ad-p53WT viral particles directly into the tumour. The mice treated with the combination therapy survived longer than animals treated with cisplatin or adenovirus alone. Pronounced inhibition of tumour development and high levels of apoptosis were apparent in tumour biopsy samples from the mice treated with the combination therapy compared with the control groups.

4.2. Pro-drug-Activating Enzymes

Virally directed enzyme pro-drug therapy (VDEPT) is based on the intro-duction into a cell (using viral vectors) of a gene encoding a foreign enzyme, which converts a relatively non-toxic agent (the pro-drug) into an active cytotoxic compound (suicide gene therapy) (Figure 3). Several enzy-mes have been used including HSV-TK and the *Escherichia coli*-derived cytosine deaminase and nitroreductase (*ntr*) enzyme genes. HSV-TK phos-phorylates the antiviral agent ganciclovir to an intermediate (ganciclovir monophosphate) which is then phosphorylated by cellular enzymes to ganciclovir triphosphate, a potent inhibitor of DNA synthesis [50]. Cells expressing HSV-TK are extremely sensitive to ganciclovir whereas non-expressing cells are resistant, leading to a large therapeutic index. Cytosi-ne deaminase converts the non-toxic pro-drug 5-fluorocytosine to the cyto-toxic agent 5-fluorouracil [51], whereas the *ntr* enzyme [52] reduces the non-toxic pro-drug CB1954 (5-[aziridin-1-yl]-2,4-dinitrobenzamide) to a powerful bifunctional alkylating agent (5-[aziridin-1-yl]-4-hydroxyl-

VIRALLY DIRECTED ENZYME PRODRUG THERAPY (VDEPT)

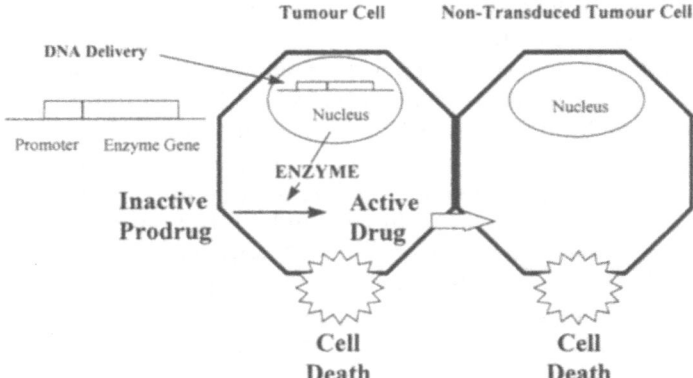

Figure 3. Principle of VDEPT: a therapeutic DNA construct is introduced into a tumour cell. The presence of tumour-specific transcription factors allows transcription and translation of the gene to produce the enzyme which converts the pro-drug to its active form, causing cell death. A bystander effect is observed with the active form of the drug killing a neighbouring untrans-duced cell.

amino-2-nitrobenzamide) [53]. An important feature of the enzyme-pro-drug approach is the so-called bystander effect in which active drugs can diffuse from transduced cells containing the activating enzyme, causing the death of untransduced cells in the vicinity [53]. This is a very important phenomenon because it is unlikely that, with levels of gene delivery cur-rently, attainable, every tumour cell will be transduced with the pro-drug-activating enzyme.

An adenoviral vector containing HSV-TK has been used to transduce human NSCLC and malignant mesothelioma cell lines *in vitro*. Increased sensitivity to ganciclovir and a significant bystander effect was observed in mixing experiments, whereby transduced and non-transduced cells were mixed in varying proportions before exposure to ganciclovir [54].

Cell type-specific regulation of HSV-TK linked to the CEA promoter has been demonstrated in human lung cancer cells both *in vitro* and *in vivo*. A CEA-producing cell line (A549) and a CEA-negative line (CADO-LC9) were transfected with CEA–HSV-TK and then exposed to ganciclovir. The transfected A549 cells were more than 1000 times as sensitive to ganciclovir as the parental cells, whereas the transfected CEA-negative cell line CADO-LC9 was still resistant. Significant regression of HSV-TK-expressing A549 tumours in nude mice was observed after treatment with ganciclovir [55].

Cell-specific gene expression has also been achieved using a synthetic promoter based on multiple repeats of the MYC-MAX response element. SCLC is highly aggressive, characterized by rapid tumour growth, invasion and metastases. Many SCLCs are sensitive to initial chemotherapy but relapse rapidly and become resistant to further treatment [56]. Up to 83% of SCLCs have been shown to overexpress members of the MYC family of proto-oncogene proteins and tumours overexpressing MYC are associated with a poor prognosis [57]. It has previously been demonstrated that the MYC family proteins form heterodimers with MAX protein [58] and that MYC-MAX dimers bind specifically to the nucleotide sequence CACGTG to activate gene transcription [59].

Based on this finding a synthetic promoter has been developed to drive suicide gene expression in SCLCs overexpressing the MYC family of pro-teins [38]. Four repeats of the MYC-MAX response element were joined to the HSV-TK promoter, and cloned in a catalase (CAT) receptor vector. The reporter construct (pMTK-CAT) was transfected into SCLC cell lines expressing different levels of MYC. In cells overexpressing MYC, pMTK-CAT expression was 9.5-fold greater than the control vector pSV2-CAT, but it was only 3.0% of pSV2-CAT in the MYC-negative cell lines. SCLC cell lines transfected with MYC-MAX HSV-TK expression plasmids were up to 500 times more sensitive to ganciclovir than the parental cells *in vitro*. The transfected and parental cells were then implanted into nude mice; tumours expressing TK regressed significantly when treated with ganciclovir and significant bystander killing was observed in mixing experiments with tumours made up of varying proportions of parental and transduced cells.

4.3. Immunological Approaches

The development of a tumour vaccine, which would provoke an immune response specifically directed against tumour cells, is an attractive proposition for cancer therapy [60]. Systemic immune stimulation with high-dose (IL-2) is highly toxic and has limited efficacy [61, 62], resulting partly from the short half-life of the protein. TNF produces marked antitumour responses in mice but has been disappointing clinically, as a result of the toxic effects of TNF in humans at concentrations above 500 µg/m², which is at least 10-fold lower than the dose tolerated by mice [63]. The antitumour immune response of the host can be improved by modification of tumour cells to express cytokines such as IL-2, IL-4, TNFα, interferon-γ or granulocyte-macrophage colony-stimulating factor (GM-CSF). The expression of such cytokines within transduced tumour cells would lead to increased local cytokine production, which may increase immunogenicity, and provoke a systemic immune response which may aid in the destruction of circulating tumour cells, thereby reducing metastatic potential and resulting in an improved clinical response. Enhanced expression of MHC class I and II molecules on tumour cells can also be achieved by overexpression of cytokine genes or direct transfection of MHC genes [64]. In animal models non-immunogenic tumours have been engineered to express cytokines or members of the MHC complex and stimulation of an immune response was observed [65, 66]. Several investigators have inserted the IL-2 gene into animal tumours which, after implantation, have conferred antitumour immunity on the host [67, 68]. Tumour-infiltrating lymphocytes (TILs) could serve as a good delivery system of IL-2 to human tumours, the rationale being that the active secretion of IL-2 in the vicinity of the tumour could increase the number of cytotoxic T cells against the tumour and reduce systemic toxicity [69, 70].

A recent phase I clinical trial [71] has used IL-2 gene therapy to treat 10 patients with advanced lung cancer with malignant pleural effusions. TILs were obtained from pleural effusions, expanded in vitro and transduced with a recombinant retrovirus based on Moloney murine leukaemia virus (MMLV) containing the human IL-2 cDNA. The transduced TILs were returned to the chest cavity and 2×10^5 IU IL-2 was injected directly. The IL-2 treatment was then repeated daily for 1–2 weeks and the whole procedure repeated 2 weeks later. Six of ten patients did not reaccumulate their pleural effusions for at least 4 weeks after treatment, two remained effusion free for up to 2 weeks, and there was no response observed in the other two patients. In one patient the size of the primary tumour was reduced significantly after the IL-2 gene therapy. Phase II and III trials are being planned for this treatment.

Another phase I trial is currently under way using tumour cells transfected with IL-2 in patients with limited stage SCLC [72]. Patient's tumour cells are harvested, expanded in vitro, transfected using liposomes complexed with a vector containing the human IL-2 cDNA, irradiated, and then returned to the patient. The results of this study still have to be published.

An alternative immunological approach has been developed by modifying tumour cells to express IL-6 and *E. coli* cytosine deaminase [73]. This strategy was based on previous findings that transduction of the murine fibrosarcoma cell line 205 with IL-6 (205-IL-6) reduced tumorigenicity and increased immunogenicity [74], and that transduction of 205 with *E. coli* cytosine deaminase followed by treatment with 5-fluorocytosine resulted in cell death [75]. The hypothesis was that cells secreting IL-6 would induce an antitumour effect and could then be destroyed by administration of 5-fluorocytosine. Wild-type 205 is very aggressive and will form tumours in normal syngeneic mice; however, 205-IL-6-CD failed to form tumours in such mice and was then used to immunize mice that had pre-existing wild-type 205 pulmonary metastases, resulting in prolonged survival, compared with immunization with 205-IL-6 or 205-CD alone, and tumour cure in some of the mice. This study demonstrates that genetic modification of a poorly immunogenic tumour with a cytokine and a suicide gene (mice were not treated with 5-fluorocytosine) can produce an effective autologous tumour vaccine in animals with small metastatic tumour burdens. This observation may also help in the understanding of the bystander effect. Although it has been demonstrated that there is transfer of activated toxins from the genetically modified cells to wild-type cells *in vitro* [76, 77], it has recently been shown that suicide gene products are potentially immunogenic and may help induce an antitumour response [75].

4.4. Antisense Oligodeoxynucleotides

Antisense oligodeoxynucleotides are small synthetic pieces of single-stranded DNA or a chemical analogue, which are complementary to specific cellular DNA or RNA sequences [78]. The binding of these oligonucleotides to their target sequences inhibits transcription or translation of the target gene. Several studies have demonstrated antiproliferative effects of antisense oligonucleotides on lung cancer cell lines, including sequences binding to *p53* [79], c-*my* [80], L-*myc* [81], c-*kit* [82], IL-8 receptor [83] and cyclin D1 [84]. Insulin-like growth factors (IGFs) are often essential for the maintenance of the malignant phenotype, and the IGF-I receptor is often overexpressed in lung cancer. Transfection of cell lines with an adenoviral vector expressing antisense to the IGF-I receptor caused a reduction in the number of receptors and a decrease in tumorigenicity. Administration of the adenovirus to nude mice carrying H460 xenografts prolonged survival compared with mice treated with a receptor virus [85].

Activation of the *ras* oncogene is a common event in the pathogenesis of lung cancer. It has been demonstrated that the introduction of an antisense

K-*ras* fragment was able specifically to inhibit expression of mutant K-*ras* protein in H460a human NSCLC cells, resulting in a reduction of cell proliferation and tumorigenicity in nude mice [86]. The antisense K-*ras* was then cloned into a retroviral vector and packaged in GP + envAM12 cells. Transduction of H460a cells with the viral supernatant resulted in a 10-fold reduction in proliferation and specific inhibition of the mutant K-*ras* p21 protein expression [87]. In an *in vivo* study nude mice were inoculated with H460a cells, and viral supernatants from control retrovirus, antisense K-*ras* virus or sense K-*ras* virus were injected intratracheally for 3 days. At postmortem examination, 30 days after inoculation of tumour cells, 90% of the control mice had tumours compared with only 13% of the mice treated with the antisense K-*ras* virus [88]. The antisense K-*ras* retrovirus is now being used in clinical trials for NSCLC.

4.5. Ribozymes

Ribozymes are catalytic RNA molecules that cleave specific messenger RNAs; ribozymes can be introduced directly into cells using liposomes or cloned into viral vectors. The catalytic sequence can be designed to cleave a specific target sequence by incorporating flanking sequences that are complementary to the target RNA. Retrovirus-mediated transduction of human H226Br human lung cancer cells, with an anti-*p53* ribozyme designed to cleave unspliced *p53* mRNA, has been shown to suppress cell growth *in vitro* [89].

5. Conclusion

Gene therapy offers exciting new prospects for the treatment of lung cancer, although only intensive investigation will determine which of the gene therapy approaches described will turn out to be the most efficacious. There are now over 100 clinical trials in progress using gene therapy as a treatment of cancer and eight clinical trials are under way for the treatment of lung cancer (Table 1). The trials use various methods of gene delivery, but by far the most common method of gene transfer is retroviral transduction, which is being used in about 70% of the clinical protocols for cancer. Most of the trials are still at the phase I stage and the results have not yet been fully published. Preliminary findings have been encouraging and most protocols appear to be safe with few adverse side effects being reported. It is far too early to assess the therapeutic efficacy of gene therapy; most of the trials to date are in patients with advanced disease and major difficulties lie in adapting an approach that works *in vitro* to give a clinically significant response *in vivo*. Careful monitoring of the scientific endpoints of the trials, even with poor clinical results, is essential to interpret

Table 1. Clinical protocols using gene therapy for the treatment of lung cancer

Nucleic acid transferred	Method of gene transfer
βGAL cDNA (marker study)	Adenovirus
IL-2 cDNA	Adenovirus
IL-2 cDNA	Retrovirus
IL-2 cDNA	Lipofection
p53 cDNA	Adenovirus
p53 cDNA	Retrovirus
K-ras antisense	Retrovirus
HLA-B7/β_2-microglobulin	Lipofection

findings and allow the refinement of strategies and vectors. The National Institutes of Health (Bethesda, USA) have set up a panel of experts to provide recommendations regarding future gene therapy trials, which has emphasized three key areas of research that need to be developed. The first is the refinement of vectors and an understanding of the vector–host interactions. Vectors need to be improved to maintain an adequate level of cell-specific or tissue-specific gene expression. The second is to increase the basic understanding of disease pathogenesis and pathophysiology to aid the development of new treatment strategies. The final recommendation is the development of appropriate animal models in which to test strategies before clinical trials, as some phase I trials in the USA have been established on the basis of few animal data.

In addition to the strategies outlined, it is conceivable that radical new methods of gene delivery or targeting may be developed. Examples of new approaches include the use of replication-competent viruses, lytic viruses, and the possibility of modifying retroviral envelope proteins or adenoviral fibre protein to allow cell-specific targeting.

The number of gene therapy protocols and clinical trials is increasing rapidly and, with a better understanding of the basic scientific principle involved, the data obtained over the coming years should, it is hoped, determined whether gene therapy provides a significant advantage over traditional methods of treatment for lung cancer and which approaches and methods of gene delivery will be most beneficial.

References

1 Boring CC, Squires TS, Tong T (1992) Cancer statistics. Cancer J Clin 42: 19–38
2 Goyette MC, Cho K, Fasching CL et al. (1992) Progression of colorectal cancer is associated with multiple tumor suppressor gene defects but inhibition of tumorigenicity is accomplished by correction of any single defect via chromosome transfer. Mol Cell Biol 12: 1387–1395
3 Takahashi T, Carbone D, Takahashi T et al. (1992) Wild-type but not mutant p53 suppresses the growth of human lung cancer cells bearing multiple genetic lesions. Cancer Res 52: 2340–2343

4 Donahue RE, Kesseler SW, Bodine D et al. (1992) Helper virus-induced T cell lymphoma in non-human primates after retroviral mediated gene transfer. *J Exp Med* 176: 1125–1135

5 Markowitz D, Goff S, Bank A (1988) Construction and use of a safe and efficient amphotropic packaging cell line. *Virology* 167: 400–406

6 Bartholomew RM, Esser AF, Muller-Eberhard HJ (1978) Lysis of oncornaviruses by human serum: Isolation of the viral complement (C1) receptor and identification as p15C. *J Exp Med* 147: 844–853

7 Cossett FL, Takeuchi Y, Battini JL et al. (1995) High-titre packaging cells producing recombinant retroviruses resistant to human serum. *J Virol* 69: 7430–7436

8 Wold WSM, Gooding LR (1991) Region E3 of adenovirus: a cassette of genes involved in host immunosurveillance and virus-cell interactions. *Virology* 184: 1–8

9 Kochanek S, Clemens PR, Mitani K et al. (1996) A new adenoviral vector: Replacement of all viral coding sequences with 28 kb of DNA independently expressing both full-length dystrophin and beta-galactosidase. *Proc Natl Acad Sci USA* 93: 5731–5736

10 Russel DM, Miller AD, Alexander IE (1994) Adeno-associated virus vectors preferentially transduce cells in S phase. *Proc Natl Acad Sci USA* 91: 8915–8919

11 Halbert CL, Alexander IE, Wolgamot GM, Miller AD (1995) Adeno-associated virus vectors transduce primary cells much less efficiently than immortalized cells. *J Virol* 69: 1473–1479

12 Clinical Protocols (1995) *Cancer Gene Ther* 2: 225–234

13 Huang Q, Vonsattel JP, Schaffer PA et al. (1992) Introduction of a foreign gene (*Escherichia coli lacZ*) into rat neostriatal neurons using herpes simplex virus mutants: a light and electron microscopy study. *Exp Neurol* 115: 303–316

14 Breakefield XO (1993) Gene delivery into the brain using virus vectors. *Nature Genet* 3: 187–189

15 McKie EA, MayLean AR, Lewis AD et al. (1996) Selective *in vitro* replication of herpes simplex virus type 1 (HSV-1) ICP34.5 null mutants in primary human CNS tumours–evaluation of a potentially effective clinical therapy. *Br J Cancer* 74:745–752

16 Kucharczuk JC, Randazzo B, Chang MY et al. (1997) Use of a "replication-restricted" herpes virus to treat experimental human malignant mesothelioma. *Cancer Res* 57: 466–471

17 Wolff JA, Malone RW, Williams P et al. (1990) Direct gene transfer in mouse muscle *in vivo*. *Science* 247: 1465–1468

18 Neumann E, Schaefer-Ridder M, Wang Y, Hofschneider PH (1982) Gene transfer into mouse lyoma cells by electroporation in high electric fields. *EMBO J* 1: 841–845

19 Yang N-S, Burkholder J, Roberts B et al. (1990) *In vitro* and *in vivo* gene transfer to mammalian somatic cells by particle bombardment. *Proc Natl Acad Sci USA* 87: 9568–9572

20 Felgner PL, Gadek TR, Holm M et al. (1987) Lipofection: a highly efficient liposome-mediated DNA-transfection procedure. *Proc Natl Acad Sci USA* 84: 7413–7417

21 Farhood H, Bottega R, Epand RM et al. (1992) Effect of cationic cholesterol derivatives on gene transfer and protein. *Biochim Biophys Acta* 1111: 239–246

22 Tursz T, Cesne AL, Baldeyrou P et al. (1996) Phase I study of a recombinant adenovirus-mediated gene transfer in lung cancer patients. *J Natl Cancer Instit* 88: 1857–1863

23 Roth JA, Nguyen D, Lawrence DD et al. (1996) Retrovirus-mediated wild-type p53 gene transfer to tumors of patients with lung cancer. *Nature Med* 2: 985–991

24 Kun LE, Gajjar A, Muhlbauer M et al. (1995) Stereotactic injection of herpes simplex thymidine kinase vector producer cells (PA317-G1Tk1SvNa.7) and intravenous ganciclovir for the treatment of progressive or recurrent primary supratentorial pediatric malignant brain tumors. *Hum Gene Ther* 6: 1231–1255

25 Klatzmann D (1996) Gene therapy for metastatic malignant melanoma: evaluation of tolerance to intratumoral injection of cells producing recombinant retroviruses carrying the herpes simplex virus type 1 thymidine kinase gene, to be followed by ganciclovir administration. *Hum Gene Ther* 7: 255–267

26 Wu GY, Wilson JM, Shalaby F et al. (1991) Receptor mediated gene delivery *in vivo*-partial correction of genetic analbuminemia in Nagrase rats. *J Biol Chem* 266: 14338–14342

27 Culver KW, Ram Z, Wallbridge S et al. (1992) *In vivo* gene transfer with retroviral vector-producer cells for treatment of experimental brain tumors. *Science* 256: 1550–1552

28 Shinkai T, Saijo N, Tominaga K et al. (1986) Serial plasma carcinoembryonic antigen measurement for monitoring patients with advanced lung cancer during chemotherapy. *Cancer* 57: 1318–23

29 Benchimol S, Fuks A, Joth S et al. (1989) Carcinoembryonic antigen, a human tumour marker, functions as an intercellular adhesion molecule. *Cell* 57: 327–334

30 Thompson JA, Grunert F, Zimmermann W (1991) Carcinoembryonic antigen gene family: Molecular biology and clinical perspectives. *J Clin Lab Anal* 5: 344–366

31 Richards CA, Wolberg AS, Huber BE (1993) The transcriptional control region of the human carcinoembryonic antigen gene: DNA sequence and homology studies. *DNA Sequence* 4: 185–196

32 Balague C, Gambus G, Carrato C et al. (1994) Altered expression of MUC2, MUC4 and MUC5 mucin genes in pancreas tisue and cancer cell lines. *Gastroenterology* 106:1054–1061

33 Hollingsworth MA, Strawhecker JM, Caffrey TC, Mack DR (1994) Expression of MUC1, MUC2, MUC3 and MUC4 mucin messenger RNAs in human pancreatic and intestinal tumour cell lines. *Int J Cancer* 57: 198–203

34 Leung HY, Hughes CM, Kloppel G et al. (1994) Localisation of fibroblast growth factors and their receptors in pancreatic adenocarcinoma by *in situ* hybridisation. *Int J Oncol* 4: 1219–1223

35 Yarden Y, Weinberg RA (1989) Experimental appraoches to hypothetical hormones-detection of a candidate ligand of the neu proto-oncogene. *Proc Natl Acad Sci USA* 86: 3179–3183

36 Huber BE, Richards CA, Krenitsky TA (1991) Retroviral-mediated gene transfer for the treatment of hepatocellular carcinoma: an innovative approach for cancer therapy. *Proc Natl Acad Sci USA* 88: 8039–8043

37 Kuriyama M (1986) Prostata-specific antigen in prostate cancer. *Int J Biol Markers* 1:67–76

38 Kumagai T, Tanio Y, Osaki T et al. (1996) Eradication of Myc-overexpressing small cell lung cancer cells transfected with herpes simplex virus thymidine kinase gene containing Myc-Max response elements. *Cancer Res* 56: 354–358

39 Debbas M, White E (1993) Wild-type p53 mediates apoptosis by E1A, which is inhibited by E1B. *Genes Devel* 7: 546–554

40 Bischoff JR, Kirn DH, Williams A et al. (1996) An adenovirus mutant that replicates selectively in p53-deficient human tumor cells. *Science* 274: 373–376

41 Heise C, Sampson-Johannes A, Williams A et al. (1997) ONYX-015, an E1B attenuated adenovirus, causes tumor-specific cytolysis and antitumoral efficacy that can be augmented by standard chemotherapeutic agents. *Nature Med* 3: 639–645

42 Takahashi T, Takahashi T, Suzuki H et al. (1991) The p53 gene is very frequently mutated in small-cell lung cancer with a distinct nucleotide substitution pattern. *Oncogene* 6: 1775–1778

43 Brambilla E, Gazzeri S, Moro D et al. (1993) Immunohistochemical study of p53 in human lung carcinomas. *Am J Pathol* 143: 199–210

44 Liu TJ, Zhang WW, Taylor DL et al. (1994) Growth suppression of human head and neck cancer cells by the introduction of a wild-type p53 gene via a recombinant adenovirus. *Cancer Res* 54: 3662–3667

45 Aisenberg AC, Wilkes BM, Jacobson JQ (1988) The bcl-2 gene is rearranged in many diffuse B-cell lymphomas. *Blood* 71: 969–972

46 Fontanini G, Vignati S, Bigini D et al. (1995) Bcl-2 protein: a prognostic factor inversely correlated to p53 in non-small-cell lung cancer. *Br J Cancer* 71: 1003–1007

47 Cai DW, Mukhopadhyay T, Liu Y et al. (1993) Stable expression of the wild-type p53 gene in human lung cancer cells after retrovirus-mediated gene transfer. *Hum Gene Ther* 4: 617–624

48 Fujiwara T, Cai DW, Georges RN et al. (1994) Therapeutic effect of a retroviral wild-type p53 expression vector in an orthotopic lung cancer model. *J Natl Cancer Instit* 86: 1458–1462

49 Nyguyen DM, Spitz FR, Yen N et al. (1996) Gene therapy for lung cancer: enhancement of tumor suppression by a combination of sequential systemic cisplatin and adenovirus-mediated p53 gene transfer. *J Thorac Cardiovasc Surg* 112: 1372–1376

50 Moolten F (1986) Tumour chemosensitivity conferred by inserted herpes thymidine kinase genes: paradigm for a prospective cancer control strategy. *Cancer Res* 46: 5276–5281

51 Haskell CM (1990) Drugs used in cancer chemotherapy. In: CM Haskell (ed). *Cancer treatment*. 3rd edn. WB Saunders, Philadelphia, 44–101

52 Anlezark GM, Melton RG, Sherwood RF et al. (1992) The bioactivation of CB 1954. I. Purification and properties of a nitroreductase enzyme from *Escherichia coli* – a potential enzyme for antibody direct enzyme therapy (ADEPT). *Biochem Pharmacol* 44: 2289–2295

53 Knox RJ, Friedlos F, Jarman M, Roberts JJ (1988) A new cytotoxic, DNA interstrand cross-linking agent, 5-(aziridin-1-yl)-4-hydroxylamino-2-nitrobenzamide, is formed from 5-(aziridin-1-yl)-2,4-dinitrobenzamide (CB 1954) by a nitroreductase enzyme in Walker carcinoma lines. *Biochem Pharmacol* 37: 4661–4669

54 Smythe WR, Hwang HC, Amin KM et al. (1994) Use of recombinant adenovirus to transfer the herpes simplex virus thymidine kinase (HSVtk) gene to thoracic neoplasms: an effective *in vitro* drug sensitization system. *Cancer Res* 54: 2055–2059

55 Osaki T, Tanio Y, Tachibana I et al. (1994) Gene therapy for carcinoembryonic antigen-producing human lung cancer cells by cell type-specific expression of herpes simplex virus thymidine kinase gene. *Cancer Res* 54: 5258–5261

56 Grilli R, Oxman AD, Julian JA (1993) Chemotherapy for advanced non-small-cell lung cancer: how much benefit es enough? *J Clin Oncol* 11: 1866–1872

57 Johnson BE, Makuch RW, Simmons AD et al. (1988) myc family DNA amplification in small cell lung cancer patients' tumors and corresponding cell lines. *Cancer Res* 48: 5163–5166

58 Muhle-Goll C, Nilges M, Pastore A (1995) The leucine zippers of the HLA-LZ proteins Max and c-Myc preferentially form heterodimers. *Biochemistry* 34: 13544–13564

59 Fisher F, Crouch DH, Jayaraman PS et al. (1993) Transcription activation by Myc and Max: flanking sequences target activation to a subset of CACGTG motifs *in vivo*. *EMBO J* 12: 5075–5082

60 Pardoll DM (1993) Cancer vaccines. *Immunol Today* 14: 310–316

61 Sivanandham M, Scoggin SD, Sperry RG, Wallack MK (1992) Prospects for gene therapy and lymphokine therapy for metastatic melanoma. *Ann Plastic Surg* 28: 114–118

62 Dillman RO (1994) The clinical experience with interleukin-2 in cancer therapy. *Cancer Biother* 9: 183–209

63 Lejeune F, Lienard D, Eggermont A et al. (1994) Rationale for using TNF alpha and chemotherapy in regional treatment of melanoma. *J Cell Biochem* 56: 52–61

64 James RF, Edwards S, Hui KM et al. (1991) The effect of class II gene transfection to the tumorigenicity of the H-2K negative mouse leukemia cell line. *Immunology* 72: 213–218

65 Dranoff G, Jaffe E, Lazenby A et al. (1993) Vaccination with irradiated tumor cells engineered to secrete murine granulocyte-macrophage colony-stimulating factor stimulates potent, specific and long-lasting anti-tumor immunity. *Proc Natl Acad Sci USA* 90: 3539–3543

66 Plautz GE, Yang Z-Y, Wu B-Y et al. (1993) Immunotherapy of malignancy by *in vivo* gene transfer into tumors. *Proc Natl Acad Sci USA* 90: 4645–4649

67 Gansbacher B, Zier K, Daniels B et al. (1990) Interleukin 2 gene transfer into tumor cells abrogates tumorigenicity and induces protective immunity. *J Exp Med* 172: 1217–1224

68 Connor J, Bannerji R, Saito S et al. (1993) Regression of bladder tumors in mice treated with interleukin 2 gene-modified tumor cells. *J Exp Med* 177: 1127–1134

69 Kasid A, Morecki S, Aebersold P et al. (1990) Human gene transfer: characterization of human tumor-infiltrating lymphocytes as vehicles for retroviral-mediated gene transfer in man. *Proc Natl Acad Sci USA* 87: 473–477

70 Culver KW, Cornetta K, Morgan R et al. (1991) Lymphoxytes as cellular vehicles for gene therapy in mouse and man. *Proc Natl Acad Sci USA* 88: 3155–3159

71 Tan Y, Xu M, Wang W et al. (1996) IL-2 gene therapy of advanced lung cancer patients. *Anticancer Res* 16: 1993–1998

72 Cassileth PA, Podack E, Sridhar K et al. (1995) Phase I study of transfected cancer cells expressing the interleukin-2 gene product in limited stage small cell lung cancer. *Hum Gene Ther* 6: 369–383

73 Mullen CA, Petropoulos D, Lowe RM (1996) Treatment of microscopic pulmonary metastases with recombinant autologous tumor vaccine expressing interleukin 6 and *Escherichia coli* cytosine deaminase suicide genes. *Cancer Res* 56: 1361–1366

74 Mullen CA, Coale MM, Levy AT et al. (1992) Fibrosarcoma cells transduced with the IL-6 gene exhibited reduced tumorigenicity, increased immunogenicity, and decreased metastatic potential. *Cancer Res* 52: 6020–6024

75 Consalvo M, Mullen CA, Modesti A et al. (1995) 5-Fluorocytosine-induced eradication of murine adenocarcinomas engineered to express the cytosine deaminase suicide gene requires host immune competence and leaves an efficient memory. *J Immunol* 154: 5302–5312

76 Bi WL, Parysek LM, Warnick R, Stambrook PJ (1993) *In vitro* evidence that metabolic cooperation is responsible for the bystander effect observed with HSV the retroviral gene therapy. *Hum Gene Ther* 4: 725–731

77 Freeman SM, Abbound CN, Whartenby KA et al. (1993) The "bystander effect": tumor regression when a fraction of the tumor mass is genetically modified. *Cancer Res* 53: 5274–5283

78 Tidd DM (1990) A potential role for antisense oligonucleotide analogues in the development of oncogene targeted chemotherapy. *Anticancer Res* 10: 1169–1182

79 Mukhopadhyay T, Roth JA (1996) Functional inactivation of p53 by antisense RNA induces invasive ability of lung carcinoma cells and downregulates cytokeratin synthesis. *Anticancer Research* 16: 1683–1689

80 Saijo Y, Uchiyama B, Abe T et al. (1997) contigous four-guanosine sequence in c-myc antisense phosphorothioate oligonucleotides inhibits cell growth on human lung cancer cells: possible involvement of cell adhesion inhibition. *Jpn J Cancer Res* 88: 26–33

81 Dosaka-Akita H, Akie K, Hiroumi H et al. (1995) Inhibition of proliferation by L-*myc* antisense DNA for the translational initiation site in human small cell lung cancer. *Cancer Res* 55: 1559–1564

82 Yamanishi Y, Maeda H, Hiyama K et al. (1996) Specific growth inhibition of small-cell lung cancer cells by adenovirus vector expressing antisense c-*kit* transcripts. *Jpn J Cancer Res* 87: 534–42

83 Olbina G, Cieslak D, Ruzdijic S et al. (1996) Reversible inhibition of IL-8 receptor B mRNA expression and proliferation in non-small cell lung cancer by antisense oligonucleotides. *Anticancer Res* 16: 3525–3530

84 Schrump DS, Chen A, Consoli U (1996) Inhibition of lung cancer proliferation by antisense cyclin D. *Cancer Gene Ther* 3: 131–135

85 Lee CT, Wu S, Gabrilovich D et al. (1996) Antitumor effects of an adenovirus expressing antisense insulin-like growth factor I receptor on human lung cancer cell lines. *Cancer Res* 56: 3038–3041

86 Mukhopadhyay T, Tainsky M, Cavender AC, Roth JA (1991) Specific inhibition of K-ras expression and tumorigenicity of lung cancer cells by antisense RNA. *Cancer Research* 51(6): 1744–1748

87 Zhang Y, Mukhopadhyay T, Donehower LA et al. (1993) Retroviral vector-mediated transduction of K-ras antisense RNA into human lung cancer cells inhibits expression of the malignant phenotype. *Hum Gene Ther* 4: 451–60

88 Georges RN, Mukhopadhyay T, Zhang Y et al. (1993) Prevention of orthotopic human lung cancer growth by intratracheal instillation of a retroviral antisense K-ras construct. *Cancer Res* 53: 1743–1746

89 Cai DW, Mukhopadhyay T, Roth JA (1995) Suppression of lung cancer cell growth by ribozyme-mediated modification of p53 pre-mRNA. *Cancer Gene Ther* 2: 199–205

Index

activator protein-1 (AP-1)   50
adhesion molecule   132
adhesion molecule, immunoglobulin-like
   136
β_2-adrenergic receptor   32
β-adrenergic receptor kinase (βARK)   111
β-adrenoreceptor   32, 101
β-agonist, mechanism of action of   101
airway epithelium   146
allergen   92
allergen Bla g 1   153
allergen Fel d 1   153
allergen Per a 1   153
antigen-presenting cell   145
α_1-antitrypsin deficiency   6
asthma   72, 85, 145
asthma, nocturnal   32
asthma, non-atopic   93
atopy   86

biopsy, bronchial   88

CAAT/enhancer-binding protein   53
cAMP response element (CRE)   108
cAMP response element binding protein
   (CREB)   55, 108
cancer   183
candidate gene   25
CC chemokine   33
cell adhesion, epithelial   155
c-erbAβ proto oncogene   172
chemoattractant   126
chemokine   33, 87, 126
chromosome 3p   166
chromosome 12   28
c-myc   166
crossing over   24
cysteine proteinase   147
cystic fibrosis   5
cytokine   32, 85
cytokine cluster   26

Der p 1   150
disease, inflammatory   13
disease, pulmonary infectious   15
disease, pulmonary vascular   16
DNA delivery system, non-viral   184
drug interaction   63

enzyme pro-drug therapy, virally-directed
   (VDEPT)   192
eosinophil   125
eotaxin   33, 129

gene targeting   187
gene therapy   1, 183

glucocorticoid receptor (GR)   56
glucocorticoid response element (GRE),
   consensus sequence of   116
glucocorticoid therapy   88
G-protein   107
granulocyte macrophage-colony stimulating
   factor (GM-CSF)   71, 87
granulocyte macrophage-colony stimulating
   factor, gene regulation of   73

HER-2/neu   166
high affinity receptor for IgE (FcεRIβ),
   β-chain of   27
house dust mite (HDM)   145
H-ras   166
human β-receptor gene, polymorphism of
   119
human genome screen   33
human leukocyte antigen (HLA)   28
hypermethylation   174
hyperresponsiveness, bronchial   85

immunocytochemistry   91
immunoglobulin E (IgE)   86
immunoglobulin M (IgM)   85
inflammation, steroid-resistant   59
in situ hybridisation   89
integrin   136
interleukin 3 (IL-3)   71
interleukin 3, gene regulation of   76
interleukin 4 (IL-4)   71, 86
interleukin 4, gene regulation of   75
interleukin 5 (IL-5)   71, 86
interleukin 5, gene regulation of   77
interleukin 13 (IL-13)   71, 86

JAK/STAT family   53

lavage, bronchoalveolar (BAL)   88, 129
linkage, genetic   24
lod score   24
lung cancer   9, 165
lung tumour   183

macrophage inflammatory protein-1β
   (MIP-1β)   33
malignancy, thoracic   9
mast cell   90
mesothelioma, malignant   9
mouse genomic screen   34
mucosa, bronchial   85

non-small cell lung cancer (NSCLC)   166
nonviral vector system   4
nuclear factor kappa B (NF-κB)   46
nuclear factor kappa B inhibitor   62

oncogene   168

*p*53 gene   166
papain   147
permeability, epithelial   155
positional cloning   24
promoter, tumour-specific   188
α_1-proteinase inhibitor   151

radioallergosorbent test (RAST)   93
raf   166
RANTES   33
β-receptor, desensitization of   111
β-receptor, down-regulation of   111
recruitment, eosinophil   87
response, inflammatory   125
retinoblastoma   166

selectin   133
serine proteinase   152
skin-prick test   93
small cell lung cancer (SCLC)   166
surfactant protein B deficiency   8

T cell   71, 85
T cell, nuclear factor of acitvated   59
T cell receptor (TCR)   28
Th1 cell   91
Th2 cell   71, 91
transcription factor, specific   45
transcription factor, therapeutic implications
   61
transcription factor, ubiquitous   45
transcription machinery, basal   44
transition mutation   167
tuberculin   92
tumour necrosis factor α (TNF-α)   33
tumour suppressor gene expression,
   restoration of   190
tumour vaccine   194
tyrosine phosphorylation   173

VCAM-1   135
vector, adenoviral   4, 184
vector, retroviral   3, 184
vector, viral   184
virus, adeno-associated (AAV)   4
VLA-4   135

RPP
Respiratory Pharmacology and
Pharmacotherapy

Clinical and Biological Basis of Lung Cancer Prevention

Martinet Y., et al. (Ed.)

Lung cancer is a disease with pandemic public health implications as it is now the leading cause of cancer mortality throughout the world. This book results from two recent International Association for the Study of Lung Cancer (IASLC) Workshops on lung cancer prevention. It strikes a balance between considering public health approaches to tobacco control and population-based screening, advances in clinical evalua-tion of chemoprevention approaches, and the biology of lung carcinogenesis.

Indeed, while the science of smoking cessation is evolving as new pharmacological tools are moving into clinical evaluation, the current impact of molecular diagnostics is profound. The rapidly-evolving diagnostic technologies are revolution-izing basic scientific investigation of cancer, and this trend is expected to soon spill over into the clinical practice of medicine. The evolution of economical diagnostic platforms to allow for direct bronchial epithelial evaluation in high-risk populations promises to improve the diagnos-tic lead-time for this disease. The hope is that enough progress will occur to permit lung cancer

detection in advance of clinical cancer so that the disease can be addressed early on, while it is still confined to the site of origin.

Chemoprevention, which is designed to intervene in the early phase of carcinogenesis prior to any subjective clinical manifestation of a cancer, is also generating greater research interest. Moreover, the benefit of aerosolized adminis-tration of chemoprevention agents over conven-tional oral administration has strong appeal and may result in the reduction of the incidence of cancer when combined with new diagnostic technologies.

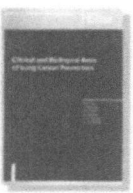

RPP – Respiratory Pharmacolo-gy and Pharmacotherapy
MartinetY., et al. (Ed.)
Clinical and Biological Basis of Lung Cancer Prevention
1997. 344 pages. Hardcover
ISBN 3-7643-5778-9

BioSciences with Birkhäuser

(Prices are subject to change without notice. 10/98)

For orders originating from all over the world except USA and Canada:

Birkhäuser Verlag AG
P.O. Box 133
CH-4010 Basel / Switzerland
Fax: +41 / 61 / 205 07 92
e-mail: orders@birkhauser.ch

For orders originating in the USA and Canada:

Birkhäuser Boston, Inc.
333 Meadowland Parkway
USA-Secaucus, NJ 07094-2491
Fax: +1 / 201 348 4033
e-mail: orders@birkhauser.com

Birkhäuser

MCBU
Molecular and Cell Biology Updates

Molecular Aspects of Cancer and its Therapy

Mackiewicz A.,
University School of Medical Sciences, Poland /
Sehgal P.B.,
New York Medical College, Valhalla, NY (Ed.)

This book highlights recent progress in the molecular, cellular and immunological mechanisms that contribute to the pathophysiology of cancer and the design of therapeutic modalities based upon these molecular insights. Areas of particular emphasis include cancer immunology and the immunotherapy of cancer, the role of cytokines in modulating the social behaviour of cancer cells, the genetic alterations that characterize human cancer and metastasis, and a consideration of the more experimental approaches to cancer therapy, including gene therapy using expression vectors for cytokines and their receptors, antisense RNA therapy, and anti-idiotypic antibody immunization.

This volume serves to introduce the general reader as well as the cancer specialist to personalized perspectives of particular topics in cancer research by leading research groups in the field. The combination of a „reviews"-approach with a more research-oriented approach in discussions of specific research topics provides a stimulating and forward-looking volume which serves to update selected aspects of cancer research today. This combination will be useful to both the beginner as well as the more advanced biomedical scientist.

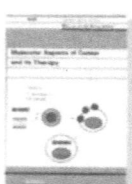

MCBU – Molecular and Cell Biology Updates
Mackiewicz A., et al. (Ed.)
Molecular Aspects of Cancer and its Therapy
1998. 240 pages. Hardcover
ISBN 3-7643-5724-X

BioSciences with Birkhäuser

(Prices are subject to change without notice. 10/98)

For orders originating from all over the world except USA and Canada:

Birkhäuser Verlag AG
P.O. Box 133
CH-4010 Basel / Switzerland
Fax: +41 / 61 / 205 07 92
e-mail: orders@birkhauser.ch

For orders originating in the USA and Canada:

Birkhäuser Boston, Inc.
333 Meadowland Parkway
USA-Secaucus, NJ 07094-2491
Fax: +1 / 201 348 4033
e-mail: orders@birkhauser.com

Birkhäuser

MCBU
Molecular and Cell Biology Updates

Cell Growth and Oncogenesis

Bannasch P.,
Deutsches Krebsforschungszentrum,
Heidelberg,Germany /
Kanduc D., Papa S.,
University of Bari /
Tager J.M.,
University of Amsterdam, The Netherlands (Ed.)

Rapid progress has been made in our understanding of the molecular mechanisms of cell growth and oncogenesis during the past decade. This book comprises recent results on the regulation of cell growth in normal and neoplastic tissues by growth factors including hormones, and by the activation and inactivation of oncogenes and tumor suppressor genes, respectively. Special attention has been given to the presentation of the frequently neglected close correlation between changes in signal transduction and metabolism pathways during oncogenesis.

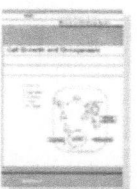

MCBU – Molecular and Cell Biology Updates
Bannasch P., et al. (Ed.)
Cell Growth and Oncogenesis
1998. 314 pages. Hardcover
ISBN 3-7643-5727-4

BioSciences with Birkhäuser

(Prices are subject to change without notice. 10/98)

For orders originating from all over the world except USA and Canada:

Birkhäuser Verlag AG
P.O. Box 133
CH-4010 Basel / Switzerland
Fax: +41 / 61 / 205 07 92
e-mail: orders@birkhauser.ch

For orders originating in the USA and Canada:

Birkhäuser Boston, Inc.
333 Meadowland Parkway
USA-Secaucus, NJ 07094-2491
Fax: +1 / 201 348 4033
e-mail: orders@birkhauser.com

Birkhäuser

Methods in Pulmonary Research

Uhlig S.,
Forschungszentrum Borstel, Germany /
Taylor A.E.,
University of Southern Alabama, Mobile, AL,
USA (Ed.)

Methods in Pulmonary Research presents a comprehensive review of methods used to study
physiology and the cell biology of the lung. The book covers the entire range of techniques from
those that require cell cultures to those using in vivo experimental models.
Up-to-date techniques such as intravital microscopy are presented. Yet standard methods such as
classical short circuit techniques used to study tracheal transport are fully covered. This book will
be extremely useful for all who work in pulmonary research, yet need a practical guide to
incorporate other established methods into their research programs. Thus the book will prove to
be a valuable resource for cell biologists who wish to use organs in their research programs as
well biological scientists who are moving their research programs into more cell related phenom-
ena.

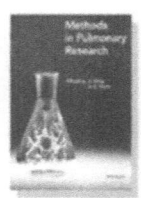

Uhlig S., Taylor A.E. (Ed.)
**Methods in Pulmonary
Research**
1998. 544 pages. Hardcover
ISBN 3-7643-5427-5

BioSciences with Birkhäuser

(Prices are subject to change without notice. 10/98)

For orders originating from all over the
world except USA and Canada:

For orders originating in the USA and
Canada:

Birkhäuser Verlag AG
P.O. Box 133
CH-4010 Basel / Switzerland
Fax: +41 / 61 / 205 07 92
e-mail: orders@birkhauser.ch

Birkhäuser Boston, Inc.
333 Meadowland Parkway
USA-Secaucus, NJ 07094-2491
Fax: +1 / 201 348 4033
e-mail: orders@birkhauser.com

Birkhäuser